CONTENTS

PREFACE

Sleep breathing disorders represent one of the most important factors that influence prognosis in critical patients, directly as an initial cause or indirect process that deteriorates after admission to the Intensive Care Units. Despite this known association, there is little scientific information in key practical questions. For example, how does one approach and diagnose sleep breathing disorders in critical care medicine? How can one measure these associations in patients under non-invasive and invasive mechanical ventilation? During weaning from mechanical ventilation, extubation process, or prevention extubation failure, and finally, their association with short and long term prognosis in medical and postoperative critically patients. In this scenario, they are of great interest to understand these associations.

In this book, the authors analyze the rationale for diagnosis and treatment in critically mechanically ventilated, from non-invasive, invasive and weaning from mechanical ventilation process, treatments, protocols and follow-up patients' recommendations. The high prevalence of sleep breathing disorders, increment critically mechanical ventilated patients, new forms of invasive and non-invasive mechanical ventilation justify as multidisciplinary perspective this book, useful for pulmonologists, critical care and anesthesiologist.

Chapter 1 - Sleep disordered breathing is the most common sleep disease, and obstructive sleep apnea is the most common disorder among the sleep disordered breathing. Comorbid conditions in critically ill patients (mechanically ventilated) in ICU may effect both the primary reason of ICU stay and outcome. Obstructive sleep apnea is not one of the known comorbid conditions among the patients who are treated in ICU. Diabetes mellitus, hypertension and other respiratory diseases rather than sleep disordered breathing are known conditions, however, OSA are not among those. Prevalence of sleep disordered breathing varies from 10% to 20% in mechanically ventilated patients. Sleep disordered breathing is one of the main reasons for hypercapneic respiratory problems, therefore it is important to be aware of sleep disordered breathing in mechanically ventilated patients, otherwise there may be delay in extubation or discharge from ICU. The prevalence of OSA is 10% in women, and 15-20% in men. Few retrospective studies reported the prevalence of OSA as 10 to 20%. There are many people undiagnosed with OSA. Therefore previously reported prevalence of OSA in mechanically ventilated patients don't reflect the real prevalence. Prospectively well-designed new studies can report the real prevalence of OSA in mechanically ventilated patient.

Chapter 2 - The interaction between the mechanical ventilator and a patient with sleep disordered breathing is a complex process. Factors such as body mass index, etiology of sleep disordered breathing, pulmonary pathology, and environmental factors all play a role. Sleep is a difficult entity to study in the Intensive Care Unit (ICU) due to the critical nature of illness and disruptions in sleep architecture, staging, and circadian rhythm. Factors such as body position, medications, and volume status all impact the mechanically ventilated patient with sleep disordered breathing. Hypoventilation disorders and central sleep apnea are also important factors to consider during mechanical ventilation as there may be complications that arise from the intubation and extubation process as well as the duration of time on the ventilator.

Chapter 3 - The respiratory muscle pump consists of primary inspiratory muscles, of which the diaphragm is the predominant contributor. Many patients develop sleep-disordered breathing. This is predominantly in the form of obstructive sleep apnoea, which imposes a load on the respiratory muscle pump, but can also be caused by a variety of conditions that either reduce the capacity of the respiratory muscle pump (neuromuscular conditions) or increase the load (airway obstruction, obesity) leading to nocturnal hypoventilation.

Chapter 4 - Upper Airways anatomical abnormalities play a central role in OSA pathophysiology. Upper Airways clinical examination represents an essential step in the evaluation of an OSA patient. Awake and sleep/sedation endoscopic examination provide analysis of the site, grade and pattern of Upper Airways collapsibility. Drug-Induced Sleep Endoscopy has been found to be useful for anatomical assessment of Upper Airways and treatment option selection in OSA patients. Adeno-Tonsillar hypertrophy is the most important anatomical abnormality for pediatric OSA. Customized, multidisciplinary, combined therapy represents the treatment option for achieving the best outcomes. In this chapter, the authors are mainly discussing the UA anatomical features in relation to OSA pathophysiology in the adult and pediatric OSA patients, as well as study the impact of UA anatomical characteristics in the treatment of an OSA patient.

Chapter 5 - Sleep related breathing disorders (SRBDs) can be diagnosed using various devices commonly categorised into Type I-IV studies. These are classified according to; the number of parameters, whether they require an attending sleep technologist and their setting. Type I and II studies combine 7 channels including respiratory parameters and electroencephalogram (EEG), to give the most accurate respiratory analysis. However, these may be impractical in a standard critical care setting. Type III and IV studies are both portable and easier to set up. Type III devices measure respiratory parameters only and can provide information on the type of SRBD. Type IV devices measure 1-2 parameters, but cannot differentiate the nature of the SRBD. Both devices may underestimate the severity of the SRBD as they do not directly measure sleep. Peripheral arterial tonometry (PAT) is easy to use and offers an indirect measure of sleep, without EEG, but has limited evidence in the critical care setting. Finally, CO_2 monitoring can be used in conjunction with these studies to help assess hypoventilation.

Chapter 6 - Attended in-laboratory polysomnography remains the gold standard method for diagnosing sleep-related breathing disorders. However, it is expensive, time-consuming, and requires expert technical input to assure the quality of the measurement. Therefore alternative diagnostic tests may be required in the general ward and critical care environments. Unattended polysomnography is increasingly used in the home, as well as in the hospital environment, and has a high degree of correlation with the results of attended in-laboratory polysomnography. Portable respiratory polygraphy is an alternative that allows diagnosis of both obstructive and central events during nocturnal recording, but is limited by the inability to detect sleep stage, and tends to underestimate the apnoea-hypopnoea index. Nocturnal pulse oximetry and transcutaneous capnography is useful for screening for patients in whom there is a high index of suspicion for sleep-disordered breathing and can detect response to treatment. Capnography is particularly helpful for those patients requiring ventilator support for sleep hypoventilation syndromes. Technologies such as peripheral arterial tonometry are helpful in diagnosing patients with sleep-disordered breathing. However, in cases where unattended, portable modalities used to screen patients with suspected sleep-related breathing disorders give negative or inconclusive results, then attended laboratory polysomnography should be deployed."

Chapter 7 - Chronic hypoventilation affects patients with disorders on any level of the respiratory system. Obesity hypoventilation syndrome (OHS), COPD, neuromuscular diseases and congestive heart failure are most frequent causes of respiratory failure and hypoventilation worsens during sleep in these diseases. Optimal treatment of patients with chronic hypoventilation with NIV crucially depends on the underlying pathophysiological mechanisms. Treatment of chronic hypercapnic respiratory failure with noninvasive ventilation improves daytime dyspnea, PaCO2, hypersomnolence, exacerbations, readmissions and survival.

Chapter 8 - Intermittent hypoxia is the key pathophysiological feature linking obstructive sleep apnoea (OSA) with vascular damage. Severe intermittent hypoxia results in sympathetic overdrive and oxidative stress which promote systemic hypertension and endothelial dysfunction. Continuous positive airway pressure (CPAP) improves endothelial function and can reduce blood pressure in OSA. OSA and other types of sleep-disordered breathing might be aggravated in the critically ill patient in the intensive care unit, e.g., due to hypervolemia or impaired vigilance. The cardiovascular consequences of OSA, e.g., blood pressure surges or disturbed cardiac repolarisation, might be particularly disadvantageous in the critically ill patient. However, there is no data to support either diagnostic approaches nor treatment with CPAP in suspected OSA in critically ill patients to reduce the length of stay in the intensive care unit or improve the short-term outcome.

Chapter 9 - Patients with obstructive sleep apnea (OSA) suffer from increased risk of developing cognitive and functional deficits. Significant links between OSA and several major neuropsychiatric and neurologic disorders have been proposed, and the treatment with continuous positive airway pressure (CPAP) appears to ameliorate some of these risks. Future studies will determine which cognitive domains and the associated illness-driven pathomechanisms are best targeted with various combinations of CPAP treatments.

Chapter 10 - The effects of obstructive sleep apnea (OSA) treatment by means of continuous positive airway pressure (CPAP) are numerous and diverse. In fact restoring the normal breathing pattern and oxygen saturation throughout the night by treating apneas and hypopneas can resolve multiple OSA-related consequences involving different human organ systems. Some of these effects are well known such as those on the cardiovascular system: treating intermittent hypoxia allows to reduce the sympathetic nervous activation that triggers renin-angiotensin-aldosterone system, responsible of the development of arterial hypertension and, ultimately, of chronic kidney disease. Others are less studied such as the effect of CPAP on the progression of non-alcoholic fatty liver disease (NAFLD). In the present chapter the authors will discuss in depth the consequences of CPAP treatment in patients with OSA and cardiac, renal and hepatic co-morbidities.

Chapter 11 - High flow therapy is a novel treatment that delivers warm, humidified air at a high flow. High flow therapy has numerous beneficial physiological effects and is now validated for the management of severe acute respiratory failure. Its use in the home setting is feasible. However, to date, the use of high flow therapy during sleep has only been shown to be effective for the management of obstructive sleep apnea in children.

Chapter 12 - Non-invasive ventilation delivers differential positive airways pressures during inspiration and expiration. It may be applied in the management of obesity hypoventilation syndrome, with or without severe obstructive sleep apnoea, and sleep-disordered breathing that occurs in association with chronic obstructive pulmonary disease and neuromuscular disease, including motor neurone disease, muscular dystrophies and chest wall deformities. Nocturnal application of NIV in these settings may effectively abolish nocturnal hypoventilation and can improve patient-reported outcomes, including sleepiness and health status, and reduce healthcare utilisation. NIV should be delivered by trained specialists. Patients should be collaboratively involved in decisions relating to interfaces and ventilator settings and provided with access to technical support. All patients should undergo regular clinical follow-up at a specialist ventilation unit. This may be conducted in the outpatient department or, where resources permit, outreach services can deliver home-based care to patients unable to attend hospital appointments.

Chapter 13 - Sleep-related disorders are life-threatening conditions. The optimal level of treatment should be decided in a sleep laboratory.Side effects directly influencing the patient's adherence to treatment are known. Unintentional leaks are very common in NIV. Leakage may be absent or minimum when the patient is awake, but may worsen during sleep as a result of the loss of voluntary control and reduced muscle tone. Every effort should be made to minimise air leaks, maximise patient comfort and optimise patient-ventilator interaction. The interface is of predominant relevance for adherence to NIV therapy. A variety of masks are now accessible, and producers continue to improve mask design. During NIV, a variable resistance developed by the Upper Airway (UA) is included between the ventilator and the lungs. The UA may change its opposition to airflow, compromising the delivery of an adequate tidal volume to the lungs. Intermittent obstruction of the UA is prevalent during NIV and may be correlated or to obstructive events at the oropharyngeal level.

Chapter 14 - Obesity hypoventilation syndrome (OHS) is defined by the presence of hypercapnia in an obese patient with sleep-disordered breathing. Obesity influences respiratory physiology by decreasing compliance of the respiratory system and reducing lung volumes. In addition, respiratory centres' responses are blunted. Patients with OHS most often present with acute hypercapnic failure with the need for noninvasive ventilation (NIV) or in sleep centres with typical symptoms of obstructive sleep apnea (OSA). An important feature of OHS is increased cardiometabolic morbidity and mortality. NIV is the initial treatment of acute hypercapnic respiratory failure (AHRF). When used in the correct patient by a skilled NIV team in a proper fashion NIV is successful in the majority of obese patients with AHRF. In a chronic setting, patients with OHS should be treated according to sleep study results. When severe OSA is present, continuous positive airway pressure (CPAP) is the first choice of treatment, if adequate physiological and clinical responses can be achieved. The rest of the patients should be treated with home NIV.

Chapter 15 - Sleep-related breathing disorders are a frequent phenomenon in patients with neuromuscular diseases. There are many mechanisms which predispose the occurrence of respiratory events during sleep. The principal pathomechanisms are weakness of respiratory muscles (mainly diaphragm), impaired breathing control and restriction of the chest. There are three main types of sleep-related breathing disorders: hypoventilation, central events and obstructive events. The gold standard for the diagnosis is full polysomnography, with concomitant measurement of transcutaneous partial pressure of O2 and CO2. Non-invasive ventilation is a treatment of choice and should be started in a hospital setting in order to adequately titrate the settings. Inadequate treatment is a risk factor of a worse prognosis. Tolerability of long-term non-invasive ventilation may be an issue in neuromuscular patients.

Chapter 16 - Sleep abnormalities are common problems in patients who are mechanically ventilated in the intensive care unit (ICU). Causes of sleep disturbances in ICU patients are multifactorial. Mechanical ventilation typically disturbs and disrupts sleep. The severity of the disease, the endotracheal tube, mask, nasogastric tube, aspiration, physical restraints, and mouth patches in patients undergoing mechanical ventilation cause sleep deprivation. Ventilator modes applied in mechanical ventilation also affect sleep quality and cause sleep related breathing disorders. Ventilator settings and modes affect sleep quality and can cause sleep related breathing disorders, especially if patient ventilator asynchrony exists.

Chapter 17 - Sleep related breathing disorders" are respiratory failure during sleep and associated with narrowing or closing of the upper airway in many cases. The degree of respiratory disorders ranges from a partial obstruction of the airway to apnea asssociated with recurrent hypoxemia. Sleep-related breathing disorders include: obstructive sleep apnea (OSAs) disorders, central sleep apnea (CSA) syndromes, sleep-releated hypoventilation disorders and sleep-releated hypoxemia disorder. The decrease of chest wall compliance, lung capacity(functional residual volume) in patients with sleep-related respiratory disorders may cause difficulties in airway control. This condition, these patients may require intense perioperative management because of prolonged respiratory depression potential due to residual anesthetic agents and increases concerns about the application of general anesthesia. It is important to plan a perioperative anesthesia management for potential adverse events such as airway management, difficult mask ventilation and difficult intubation. In the postoperative period, close hemodynamic monitoring, blood oxygen level and continuous positive airway pressure (CPAP) should be provided and respiratory support should be provided.

Chapter 18 - Sedation and analgesia can result in increased mechanical ventilation requirements. Careful pre-procedure planning should include a multi-disciplinary assessment of benefit balanced against risks of proposed procedures. Individualised assessment must include potential airway management issues, cardio-respiratory limitations, metabolic considerations, medication and functional issues affecting positioning for the procedure. Checklists encourage a standardised approach for best and safest peri-procedural course. Choice of sedation technique includes intermittent bolus or titrated continuous infusions selected for patient factors, ease of use and recovery profile. Planning analgesia takes into account existing pain management requirements, a multi-modal approach with local, regional and central neuraxial techniques. Routes of parenteral analgesia depend on the patient's ability absorb medications. A stepwise approach with an escalating and de-escalating regime for acute pain is employed. Careful monitoring and support of the patient, with available resuscitation equipment and expertly trained staff is mandatory.

Chapter 19 - Postoperative period is a critical process that requires careful approach for Sleep-Related Breathing Disorders (SRBDs) patients. In addition to sensitivity to post-surgical medication, complications such as cardiac, neurological and comorbidities, especially respiratory, may occure. Therefore, close follow-up and implementation of the necessary precautionary strategies in accordance with the recommendations may provide successful management of the postoperative process.

Chapter 20 - OSA/OHS is common in patients who undergo mechanical ventilation. Undiagnosed and untreated OSA/OHS is associated with increased risk of difficult intubation or extubation failure. Morbid Obesity, neck circumference >42 cm, STOP-Bang score >3, as well as craniofacial anatomical features such as retrognathia, macroglossia are also risk factors for OSA/difficult intubation. Submental ultrasound, cuff- leak test and post-extubation spirometry could be used in addition to sleep studies to identify those at high risk of upper airway collapse. Minimising opioid use, avoiding deeper level of anaesthesia, using semi-upright position post extubation and prophylactic use of PAP therapy/NIV - are likely to reduce the risk of extubation failure. In those with hypercapnic respiratory failure and/or overlap of OSA and COPD the author would recommend NIV rather than CPAP. Tracheostomy decanulation should be preceded by assessment and treatment of any upper airway pathology including OSA.

Chapter 21 - Weaning from mechanical ventilation is a key task for any intensivist. While the majority of patients will be liberated from invasive ventilation quickly, 20-30% will experience difficulty in weaning. These patients require a comprehensive physiological assessment to determine the cause of the weaning difficulty followed by a multidisciplinary approach to management. Complex weaning patients are likely to need optimisation of nutrition, physical rehabilitation and psychological health, as well as prevention of ventilator-associated pneumonias. This group of patients require a large amount of resources and are likely to require long-term care, which is best coordinated through specialist regional centres.

Chapter 22 - There is an increasing number of patients with prolonged mechanical ventilation (PMV) with associated increased health care burdens and poor long-term outcomes. Sleep-disordered breathing (SDB) is very frequent in the general population but has been studied rarely in the PMV population. Based on a limited number of studies, the prevalence of SDB, mostly OSA and sleep-related hypoxemia in patients with PMV has been as high 95%. PSG with or without a capped tracheostomy is the most comprehensive testing modality, but other methods, such as polygraphy and nocturnal oximetry, can be considered to facilitate ventilator weaning and decannulation. Patients with SDB can be successfully decannulated and transitioned to positive airway pressure (PAP) therapy. Further study is needed to determine the impact of diagnosis and treatment of SDB in the short and long-term outcomes of this population. This chapter reviews the diagnosis and treatment of SDB in patients with PMV.

Chapter 23 - Invasive mechanical ventilation via a tracheostomy tube (tracheostomy ventilation, TV) should be considered for critically ill patients with prolonged weaning course and for those with advanced chronic respiratory failure (e.g., patients with neuromuscular diseases, NMDs). Tracheostomy can be performed either with a surgical procedure or with various percutaneous dilatory procedures, the last being increasingly used in intensive care units (ICUs). In ICU patients early tracheostomy may expedite weaning and reduce sedation duration as well as the incidence of ventilator-associated pneumonia, although it is doubtful if it can also decrease mortality. Implementation of TV in patients with advanced chronic respiratory failure (commonly patients with NMDs) may lead to increased survival in some patients (e.g., younger patients with amyotrophic lateral sclerosis) although its effects on their health-related quality of life is unclear. TV in patients with chronic respiratory failure is associated with increased nursing requirements and caregiver burden.

Chapter 24 - Sleep disordered breathing disorders and in particular obstructive sleep apnoea, are very common. In fact obstructive sleep apnoea is now one of the commoner chronic respiratory condition. This condition has significant and serious implications on the health outcomes of affected individuals. It also has negative social consequences. As most adults with obstructive sleep apnoea share a bed with their partners or spouses, it will directly affect them during the night and it will also have a bearing on their overall wellbeing. The effects of sleep disordered breathing disordered will further cascade down to the family and society. The burden of sleep disordered breathing disorders is huge and going forwards specialist clinics are unlikely to be able to cope with health demands of the affected individuals. A joint collaborative approach with primary care might be needed.

In: Sleep Medicine in Critical Care
Editors: Antonio M. Esquinas et al.
ISBN: 978-1-53617-768-8

Chapter 1

PREVALENCE OF SLEEP-DISORDERED BREATHING (SDB) IN PATIENTS WITH MECHANICAL VENTILATION

Baran Balcan*[*], *MD
Department of Pulmonary Medicine and Intensive Care,
Marmara University, Istanbul, Turkey

ABSTRACT

Sleep disordered breathing is the most common sleep disease, and obstructive sleep apnea is the most common disorder among the sleep disordered breathing. Comorbid conditions in critically ill patients (mechanically ventilated) in ICU may effect both the primary reason of ICU stay and outcome.

Obstructive sleep apnea is not one of the known comorbid conditions among the patients who are treated in ICU. Diabetes mellitus, hypertension and other respiratory diseases rather than sleep disordered breathing are known conditions, however, OSA are not among those. Prevalence of sleep disordered breathing varies from 10% to 20% in mechanically ventilated patients. Sleep disordered breathing is one of the main reasons for hypercapneic respiratory problems, therefore it is important to be aware of sleep disordered breathing in mechanically ventilated patients, otherwise there may be delay in extubation or discharge from ICU.

The prevalence of OSA is 10% in women, and 15-20% in men. Few retrospective studies reported the prevalence of OSA as 10 to 20%. There are many people undiagnosed with OSA. Therefore previously reported prevalence of OSA in mechanically ventilated patients don't reflect the real prevalence. Prospectively well-designed new studies can report the real prevalence of OSA in mechanically ventilated patient.

---

[*] Corresponding Author's E-mail: drbaranbalcan@gmail.com.

1. INTRODUCTION

In critically ill patients there may be more than one chronic comorbid disease which may effect the primary acute condition and outcome in intensive care unit (ICU) [1]. Additionally, the existing comorbid condition may have an impact on developing extra difficulties in treatment of primary condition of ICU stay. It was previously reported that in all sepsis patients nearly 60 % had at least one chronic condition [1]. The most common chronic comorbidities observed in ICU are Diabetes Mellitus and Hypertension, followed by chronic pulmonary diseases (chronic obstructive pulmonary disease [COPD], asthma, etc…), acute coronary syndrome, neurological diseases, trauma etc… Sleep disordered breathing does not exist among those common comorbid conditions, however, it can be counted in chronic pulmonary diseases group.

In this chapter our aim was to evaluate the prevalence of sleep disordered breathing among the mechanically ventilated ICU patients.

2. SLEEP DISORDERED BREATHING

As summarized in table 1 there is a wide range of classification of Sleep disorders. According to international classification of sleep disorders, Sleep Disordered Breathing (SDB) is the most observed sleep disorder. Sleep disordered breathing includes a wide range of disorders, mostly observed categories of obstructive sleep apnea (OSA), central sleep apnea, and sleep related hypoventilation syndrome. The mostly observed SDB is OSA and the prevalence of OSA varies according to how OSA is defined and which cut-off value has been taken for apnea-hypopnea index (AHI). In the general population based on studies, the prevalence of OSA has been expected to be 14% of men and 5% of women, consuming the cutoff AHI level as ≥ 5 events/h (hypopneas associated with 4% oxygen desaturations). Obstructive sleep apnea is characterized by partial or complete obstruction of airflow because of an abnormality in oropharynx that exist during sleep. Complete obstruction isknown as apnea (complete or 90 % airflow cessation for 10 seconds), and partial obstruction is known as hypopneas (reduction in airflow 30 % from baseline value, and 3 % decline in oxyhemoglobin saturation or arousal from sleep). If there are symptoms such as excessive daytime sleepiness (EDS), fatigue, mood abnormalities and concentration difficulties beside 5 or more events during sleep based on plysomnography (PSG) or cardiorespiratory polygraphy (CRPG), it's called Obstructive sleep apnea syndrome (OSAS), or without those symptoms, if there is more than 15 events per hour during sleep it's again called OSAS. Obstructive sleep apnea is accepted as an independent risk factor for cardiovascular morbidity and mortality [2].

Table 1. International Classification of Sleep Disorders – Third Edition (ICSD-3)

Insomnia
Sleep Related Breathing Disorders
Obstructive sleep apnea
Central Sleep Apnea
Sleep-Related Hypoventilation Disorders
Sleep-Related Hypoxemia Disorder
Central Disorders of Hypersomnolence
Circadian Rhythm Sleep-Wake Disorders
Parasomnias
Sleep Related Movement Disorders

Comorbid conditions such as Diabetes Mellitus, Hypertension, Coronary Arterial Disease, Chronic Heart Failure, Obesity, and Cerebrovascular Disease are highly observed in patients with sleep disordered breathing especially obstructive sleep apnea who are admitted to Intensive Care Unit (ICU). Patients, especially obese ones who are treated in ICU, are observed to be at high risk of hypercapneic respiratory failure, and sleep disordered breathing is identified as the reason of hypercapneic respiratory failure in those patients. Association between OSA and these co-morbid conditions is defined as a reason of increased mortality in ICU. After surgery there are difficulties in extubation of patients with OSA, and need of transfer to ICU. ICU stays and time for extubation are prolonged for patients with sleep disordered breathing [3].

3. Prevalence of OSA in ICU

In the previous literature there is not any study that evaluates the prevalence of OSA prospectively in ICU patients or in patients with mechanically ventilated. In retrospective studies the prevalence of OSA was suggested to be between 10 to 20 %.

To our best knowledge there are few studies that evaluated the prevalence of SDB in ICU patients. In a study with 15,590 patients, they evaluated OSA retrospectively. OSA was diagnosed among 7.8 % of the patients who were admitted to ICU between 2003 and 2005. For diagnosis of OSA, AHI was accepted as 5 events/hour at night in PSG. This was the first study in which prevalence of OSA was evaluated and it has been observed that OSA was common in ICU patients. However when compared to non-OSA, patients' mortality was lower in OSA group. Most of the patients with OSA areundiagnosed before admitting to ICU or before having a surgery. Anesthesiologists usually screen patients for evaluation of sleep disordered breathing, especially the patients whose Body mass index (BMI) is over 30 kg/m2. Patients with OSA may have cardiovascular complications during or after the surgery.

In another study 74,032 patients who had invasive mechanical ventilation due to respiratory infection had been evaluated retrospectively between 2009 and 2011. They observed that 10.3 % (7,601) of them had previously diagnosed Obstructive sleep apnea. They also observed that mortality of OSA patients was lower when compared to non-OSA group among the mechanically ventilated patients. Their results may suggest that respiratory tract infection with co-existing OSA may benefit from early and aggressive treatment in ICU [4].

Lindenaeuer and colleagues evaluated 250,907 pneumonia patients who were treated in 347 United States hospitals. Obstructive Sleep Apnea was observed among 15,569 (6.2 %) of the patients. 29 % of OSA patients had non-invasive mechanical ventilation support and 18 % of them had invasive mechanical ventilation. They have also suggested that OSA is a common comorbidity among patients with lower respiratory tract infection, and they have increased risk of mechanical ventilation support, they had higher rates of complications when compared to non-OSA patients, however the mortality rates were lower in OSA patients [5].

As described above the prevalence of sleep disordered breathing is between 10% and 20% among intensive care patients who need mechanical ventilation support.

4. Postoperative Prolonged Mechanical Ventilation in ICU in Obstructive Sleep Apnea Patients

There are many reasons of perioperative hypoxemia, such as sedatives given during the operation, muscle weakness, respiratory problems because of chronic pulmonary diseases, and surgical trauma, etc. There is an intermittent, nocturnal deep hypoxemia in patients with OSA, and this hypoxemia induces sympathetic activity that increases the risk of perioperative respiratory depression and difficulties in management of airway. Presence of impaired oxygenation in patients promotes longer oxygen support, longer stay of hospital, and higher need ICU support after surgeries lasting 2 or more hours. Therefore it is important to evaluate sleep disordered breathing in patients before surgeries. There may be difficulties in extubation of patients with OSA after surgeries, and those patients may need mechanical ventilation support in ICU after surgery.

Conclusion

The prevalence of OSA is 10% in women, and 15-20% in men in general population. Cardinal symptoms of OSA are loud snoring, excessive daytime sleepiness and witnessed apnea. Many people underestimate those symptoms as a sign of a disease. The real prevalence of OSA in mechanically ventilated patients is not known exactly. In few retrospective studies prevalence of OSA is between 10-20%. Those studies had results from data of previous ICD codes of the patients treated in ICU units. However there are so many patients who had undiagnosed OSA, although they had sign or symptoms of the disease previously. Therefore the estimated prevalence of OSA or sleep disordered breathing is much more than the previously reported in the literature. There should be prospectively designed studies in order to know the real prevalence of sleep disordered breathing mechanically ventilated patients.

REFERENCES

[1] Esper, A.M. and G.S. Martin, The impact of comorbid [corrected] conditions on critical illness. *Crit. Care Med.*, 2011. 39(12): p. 2728-35.

[2] Kapur, V.K., et al., Clinical Practice Guideline for Diagnostic Testing for Adult Obstructive Sleep Apnea: An American Academy of Sleep Medicine Clinical Practice Guideline. *Journal of clinical sleep medicine: JCSM*: official publication of the American Academy of Sleep Medicine, 2017. 13(3): p. 479-504.

[3] Bolona, E., P.Y. Hahn, and B. Afessa, Intensive care unit and hospital mortality in patients with obstructive sleep apnea. *Journal of critical care*, 2015. 30(1): p. 178-180.

[4] Jean, R.E., et al., Obstructive sleep apnea and acute respiratory failure: An analysis of mortality risk in patients with pneumonia requiring invasive mechanical ventilation. *J. Crit. Care*, 2015. 30(4): p. 778-83.

[5] Lindenauer, P.K., et al., Prevalence, treatment, and outcomes associated with OSA among patients hospitalized with pneumonia. *Chest*, 2014. 145(5): p. 1032-1038.

In: Sleep Medicine in Critical Care
Editors: Antonio M. Esquinas et al.
ISBN: 978-1-53617-768-8

Chapter 2

INTERACTION OF SLEEP-DISORDERED BREATIIING AND MECHANICAL VENTILATION

Gabriel Anders[1,*] and Peter C. Gay[2,†]
[1]DO, MHA, MBA, Pulmonary Critical Care Fellow,
Division of Pulmonary, Sleep, and Critical Care Medicine,
University of Missouri-Kansas City, MO, US
[2]MD, Professor of Medicine, Mayo Clinic Center for Sleep Medicine,
Division of Pulmonary and Critical Care Medicine,
Mayo Clinic, MN, US

ABSTRACT

The interaction between the mechanical ventilator and a patient with sleep disordered breathing is a complex process. Factors such as body mass index, etiology of sleep disordered breathing, pulmonary pathology, and environmental factors all play a role. Sleep is a difficult entity to study in the Intensive Care Unit (ICU) due to the critical nature of illness and disruptions in sleep architecture, staging, and circadian rhythm. Factors such as body position, medications, and volume status all impact the mechanically ventilated patient with sleep disordered breathing. Hypoventilation disorders and central sleep apnea are also important factors to consider during mechanical ventilation as there may be complications that arise from the intubation and extubation process as well as the duration of time on the ventilator.

* Corresponding Author's E-mail: andersgi@umkc.edu.
† Corresponding Author's E-mail: pgay@mayo.edu.

Keywords: Sleep Disordered Breathing, Obstructive Sleep Apnea, Intensive Care Unit, Positive End-Expiratory Pressure, Minute Ventilation

Sleep-disordered breathing (SDB) presents a special issue with the interaction of mechanical ventilation and is not often explored in the literature. Sleep-disordered breathing is an all-encompassing term that describes both acute and chronic conditions that impact breathing during periods of altered consciousness. The most common type of SDB is obstructive sleep apnea (OSA). Prevalence statistics from the Wisconsin Sleep Cohort Study found that 10% of men aged 30-49 and 17% of men aged 50 - 70 had at least moderate obstructive sleep apnea (Peppard 2013). Additionally, 3% of women aged 30-49 and 9% of women aged 50 - 70 had at least moderate obstructive sleep apnea (Peppard 2013).

Sleep disruptions in the Intensive Care Unit (ICU) is commonplace due to the acute and critical nature of the care provided. It was found that in critically ill patients, a loss of normal sleep architecture frequently occurs with a normal sleep EEG being replaced with diffuse slowing (S. Parthasarathy 2004). This can result in loss of normal sleep stages and cause sleep to be unrefreshingnonrestorative. Sleep disruptions in the ICU were found to be due to sounds elevations (21%) and patient care activities (7%), however the majority of sleep disruptions were not readily explained (68%) (S. Parthasarathy 2004).

Patients in the ICU are more predisposed to have SDB whether or not they are being mechanically ventilated. Breathing patterns in the ICU can be complicated by body position, comorbidities, and medications provided. Central Sleep Apnea and hypoventilation are two common conditions also noted in the ICU which have significant complications if not addressed effectively. Hypoventilation and failed extubation are additional complicating concerns worth discussing further when evaluating the interaction of sleep-disordered breathing and mechanical ventilation as discussed described in more detail below.

In the ICU particularly, the positioning of patients promotes obstructive sleep apnea making apneic events more common. As previous studies have shown, obstructive sleep apnea can be worse in the supine position especially if the phenotype of OSA is positional in nature as is the case for most patients. Most ICU patients are in the supine position for the majority of the time. The ICU care-team should anticipate potential difficult airway anatomy and take measures to limit the potential of airway obstruction such as minimizing opioid and sedative medications if possible, in the non-intubated patient, utilize non-supine positioning in the appropriate patient, incline the patient's bed, and utilize positive airway pressure in patients who are appropriate candidates (Malish n.d.).

Pharmacotherapy in the ICU is one of the most important factors in developing or exacerbating pre-existing SDB. Although medications such as opioids or benzodiazepines cannot be avoided, the care-team should be prepared if SDB should develop. Patients who have Continuous Positive Airway Pressure therapy at home may require different settings in the hospital due to fluid shifts, body position, and sedative medication (Chung 2016). Patients with OSA have been shown to have a narrow oropharynx and unfavorable anatomy that predisposes it to collapse under such additional confounding conditions (Malish n.d.).

The majority of patients in the ICU have significant disturbances in sleep. Sleep is interrupted due to the nature of treatments in the ICU, noise, and the critical nature of illnesses (Elliott 2013). As sleep in the ICU is significantly fragmented, it is difficult to specifically quantify. When patients in the ICU were studieds with polysomnography, it was found that the median total sleep time was five hours and was mainly comprised of stage N1 and N2 sleep with very little N3 or REM sleep with sound levels reaching 53.95 dB during the day and 50.20 dB during the night (Elliott 2013). The circadian rhythm of ICU patients is the most profoundly impacted sleep disorder regardless if a patient is mechanically ventilated.

It is intrinsically difficult to study patient's sleep in an ICU setting because of multiple factors. Loud alarms, frequent nursing cares, life-threatening illnesses, multiple intravenous drips, sedating medications, and poor sleep hygiene practices are among the few factors that make this difficult. Depending on the objectives of the investigator in studying sleep in the ICU, multiple tests may be performed. The circadian rhythm of ICU patients is the most profoundly impacted sleep disorder regardless if a patient is mechanically ventilated.

Actigraphy and urinary melatonin studies may be used in the evaluation of circadian rhythm and sleep schedules of ICU patients (Pisani 2015). Studies have shown that in septic ICU patients, there were significantly abnormal urinary melatonin level which may impact the circadian rhythm and effect the underlying physiology of sleep (Mundigler 2002). These and other techniques have revealed profound and very prolonged sleep disruption in medical and post-surgical patients especially in those undergoing cardiac procedures (Redeker 1996). One study showed that no patient who was admitted to the ICU had normal sleep (Cooper 2000). Full or limited polysomnograms may also be used in the ICU to evaluate sleep disordered breathing and efficacy of interventions to treat sleep disordered breathing (Pisani 2015). Questionnaires may also be a useful tool in studying sleep in the ICU (Pisani 2015).

If a patient does reach the point in their critical illness that they require invasive or non-invasive mechanical ventilation, the interaction of diagnosed or undiagnosed sleep disordered breathing and the ventilator is an important consideration. For OSA, which is the most common SDB condition, there are only a few considerations in regard to mechanical ventilation. As the obstruction in the oropharynx is bypassed by an endotracheal tube, OSA is essentially eliminated from the equation. However, the comorbidities of OSA are still present such as obesity and a potential resultant restrictive lung process due to excessive body mass. For this reason, patients may require a higher initial Positive End-Expiratory Pressure (PEEP) to help recruit more alveoli for gas exchange and overcome the atelectasis that is present due to the obesity and lung restriction. These patients may also require a higher Minute Ventilation (MV). For patient using non-invasive ventilation, this does not bypass the oropharynx and thus does not eliminate sleep disordered breathing. Patients using this modality may also need a high PEEP or Expiratory Positive Airway Pressure. In the ICU, both invasive and non-invasive mechanical ventilation are effective tools in treating multiple conditions, but non-invasive ventilation can be a useful bridge to avoid mechanical ventilation in some cases such as in exacerbations of heart failure and COPD.

Patients with OSA have intrinsically more difficult and high-risk airways (Rudra 2008). If a patient with an already compromised airway due to sleep disordered breathing develops a critical illness such as acute respiratory failure, acute encephalopathy, or stroke, the situation can rapidly deteriorate. Respiratory compromise in hospitalized patients is now a recognized entity under increased scrutiny. This has been defined as "a deterioration in respiratory function in which there is a high likelihood of decompensation into respiratory failure or death but for which timely specific interventions (enhanced monitoring or therapies) might prevent or mitigate decompensation" (Morris 2017). Patients with OSA have intrinsically more difficult and high-risk airways (Rudra 2008). If a patient with an already compromised airway due to sleep disordered breathing develops a critical illness such as acute respiratory failure, acute encephalopathy, or stroke, the situation can rapidly deteriorate. A respiratory insult may result in acute respiratory failure for a patient with OSA while a patient without OSA may recover without needing invasive or noninvasive support. Patients with pre-existing SDB are more likely to acutely decompensate when compared to those without SDB and it is important to note that most but not all patients with OSA are typically more difficult to intubate (Rudra 2008).

In mechanically ventilated patients with advanced heart failure, there may be a tendency to see Central Sleep Apnea/Cheyne–Stokes Respiration (CSA/CSR) in patients who are actively breathing on the ventilator. Patients who are passive or paralyzed on the ventilator will not have this breathing pattern as it is only seen with the patient's intact active intrinsic respiratory rhythm. There has been no clear data reported to show that mechanical ventilation alone increases mortality if CSR is present. It is still controversial whether CSR associated with severe heart failure is an independent predictor of adverse events (Yumino 2008). If CSR pattern of breathing is noted, it should be investigated as to why it is presentpresent, and an echocardiogram is often helpful.

The ventilator settings may also result in patient ventilator dyssynchrony causing further breathing complications. It has long been known that the patient receiving excessive pressure support may actually promote periodic breathing in patients on mechanical ventilation and that a backup rate may be necessary to reduce this complicating patient ventilator interaction. In a study by Parthasarathy et al., patients transitioning in and out of sleep were much more prone to irregular breathing patterns and fluctuation in end-tidal CO2 during pressure support than during assist-control ventilation. They concluded that higher pressure support levels induced hyperventilation which causes hypocapnia and in the absence of a backup rate and wakefulness drive, central apneas and sleep fragmentation occurred, especially in patients with heart failure (S. e. Parthasarathy 2002).

Both CPAP and bilevel PAP (BPAP) therapy lead to more favorable outcomes when treating stable chronic heart failure from ischemic or idiopathic causes in patients with CSR with an overall goal of reducing SDB and patient compliance in this study was favorable (Köhnlein 2002). Caution should be exercised however as CPAP or BPAP may worsen CSA in some patients as well described in patients with CSA or Complex Sleep Apnea (K. e. Johnson 2005). In the CAT-HF trial, Adaptive Servo Ventilation (ASV) did not change the overall cardiovascular outcomes at 6 months in the overall analysis of hospitalized heart failure patients with sleep apnea although the study was ended prematurely following the results of the SERVE-HF trial (O'Connor 2017).

It is still not clear what the specific mechanism is explaining increased mortality in the ASV group in patients with reduced ejection fraction. Subgroup analysis in the CAT-HF trial, however, suggested a positive effect of ASV in patients with a preserved ejection fraction. There will need to be further studies investigating this issue of outcomes of using ASV in patients with heart failure. The overall focus of treatment, however, is firstly optimizing the patient's volume status and comorbidities as this has been shown to help reduce CSR and improve sleep quality (Köhnlein 2002) so the best proven treatment of CSR is to treat the underlying condition. The heart failure in CSR patients with volume overload causes increased pulmonary vagal afferent traffic related to pulmonary venous congestion which causes hyperventilation and PaCO2 levels drop below the apneic threshold. This causes increased sympathetic activity and an increased circulatory delay (Bradley 1992).

In a patient with sleep disordered breathing, it is a common occurrence to have concomitant hypoventilation. Conditions causing hypoventilation will increase the likelihood of going into respiratory failure. Sleep related hypoventilation disorders such as obesity hypoventilation syndrome, sleep related hypoventilation due to a substance or medical disorder and more rarely, idiopathic central alveolar hypoventilation, congenital central alveolar hypoventilation syndrome are all possibilities in ICU patients. If patients sustain an additional pulmonary insult and are then mechanically ventilated, they may require higher minute ventilation and more assistance to recruit collapsed alveoli than those without a primary disorder of hypoventilation. Airway pressures should be monitored carefully so they do not exceed recommended levels necessary to support lung protective strategies when attempting to adequately ventilate the patient.

When a patient is weaned from a prolonged course on the ventilator, studies have shown that there is a high prevalence of SDB disorders (Diaz-Abad 2012). The patients in this cohort study were mainly found to have obstructive apneas and had the majority of their obstructive apneas resolve with PAP during a subsequent titration study (Diaz-Abad 2012). Also, when weaning from the ventilator, consideration should also be given to a trial of positive pressure at the time of extubation to avoid reintubation. Patients who have conditions predisposing them to hypoventilation such as post-bariatric surgery patients will require extra care upon liberating from the ventilator. This can be accomplished by extubating and directly placing patients on non-invasive ventilation (Ferrer 2006). Additionally, studies have shown that giving non-invasive ventilation immediately after extubation significantly improves spirometric lung function at 1 hour and 1 day postoperatively compared with continuous positive airway pressure started in the PACU specifically in the morbidly obese population of undergoing laparoscopic bariatric surgery (Neligan 2010).

It would be prudent to have a mechanism in place in the hospital setting to screen patients for sleep disordered breathing, diagnose the issue, and start treatment before any critical situations arise. Questionnaires such as the STOPBANG survey are proven to accurately predict the likelihood of severe OSA and are routinely employed now during the hospital admission process. The obstacles to these recommendations are availability of staff to perform screenings, difficulty arranging and performing successful inpatient sleep studies at most institutions, and lack of sleep medicine providers. There is also variable support for the successful introduction of CPAP in post-operative patients (Chung 2016).

Finally, a standardized protocol for hospital management of patients with sleep disordered breathing can help avoid oversite of worthwhile or necessary future diagnostics and therapeutics (Gay 2010). Some patients may benefit from hospital-based sleep study and PAP equipment availability before leaving the hospital. The presence of hypercapnia or markedly abnormal overnight oximetry may be good indicators of potential need for pre-discharge management. Many institutions have developed hospital basedhospital-based sleep consultative services but optimal care pathways require further investigation.

We have reviewed many aspects of the unique considerations with the interaction of sleep disordered patients with mechanical ventilation. Sleep is inherently disrupted in the ICU environment and especially difficult in those SDB patients struggling to maintain adequate gas exchange. Routine aspects of SDB patient care such as body position and requirements for sedative medications in the ICU lead to precarious clinical situations and all increase the chance for serious respiratory compromise. The astute clinician aware of the potential complications seen in SDB patients undergoing mechanical ventilation will make the best decisions for the optimal management during and subsequent to any hospitalized event.

KEY POINTS

1. SDB can complicate ICU care by placing the patient at higher risk for decompensation and a longer recovery time with higher risk or reintubation and prolonged mechanical ventilation
2. Although the oropharyngeal obstruction is alleviated with endotracheal intubation, patient may still require more PEEP and a higher MV
3. Patients with existing syndromes of hypoventilation will require higher ventilators setting with an increased MV and higher PEEP
4. Syndromes causing CSA/CSR are not as clearly defined in the literature when the patient is on mechanical ventilation. Care should be given not to over ventilate these patients and to treat the underlying condition.

REFERENCES

Bradley, T. 1992. "Central Sleep Apnea". *Clinical Chest Medicine,* 493 - 505.

Chung, F. et al. 2016. "CPAP in the Perioperative Setting". *Chest,* 586 - 597.

Cooper, A. 2000. "Sleep in critically ill patients requiring mechanical ventilation". *Chest,* 809 - 818.

Diaz-Abad, M., Verceles, A., Brown, J. and Scharf, S. 2012. "Sleep-Disordered Breathing May Be Under-Recognized in Patients Who Wean from Prolonged Mechanical Ventilation". *Respiratory Care*, 229 - 237.

Elliott, R., McKinley, S., Cistulli, P. and Fien, M. 2013. "Characterisation of sleep in intensive care using 24-hour polysomnography: an observational study". *Critical Care,* R46.

Ferrer, M. 2006. "Early noninvasive ventilation averts extubation failure in patients at risk: a randomized trial". *American Journal of Respiratory and Critical Care Medicine,* 164 - 170.

Gay, P. et al. 2010. "Sleep and Sleep-Disordered Breathing in the Hospitalized Patient". *Respiratory Care,* 1240 - 1254.

Johnson, D. and Johnson, K. 2012. "Obstructive Sleep Apnea and Prolonged Mechanical Ventilation". *Respiratory Care,* 326 - 327.

Johnson, K. et al. 2005. "Bilevel positive airway pressure worsens central apneas during sleep". *Chest,* 2141 - 2150.

Köhnlein, T. et al. 2002. "Assisted ventilation for heart failure patients with Cheyne-Stokes respiration". *European Respiratory Journal,* 934 - 941.

Malish, H. and Gay, P. n.d. *Perioperative care of patients with obstructive sleep apnea.*

Morris, T. et al. 2017. "Respiratory Compromise as a New Paradigm for the Care of Vulnerable Hospitalized Patients". *Respiratory Care,* 497 - 512.

Mundigler, G. et al. 2002. "Impaired circadian rhythm of melatonin secretion in sedated critically ill patients with severe sepsis". *Critical Care Medicine*, 536 - 640.

Neligan, P. et al. 2010. "Noninvasive ventilation immediately after extubation improves lung function in morbidly obese patients with obstructive sleep apnea undergoing laparoscopic bariatric surgery". *Anesthesia and Analgesia,* 1360 - 1365.

O'Connor, C. et al. 2017. "Cardiovascular Outcomes with Minute Ventilation-Targeted Adaptive Servo Ventilation Therapy in Heart Failure: The CAT-HF Trial". *Journal of American College of Cardiology,* 1577 - 1587.

Parthasarathy, S. et al. 2002. "Effect of ventilator mode on sleep quality in critically ill patients". *American Journal of Respiratory and Critical Care Medicine*, 1423 - 1429.

Parthasarathy, S. 2004. "Sleep during mechanical ventilation". *Current Opinion in Pulmonary Medicine*, 489 - 494.

Peppard, P. et al. 2013. "Increased prevalence of sleep-disordered breathing in adults". *American Journal of Epidemiology*, 1006 - 1014.

Pisani, M. et al. 2015. "Sleep in the Intensive Care Unit". *American Journal of Respiratory and Critical Care Medicine.*

Rudra, A., Chatterjee, S., Das, T., Sengupta, S., Maitra, G. and Kumar, P. 2008. "Obstructive sleep apnoea and anaesthesia". *Indian Journal of Critical Care Medicine,* 116 - 123.

Yumino, D. and Bradley, D. 2008. "Central Sleep Apnrea and Cheyne-Stokes Respiration". *Proceedings of the American Thoracic Society,* 226 - 236.

In: Sleep Medicine in Critical Care
Editors: Antonio M. Esquinas et al.
ISBN: 978-1-53617-768-8

Chapter 3

RESPIRATORY MUSCLES (INSPIRATORY, EXPIRATORY) AND SLEEP DISORDERED-BREATHING

Deeban Ratneswaran, MRCP *
and Joerg Steier, MD, PhD
King's College London, Faculty of Life Sciences and Medicine, London, UK
Lane Fox Respiratory Unit, Sleep Disorders Centre,
Guy's & St Thomas' NHS Foundation Trust, London, UK
Department of Respiratory Medicine,

ABSTRACT

The respiratory muscle pump consists of primary inspiratory muscles, of which the diaphragm is the predominant contributor. Many patients develop sleep-disordered breathing. This is predominantly in the form of obstructive sleep apnoea, which imposes a load on the respiratory muscle pump, but can also be caused by a variety of conditions that either reduce the capacity of the respiratory muscle pump (neuromuscular conditions) or increase the load (airway obstruction, obesity) leading to nocturnal hypoventilation.

* Corresponding Author. MBBS. E-mail: c.ratneswaran@gmail.com.

INTRODUCTION

The respiratory muscle pump comprises a group of muscles, which lead to ventilation. Its role is to generate both inspiration and expiration, by decreasing and increasing the intra-thoracic pressure respectively. This includes the diaphragm, abdominal muscles, chest wall muscles, shoulder and also neck muscles. Some parts of this pump are activated during inspiration, expiration, while asleep or during wakefulness, and during exercise or exertion.

Further upper airway dilator and bulbar muscles are important in maintaining the patency of the upper airway during sleep and are implicated in the development and progression of breathing disorders during sleep.

DIAPHRAGM

The diaphragm is a dome-like structure, which separates the thoracic cavity from the abdominal cavity. It is the most important muscle of respiration as it provides the greatest contribution (Mead and Loring, 1982). It is one of the *primary inspiratory muscles*, however, the diaphragm also plays a role in *passive expiration*. The diaphragm is made of 3 parts: the costal part, the crural part and a central tendon. The diaphragmatic fibres begin at the circumference of the thoracic cavity before inserting into the central tendon (a thin aponeurosis). The inferior vena cava, aorta and oesophagus pass through the diaphragm (Figure 1).

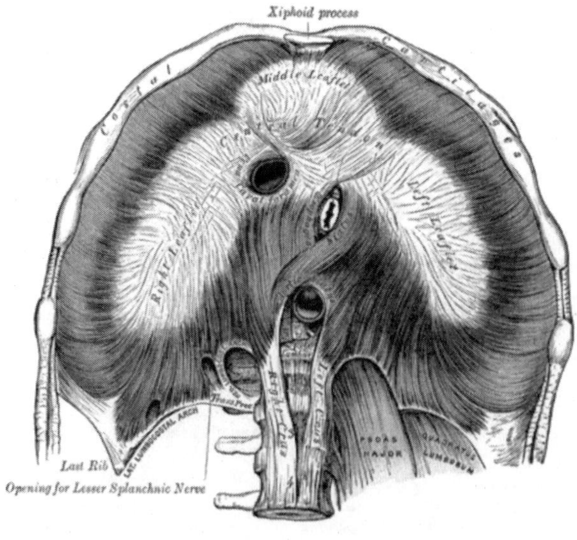

Figure 1. The human diaphragm (reproduced from Gray's Anatomy, 20th U.S. edition, originally published in 1918).

RESPIRATION

Contraction and relaxation of the diaphragm during respiration creates intra-thoracic and intra-abdominal pressure swings leading to inspiration and expiration. Contraction of the diaphragm results in caudal movement of this dome like structure, increasing the space in the thoracic cavity. The diaphragm is also responsible for lower ribcage expansion during inspiration, which supported by other *primary inspiratory muscles* such as the parasternal intercostal muscles (external intercostals and internal intercostals), increases the thoracic cavity space and results in generation of a negative intra-thoracic pressure and so inspiratory airflow. Our lungs therefore increase in size and inflate.

At times of high respiratory demand, due to respiratory dysfunction (e.g., an asthmatic attack) or high metabolic demand (e.g., exercise), this process is supported by additional *accessory inspiratory muscles* such as the sternocleidomastoid, scalene muscle groups and pectoralis minor (Figure 2).

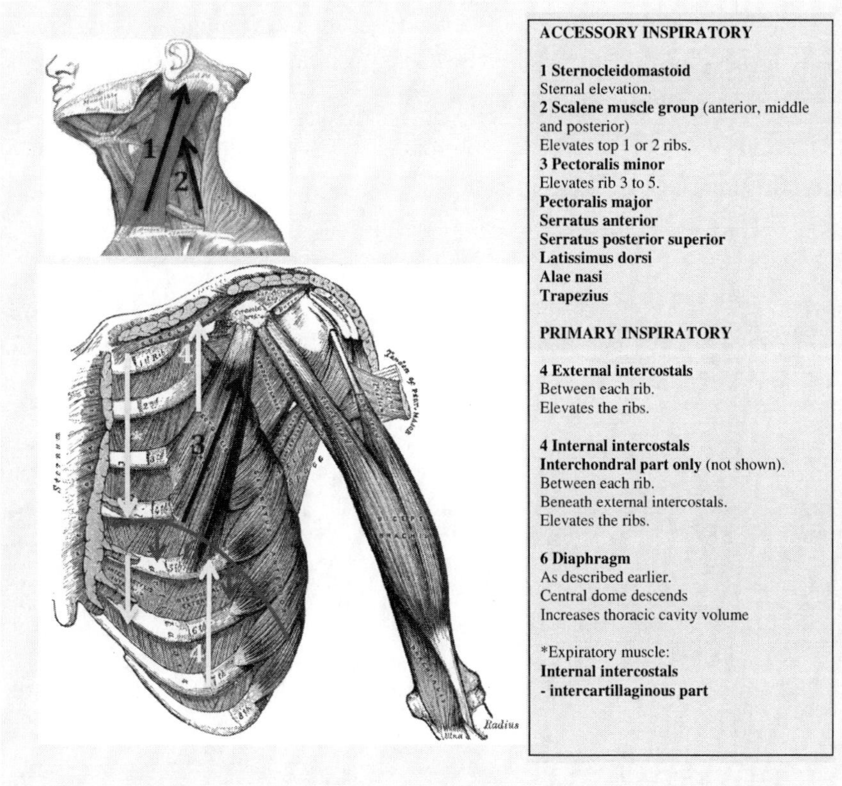

Figure 2. Muscles of inspiration (adapted from Gray's Anatomy, 20th U.S. edition, originally published in 1918). *Internal intercostal muscles, intercartillaginous part i.e., connects to the cartilage portions of each ribs. *This muscle is used in active expiration*, but is visualised here.

During inspiration, and caudal diaphragmatic movement, the curvature of the diaphragm also presses on the abdominal cavity causing an increase in the intra-abdominal cavity pressure (i.e., a positive intra-abdominal pressure). This leads to a difference in pressure between the thoracic (i.e., a negative intrathoracic pressure) and abdominal cavities - an increased transdiaphragmatic pressure.

Expiration does not normally require active muscular contraction and is a passive process. This occurs as the elastic recoil of the rib cage, diaphragm and lungs passively expire air as they return to their resting positions. In *normal* expiration, the diaphragm relaxes *passively* and returns to its cephalic position as the positive intra-abdominal pressure pushes it back towards the thoracic cavity. Therefore the lungs decrease in size and deflate in expiration as it adopts a positive intrathoracic pressure.

Muscles of Respiration

Other extra-diaphragmatic muscles also support inspiration and lung inflation, as well as expiration. These muscles include the non-diaphragmatic primary inspiratory muscles, which are the intercostal muscles (internal and external intercostal muscles), as well as accessory inspiratory muscles that are activated at times of high demand. These accessory muscles include the sternocleidomastoid, scalene muscle groups and pectoralis minor (Figure 2).

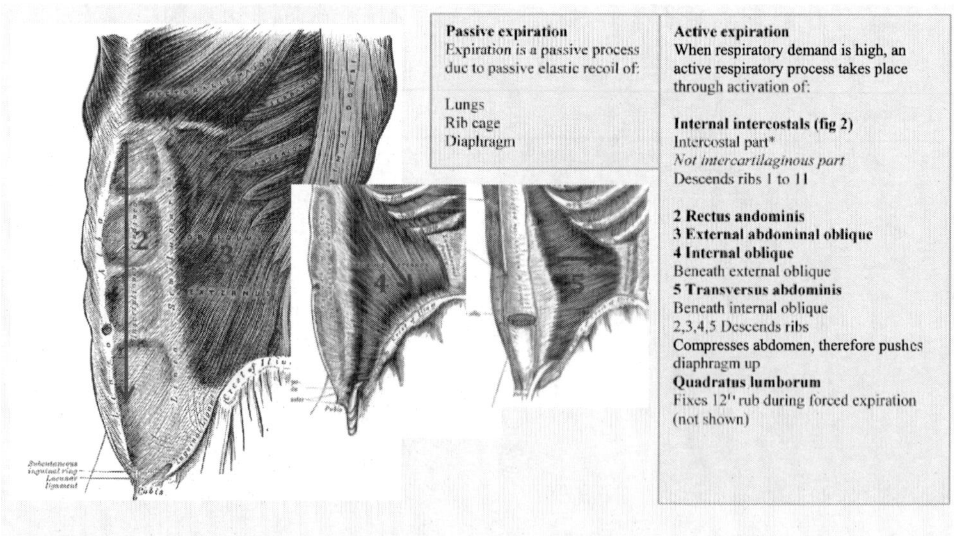

Figure 3. Muscles of expiration (adapted from Gray's Anatomy, 20th U.S. edition, originally published in 1918). *i.e., osseous part of each rib (lateral)

As well as a being a primary inspiratory muscle, the diaphragm is also a *passive expiratory muscle*, and non-volitionally allows expiration as it relaxes and returns to its cephalic position after being pushed by the positive intra-abdominal cavity pressure that exists post inspiration. Supporting expiration, there are additional non-diaphragmatic *active expiratory muscles*, which are activated during increased demand. These include the internal intercostals, rectus abdominis, internal and external abdominal oblique, transversus abdominis and quadratus lumborum (Figure 3).

Impact of Increased Load on the Respiratory Muscle Pump

Each of these muscles contribute to the overall capacity of the respiratory muscle pump, and will start to fail in efficiency where there is increased load on the respiratory system. Obesity is an important cause of increased load (Ratneswaran et al., 2018), and this additional pressure on the respiratory muscles can lead to sleep disordered breathing (Crummy et al., 2008), such as the development of the obesity hypoventilation syndrome (OHS) and obstructive sleep apnoea (OSA).

Increased load has the greatest impact around the thoracic and abdominal cavity. In the thoracic region obesity can limit the action of the external intercostals and the interchondral portion of the internal intercostals, leading to increased reliance on the *accessory inspiratory muscles*: sternocleidomastoid, scalene muscles and pectoralis minor (Figure 2). In the abdominal region, increased fat deposition around the abdominal cavity increases intra-abdominal pressure, preventing descent of the central dome of the diaphragm into the abdomen as described earlier. Reduced descent will also inhibit *forced active expiration*, which in turn reduces the effectiveness of the active expiratory muscles in expelling air from a poorly inspired lung.

Overall this can lead to slightly reduced lung volumes and a restrictive lung defect. This mechanical changes create increases in pleural pressures (Steier et al., 2010), decreases in transpulmonary pressure (Steier et al., 2014), in addition to reductions in expiratory reserve volumes (Steier et al., 2014) and functional residual capacity (Parameswaran et al., 2006), and therefore a decrease in the effective functioning of the respiratory system (Marin et al., 2005, Steier et al., 2009) compared to healthy individuals (Koenig, 2001, Pankow et al., 1998). Obese patients also develop a lower forced expiratory volume in 1 second (FEV_1) compared to non-obese subjects (Rubinstein et al., 1990, Zerah et al., 1993), which suggests an increased elastic load and that patients must deal with greater airway resistance during expiration (Figure 4).

Patients therefore have a propensity towards reduced oxygenation during sleep due to inadequate ventilation and especially during apneic and hypopneic events. Expiratory flow limitations have also been described in patients who are obese with subsequent increases in intrinsic PEEP (Pankow et al. JAP in the 90's). Therefore, there is inspiratory and expiratory ventilatory inefficiency, and this is thought to precede the obesity hypoventilation syndrome (OHS).

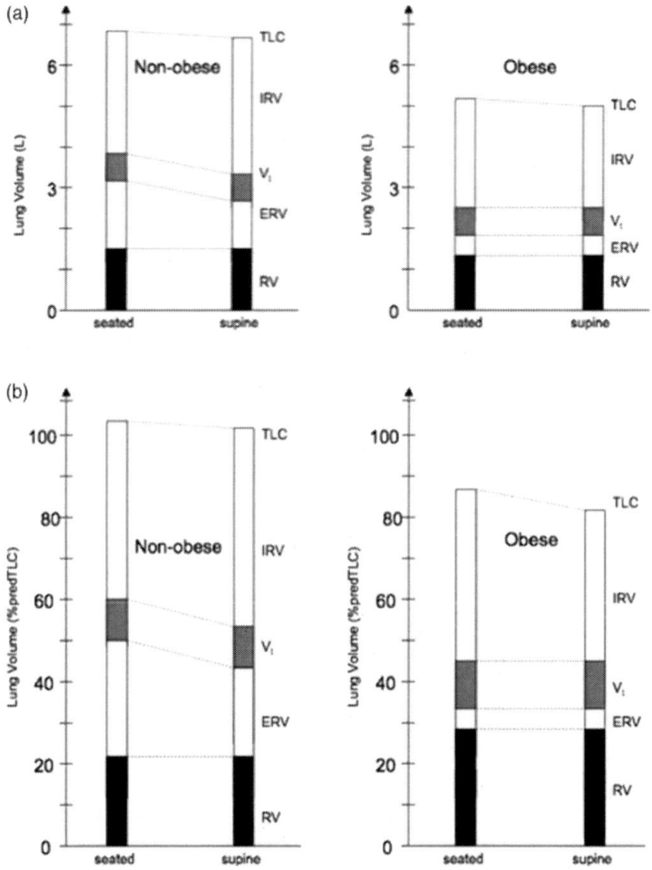

Figure 4. Simplified schematic illustration of lung volumes seated and supine in normal and obese subjects, expressed as litres (upper panel) and per cent predicted TLC (lower pane;). Parameters are derived from Tables 2 and 3. TLC, total lung capacity; IRV, inspiratory volume; V_t, tidal volume; ERV, expiratory reserve volume; RV, residual volume. (Steier et al. 2014) Reproduced with friendly permission from *Thorax*.

Obesity Hypoventilation Syndrome

Obesity hypoventilation syndrome (OHS) (Olson and Zwillich, 2005), eponymously known as the Pickwickian syndrome, after Charles Dicken's *'The Posthumous Papers of the Pickwick Club'* who's character "fat boy Joe" was thought to share its features. The author described him as "a fat and red faced boy in a state of somnolency". OHS is commonly defined as obesity with (body mass index > 30kg/m^2) and awake arterial hypercapnia ($PaCO_2$ > 45 mmHg) when other causes of hypoventilation have been excluded (Subramanian and Strohl, 1999), therefore OHS is a diagnosis of exclusion.

These patients may also develop a secondary polycythaemia. OHS shares many similar clinical features with OSA, and many of these patients with OHS also have OSA, however patients with OHS tend to be approaching severe obesity (BMI $\geq$ 40kg/m^2), with a severe OSA (Macavei et al., 2013, Mokhlesi et al., 2008). OHS patients, unlike OSA, tend to have elevated serum bicarbonate on arterial blood gas, which is indicative of their chronic hypercapnia (Rapoport et al., 1986, de Llano et al., 2005, Nowbar et al., 2004).

Patients with severe obesity (Flegal et al., 2005) and severe OSA (Young et al., 2008, Punjabi et al., 2009, Marin et al., 2005) are known to have increased morbidity and mortality with decreased health related quality of life, however OHS and hypercapnia is thought to add further additional burden. Patients with OHS have reduced quality of life (Hida, 2003, Budweiser et al., 2007a) and mortality (de Llano et al., 2005, Nowbar et al., 2004, Budweiser et al., 2007b). They also have increased health care expenses, and are at high risk of developing pulmonary hypertension and early mortality, compared to eucapnic sleep-disordered breathing (Castro-Añón et al., 2015). As the problems are directly related to an increased body habitus, weight loss can potentially reverse this disease, although patients may benefit from non-invasive ventilatory support (Royer et al., 2019).

Contributory Factors during Sleep

In normal individual mild bronchoconstriction is known to occur which can exacerbate hypoxaemia. Hypotonia of the intercostal muscles additionally occurs during sleep with atonia during REM stage of sleep (Huang et al., 2012, McSharry et al., 2014). The diaphragm also loses its tonic activity, while maintaining its phasic activity, during REM (Muller et al., 1979); and, while in the supine position during sleep, functional residual capacity also decreases (Hudgel and Devadatta, 1984). These factors are compounded by the elevated intra-abdominal pressures in obesity which significantly impact on the function on the diaphragm by increasing the load in inspiration and expiration, as well as a reduced neural respiratory drive to breathe during sleep (Ratneswaran et al., 2018) (Figure 5).

Alveolar hypoventilation also occurs during sleep in OHS (Zwillich et al., 1975) due to increased airway resistance. This is mainly due to reduced tone of the upper airway pharyngeal dilators, and this is further impacted by reduced medullary neuronal respiratory activity in sleep, which in turn leads to loss of upper respiratory muscle tonic and phasic output. During both NREM sleep and REM sleep, minute ventilation is known to fall (Douglas et al., 1982a). This fall in ventilation in OHS leads to increases in PCO_2, decreases in PO_2, and falls in arterial oxygen saturation (Lopata et al., 1979). Both the hypoxic and hypercapnic ventilatory response are known to decrease during sleep, with increasing levels of PCO2 needed to stimulate ventilation (Douglas et al., 1982b).

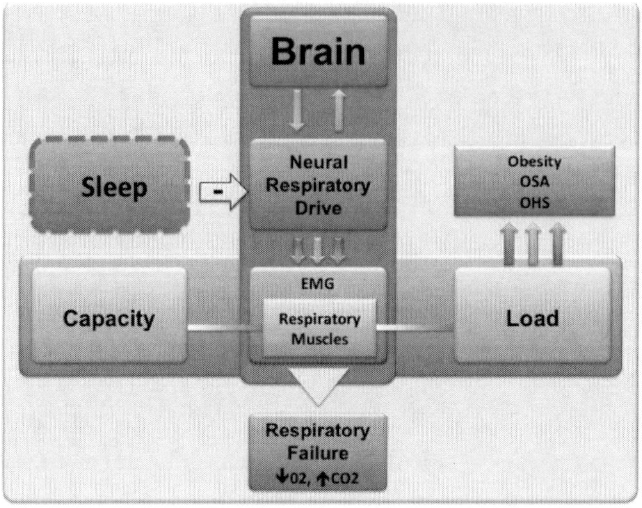

Figure 5. The load-capacity ratio of the respiratory muscle pump, simplified scheme. Multiple factors in obesity contribute to an increased load that leads to an elevated neural respiratory drive to recruit from the capacity of the respiratory muscle pump. If the elevated level of neural drive cannot be sustained (e.g., fatigue) or is influenced by other factors (e.g., sleep, drugs) an imbalance between load and capacity will develop, cause symptoms and respiratory failure when awake and sleep disordered breathing when asleep. (Ratneswaran et al., 2018) Reproduced with friendly permission from *Springer*.

Patients with OHS develop a type 2 respiratory failure due to the aforementioned load on the respiratory system and reduced ventilation efficiency. Due to the degree of severe obesity, patients are very likely to develop sleep disordered breathing and in 90% of patients with OHS this is associated with OSA, with the remaining 10% having isolated hypoventilation (Al Dabal and BaHammam, 2009, Mokhlesi, 2010). OSA typically does not cause hypercapnia as despite obesity being the predominant cause, the pathogenesis is different to that of OHS.

Obstructive Sleep Apnoea

OSA is the most common cause of sleep disordered breathing which affects 14% of adult men and 5% of adult women (Peppard et al., 2013). Patients with OSA have recurrent complete or partial collapse of the upper airway during sleep resulting in apnoeas and hypopnoeas during sleep (Remmers et al., 1978). Obesity is a significant risk factor in the development of OSA (Young et al., 1993, Peppard et al., 2013), and its prevalence is increasing due to rising levels of obesity. Obesity results in increased neck fat deposition and therefore contributes up to 50% of the pathogenesis of OSA (Dempsey et al., 2002) by creating external pressure around the neck which supports upper airway occlusion in patients with increased upper airway resistance and reduced upper airway tone.

Upper airway resistance increases during sleep due to hypotonia of the upper airway dilator muscles (Schwartz et al., 1998). These muscles include the genioglossus muscles, palatal muscles, masseter muscles, intrinsic laryngeal muscles and hyoid muscles. OSA severity is classified into mild, moderate and severe as defined by the apnoea-hypopnoea index (AHI) (Kapur et al., 2017). A large proportion of OSA remains undiagnosed (Young et al., 1997). Other pathogenic factors for obstructive sleep apnoea include increasing age, male sex, ananatomically narrow airway, in addition to variations in ventilatory control.

OSA is related to a number of pathogenic risks including hypertension (Hou et al., 2018) and endothelial dysfunction (Wang et al., 2015). Physiological and epidemiological observational studies show independent associations with adverse cardiovascular outcomes (Dong et al., 2013). OSA may also be linked to decreased vigiliance due to somnolence, and increased road traffic accidents (Ellen et al., 2006). These patients have a much reduced health related quality of life (McDaid et al., 2009) and so understanding the physiology and offering treatment is important to improve their quality of life, symptoms and reduce cardiovascular risk. Continuous positive airway pressure (CPAP) is the gold standard treatment as it abolishes the apnoes and hypopnoeas that occur due to the collapsible airway by providing a constant stream of high-pressured air to splint the airway open (Epstein et al., 2009, Sullivan et al., 1981). This helps overcome the excess load on both the respiratory muscle pump and upper airway.

CONCLUSION

The respiratory muscle pump consists of primary inspiratory muscles, of which the diaphragm is the predominant contributor. Accessory inspiratory muscles support this function. The diaphragm also allows passive expiration, but is additionally supported by active expiratory muscles when needed. Obesity increases the mechanical load on the respiratory muscles, leading to increased intra-abdominal pressures, and reduced effective ventilation. In obesity when patients are lying supine this causes an additional intrinsic PEEP, inspiratory diaphragmatic preload and a reduced operational volume for respiration close to the residual volume. Overall, the high intra-abdominal pressures and therefore reduced transpulmonary pressures in obesity result in a restrictive lung defect. In severe obesity hypoventilation can develop and this precedes the development of the obesity hypoventilation syndrome. Obesity also increases fat deposition around the neck, which in addition to decreased upper airway dilator tone results in OSA. Many patients with OHS developed sleep disordered breathing, and this is predominantly OSA.

REFERENCES

Al Dabal, L. & Bahammam, A. S. (2009). Obesity hypoventilation syndrome. *Annals of thoracic medicine*, *4*, 41.

Budweiser, S., Hitzl, A. P., Jörres, R. A., Schmidbauer, K., Heinemann, F. & Pfeifer, M. (2007a). Health-related quality of life and long-term prognosis in chronic hypercapnic respiratory failure: a prospective survival analysis. *Respiratory research*, *8*, 92.

Budweiser, S., Riedl, S. G., Jörres, R. A., Heinemann, F. & Pfeifer, M. (2007b). Mortality and prognostic factors in patients with obesity-hypoventilation syndrome undergoing noninvasive ventilation. *Journal of internal medicine*, *261*, 375-383.

Castro-Añón, O., De Llano, L. A. P., De la Fuente Sánchez, S., Golpe, R., Marote, L. M., Castro-Castro, J. & Quintela, A. G. (2015). Obesity-hypoventilation syndrome: increased risk of death over sleep apnea syndrome. *PLoS One*, *10*, e0117808.

Crummy, F., Piper, A. J. & Naughton, M. T. (2008). Obesity and the lung: 2· Obesity and sleep-disordered breathing. *Thorax*, *63*, 738-746.

De Llano, L. A. P., Golpe, R., Piquer, M. O., Racamonde, A. V., Caruncho, M. V., Muinelos, O. C. & Carro, C. A. (2005). Short-term and long-term effects of nasal intermittent positive pressure ventilation in patients with obesity-hypoventilation syndrome. *Chest*, *128*, 587-594.

Dempsey, J. A., Skatrud, J. B., Jacques, A. J., Ewanowski, S. J., Woodson, B. T., Hanson, P. R. & Goodman, B. (2002). Anatomic determinants of sleep-disordered breathing across the spectrum of clinical and nonclinical male subjects. *Chest*, *122*, 840-851.

Dong, J. Y., Zhang, Y. H. & Qin, L. Q. (2013). Obstructive sleep apnea and cardiovascular risk: meta-analysis of prospective cohort studies. *Atherosclerosis*, *229*, 489-495.

Douglas, N. J., White, D. P., Pickett, C. K., Weil, J. V. & Zwillich, C. W. (1982a). Respiration during sleep in normal man. *Thorax*, *37*, 840-844.

Douglas, N. J., White, D. P., Weil, J. V., Pickett, C. K. & Zwillich, C. W. (1982b). Hypercapnic ventilatory response in sleeping adults. *American Review of Respiratory Disease*, *126*, 758-762.

Ellen, R. L. B., Marshall, S. C., Palayew, M., Molnar, F. J., Wilson, K. G. & Man-Son-Hing, M. (2006). Systematic review of motor vehicle crash risk in persons with sleep apnea. *Journal of Clinical Sleep Medicine*, *2*, 193-200.

Epstein, L. J., Kristo, D., Strollo, Jr. P. J., Friedman, N., Malhotra, A., Patil, S. P., Ramar, K., Rogers, R., Schwab, R. J. & Weaver, E. M. (2009). Clinical guideline for the evaluation, management and long-term care of obstructive sleep apnea in adults. *J Clin Sleep Med*, *5*, 263-276.

Flegal, K. M., Graubard, B. I., Williamson, D. F. & Gail, M. H. (2005). Excess deaths associated with underweight, overweight, and obesity. *Jama*, *293*, 1861-1867.

Hida, W. (2003). Quality of life in obesity hypoventilation syndrome. *Sleep and Breathing*, *7*, 001-002.

Hou, H., Zhao, Y., Yu, W., Dong, H., Xue, X., Ding, J., Xing, W. & Wang, W. (2018). Association of obstructive sleep apnea with hypertension: A systematic review and meta-analysis. *Journal of global health*, *8*.

Huang, J., Pinto, S. J., Yuan, H., Katz, E. S., Karamessinis, L. R., Bradford, R. M., Gallagher, P. R., Hannigan, J. T., Nixon, T. & Ward, M. B. (2012). Upper airway collapsibility and genioglossus activity in adolescents during sleep. *Sleep*, *35*, 1345-1352.

Hudgel, D. W. & Devadatta, P. (1984). Decrease in functional residual capacity during sleep in normal humans. *Journal of Applied Physiology*, *57*, 1319-1322.

Kapur, V. K., Auckley, D. H., Chowdhuri, S., Kuhlmann, D. C., Mehra, R., Ramar, K. & Harrod, C. G. (2017). Clinical practice guideline for diagnostic testing for adult obstructive sleep apnea: an American Academy of Sleep Medicine clinical practice guideline. *Journal of Clinical Sleep Medicine*, *13*, 479-504.

Koenig, S. M. (2001). Pulmonary complications of obesity. *American Journal of the Medical Sciences*, *321*, 249-279.

Lopata, M., Freilich, R. A., Önal, E., Pearle, J. & Lourenço, R. V. (1979). Ventilatory control and the obesity hypoventilation syndrome. *American Review of Respiratory Disease*, *119*, 165-168.

Macavei, V. M., Spurling, K. J., Loft, J. & Makker, H. K. (2013). Diagnostic predictors of obesity-hypoventilation syndrome in patients suspected of having sleep disordered breathing. *Journal of Clinical Sleep Medicine*, *9*, 879-884.

Marin, J. M., Carrizo, S. J., Vicente, E. & Agusti, A. G. N. (2005). Long-term cardiovascular outcomes in men with obstructive sleep apnoea-hypopnoea with or without treatment with continuous positive airway pressure: an observational study. *The Lancet*, *365*, 1046-1053.

Mcdaid, C., Griffin, S., Weatherly, H., Duree, K., Van der Burgt, M., Van Hout, S., Akers, J., Davies, R., Sculpher, M. & Westwood, M. (2009). Continuous positive airway pressure devices for the treatment of obstructive sleep apnoea–hypopnoea syndrome: a systematic review and economic analysis. *NIHR Health Technology Assessment programme: Executive Summaries.* NIHR Journals Library.

Mcsharry, D. G., Saboisky, J. P., Deyoung, P., Jordan, A. S., Trinder, J., Smales, E., Hess, L., Chamberlin, N. L. & Malhotra, A. (2014). Physiological mechanisms of upper airway hypotonia during REM sleep. *Sleep*, *37*, 561-569.

Mead, J. & Loring, S. H. (1982). Analysis of volume displacement and length changes of the diaphragm during breathing. *Journal of Applied Physiology*, *53*, 750-755.

Mokhlesi, B. (2010). Obesity hypoventilation syndrome: a state-of-the-art review. *Respiratory care*, *55*, 1347-1365.

Mokhlesi, B., Kryger, M. H. & Grunstein, R. R. (2008). Assessment and management of patients with obesity hypoventilation syndrome. *Proceedings of the American Thoracic Society*, *5*, 218-225.

Muller, N., Volgyesi, G., Becker, L., Bryan, M. H. & Bryan, A. C. (1979). Diaphragmatic muscle tone. *J Appl Physiol Respir Environ Exerc Physiol*, *47*, 279-84.

National Institute for Health and Care Excellence (NICE), *Continuous positive airway pressure for the treatment of obstructive sleep apnoea/hypopnoea syndrome*. NICE Guideline [TA139]. 2016. Available from: https://http://www.nice.org.uk/guidance/ ta139/ chapter/1-Guidance [Accessed 25th March 2019].

Nowbar, S., Burkart, K. M., Gonzales, R., Fedorowicz, A., Gozansky, W. S., Gaudio, J. C., Taylor, M. R. G. & Zwillich, C. W. (2004). Obesity-associated hypoventilation in hospitalized patients: prevalence, effects, and outcome. *The American journal of medicine*, *116*, 1-7.

Olson, A. L. & Zwillich, C. (2005). The obesity hypoventilation syndrome. *The American journal of medicine*, *118*, 948-956.

Pankow, W., Podszus, T., Gutheil, T., Penzel, T., Peter, J. H. & Von Wichert, P. (1998). Expiratory flow limitation and intrinsic positive end-expiratory pressure in obesity. *Journal of Applied Physiology*, *85*, 1236-1243.

Parameswaran, K., Todd, D. C. & Soth, M. (2006). Altered respiratory physiology in obesity. *Canadian respiratory journal: journal of the Canadian Thoracic Society*, *13*, 203.

Peppard, P. E., Young, T., Barnet, J. H., Palta, M., Hagen, E. W. & Hla, K. M. (2013). Increased prevalence of sleep-disordered breathing in adults. *American journal of epidemiology*, *177*, 1006-1014.

Punjabi, N. M., Caffo, B. S., Goodwin, J. L., Gottlieb, D. J., Newman, A. B., O'connor, G. T., Rapoport, D. M., Redline, S., Resnick, H. E. & Robbins, J. A. (2009). Sleep-disordered breathing and mortality: a prospective cohort study. *PLoS medicine*, *6*, e1000132.

Rapoport, D. M., Garay, S. M., Epstein, H. & Goldring, R. M. (1986). Hypercapnia in the obstructive sleep apnea syndrome: a reevaluation of the "Pickwickian syndrome". *Chest*, *89*, 627-635.

Ratneswaran, C., Murphy, P., Hart, N. & Steier, J. (2018). Obesity, Respiratory Mechanics and Its Impact on the Work of Breathing, Neural Respiratory Drive, Gas Exchange and the Development of Sleep-Disordered Breathing. *Mechanical Ventilation in the Critically Ill Obese Patient.* Springer.

Remmers, J. E., Degroot, W. J., Sauerland, E. K. & Anch, A. M. (1978). Pathogenesis of upper airway occlusion during sleep. *J Appl Physiol*, *44*, 931-8.

Royer, C. P., Schweiger, C., Manica, D., Rabaioli, L., Guerra, V. & Sbruzzi, G. (2019). Efficacy of bilevel ventilatory support in the treatment of stable patients with obesity hypoventilation syndrome: systematic review and meta-analysis. *Sleep medicine*, *53*, 153-164.

Rubinstein, I., Zamel, N., Dubarry, L. & Hoffstein, V. (1990). Airflow limitation in morbidly obese, nonsmoking men. *Annals of internal medicine*, *112*, 828-832.

Schwartz, A. R., O'donnell, C. P., Baron, J., Schubert, N., Alam, D., Samadi, S. D. & Smith, P. L. (1998). The hypotonic upper airway in obstructive sleep apnea: role of structures and neuromuscular activity. *American Journal of Respiratory and Critical Care Medicine*, *157*, 1051-1057.

Steier, J., Jolley, C. J., Seymour, J., Roughton, M., Polkey, M. I. & Moxham, J. (2009). Neural respiratory drive in obesity. *Thorax*, *64*, 719-725.

Steier, J., Jolley, C. J., Seymour, J., Ward, K., Luo, Y. M., Polkey, M. I. & Moxham, J. (2010). Increased load on the respiratory muscles in obstructive sleep apnea. *Respiratory physiology & neurobiology*, *171*, 54-60.

Steier, J., Lunt, A., Hart, N., Polkey, M. I. & Moxham, J. (2014). Observational study of the effect of obesity on lung volumes. *Thorax*, thoraxjnl-2014-205148.

Subramanian, S. & Strohl, K. P. (1999). A management guideline for obesity-hypoventilation syndromes. *Sleep and Breathing*, *3*, 131-138.

Sullivan, C., Berthon-Jones, M., Issa, F. & Eves, L. (1981). Reversal of obstructive sleep apnoea by continuous positive airway pressure applied through the nares. *The Lancet*, *317*, 862-865.

Wang, J., Yu, W., Gao, M., Zhang, F., Gu, C., Yu, Y. & Wei, Y. (2015). Impact of obstructive sleep apnea syndrome on endothelial function, arterial stiffening, and serum inflammatory markers: an updated meta-analysis and metaregression of 18 studies. *Journal of the American Heart Association*, *4*, e002454.

Young, T., Evans, L., Finn, L. & Palta, M. (1997). Estimation of the clinically diagnosed proportion of sleep apnea syndrome in middle-aged men and women. *Sleep*, *20*, 705-706.

Young, T., Finn, L., Peppard, P. E., Szklo-Coxe, M., Austin, D., Nieto, F. J., Stubbs, R. & Hla, K. M. (2008). Sleep disordered breathing and mortality: eighteen-year follow-up of the Wisconsin sleep cohort. *Sleep*, *31*, 1071-1078.

Young, T., Palta, M., Dempsey, J., Skatrud, J., Weber, S. & Badr, S. (1993). The occurrence of sleep-disordered breathing among middle-aged adults. *New England Journal of Medicine*, *328*, 1230-1235.

Zerah, F., Harf, A., Perlemuter, L., Lorino, H., Lorino, A. M. & Atlan, G. (1993). Effects of obesity on respiratory resistance. *CHEST Journal*, *103*, 1470-1476.

Zwillich, C. W., Sutton, F. D., Pierson, D. J., Creagh, E. M. & Weil, J. V. (1975). Decreased hypoxic ventilatory drive in the obesity-hypoventilation syndrome. *The American journal of medicine*, *59*, 343-348.

In: Sleep Medicine in Critical Care
Editors: Antonio M. Esquinas et al.
ISBN: 978-1-53617-768-8

Chapter 4

THE IMPORTANCE OF UPPER AIRWAYS FEATURES IN SLEEP BREATHING DISORDERS

Andrea De Vito[1,*], Giannicola Iannella[1], Soon Sue Rene[2], Bhik Kotecha[3], Khai Beng Chong[4], Mohamed Al Ajmi[5], Muawya Bani Younes[6], Graeme Jones[7], Vinod Prabhu[7], Venkata Koka[8], Giovanni Cammaroto[1], Giuseppe Meccariello[1] and Claudio Vicini[9,10]

[1]Morgagni-Pierantoni Hospital, AUSL of Romagna, Forlì, Italy
[2]Ng Teng Fong General Hospital, Singapore
[3]Nuffield Health Brentwood, Essex, UK
[4]Tan Tock Seng Hospital, Singapore
[5]Al Nahdha Hospital, Muscat, Oman
[6]Sara Specialty Hospital, Mafraq, Jordan
[7]Glangwili General Hospital,
Hywel Dda University Health Board, Carmarthen, Wales
[8]Antoine Beclere Hospital, Clamart, France
[9]Morgagni Pierantoni Hospital, Forlì, Italy
[10]University of Ferrara, Ferrara, Italy

---

* Corresponding Author's E-mail: dr.andrea.devito@gmail.com.

Abstract

Upper Airways anatomical abnormalities play a central role in OSA pathophysiology. Upper Airways clinical examination represents an essential step in the evaluation of an OSA patient. Awake and sleep/sedation endoscopic examination provide analysis of the site, grade and pattern of Upper Airways collapsibility. Drug-Induced Sleep Endoscopy has been found to be useful for anatomical assessment of Upper Airways and treatment option selection in OSA patients. Adeno-Tonsillar hypertrophy is the most important anatomical abnormality for pediatric OSA. Customized, multidisciplinary, combined therapy represents the treatment option for achieving the best outcomes. In this chapter, we are mainly discussing the UA anatomical features in relation to OSA pathophysiology in the adult and pediatric OSA patients, as well as study the impact of UA anatomical characteristics in the treatment of an OSA patient.

Keywords: obstructive sleep apnoea, upper airways, clinical examination, drug-induced sleep endoscopy, polysomnography, sleep-breathing disorders, customized treatment

Key Points

- Upper Airways anatomical abnormalities play a central role in OSA pathophysiology
- Upper Airways examination is an essential step in the clinical evaluation of an OSA patient
- Awake and sleep/sedation endoscopic examination provide analysis of the site, grade and pattern of Upper Airways collapsibility
- Drug-Induced Sleep Endoscopy has been found to be useful for anatomical assessment of Upper Airways and treatment option selection in OSA patients
- Adeno-Tonsillar hypertrophy is the most important anatomical abnormality for paediatric OSA
- Customized, multidisciplinary, combined therapy represents the treatment option for achieving the best outcomes

Introduction

Obstructive Sleep Apnea (OSA) syndrome is a sleep-related respiratory disorder characterized by partial or complete recurrent episodes of upper airway collapse during sleep [1].

The International Classification of Sleep Disorders (ICSD-3) has defined four major categories of SDB: which encompass obstructive sleep apnea disorders (including OSA syndrome), central sleep apnea syndrome (CSA), sleep-related hypoventilation disorders and sleep-related hypoxemia disorders [1-3]. According to ICSD-3, OSA is defined as five or more episodes of apnoea and/or hypopnoea per hour of sleep with associated symptoms (e.g., excessive daytime sleepiness, fatigue, or impaired cognition) or 15 or more obstructive apnea/hypopnea events per hour of sleep regardless of associated symptoms [3-5]. Its prevalence is estimated to be between 5% to 12% of the worldwide population with a higher frequency in men [4-6].

Snoring, unrefreshed sleep, excessive daytime sleepiness (EDS), lack of concentration, impaired memory and poor quality of life are the main symptoms of OSA. OSA is recognized as a serious health hazard and an independent risk factor for motor vehicle accidents, arterial hypertension, stroke, cardiovascular diseases, cardiac arrhythmias, coronary artery disease, diabetes and cognitive dysfunction [3, 7, 8].

The most important OSA pathophysiological factors contributing to apnoea /hypopnoea events are: (1) upper airways (UA) anatomical collapsibility (UA anatomical tract); (2) inadequate responsiveness of the UA dilator muscles during sleep; (3) waking-up prematurely to airway narrowing (a low respiratory arousal threshold) and (4) oversensitive ventilatory control system (high loop gain). These factors are expressed differently in each patient, leading to different OSA pathophysiological phenotypes. Eckert et al. proposed a possible classification of OSA patients in three subgroups, based on anatomical and non-anatomical phenotypes which he named the PALM scale [6, 8]. Different possible therapeutic strategies could thereafter be introduced based on the patient's phenotype. However, PALM scale was only developed based on small clinical studies and theoretical models [6-11].

An extensive knowledge of respiratory pathophysiology is required to differentiate between OSA and other respiratory diseases (obesity-hypoventilation syndrome, chronic obstructive pulmonary diseases (COPD), chest diseases, muscular neuropathies, etc.). The latter is similarly prevalent in the general population, can cause SBD not associated with obstructive apneas (no OSA SBD), and has significant morbidity and mortality [3, 8, 10, 11].

We are mainly discussing the UA anatomical features in relation to OSA pathophysiology in the adult and pediatric OSA patients, as well as study the impact of UA anatomical characteristics in the treatment of an OSA patient in this chapter.

Adult OSA Patients

Clinical Investigation

Medical history is important in the evaluation of an OSA patient prior to ordering further test or examinations. In the approach to an adult OSA patient, the relationship of the UA abnormalities/characteristics that correlate with the OSA should be evaluated in addition to the patient's age, grade of obesity and comorbidities [12-14].

Male gender and age represent the most important non-modifiable factors in adult OSA patients. In the literature, men are more affected by OSA than women, with male-to-female ratio of OSA disorders estimated between 3:1 to 5:1 in the general population [15]. Different authors have reported that aging is positively correlated with an increase in the incidence of OSA [16, 17]. In an analysis of 427 elderly above 65 years by Ancoli et al. [18], 24% of them had an apnea/hypopnea index (AHI) of greater than 5. In another study comprising of 5615 men and women between 40 to 98 years of age, sleep apnea was found to be most frequent in subjects aged 60 years or older (approximately 50% had an AHI of 5–14, and approximately 20% had an AHI $\geq$ 15) [19].

In addition to gender and age, there are several other conditions that increase the risk of getting OSA. Obesity, use of drugs that cause muscle relaxation, endocrine disorders, smoking, and UA anatomical abnormalities are reported as the main modifiable risk factors associated with OSA [3, 4, 20].

About 80% of OSA patients are obese and obesity is an established risk factor for OSA. A very close relationship has been observed between body weight change and AHI: a 10 % weight gain has been shown to predict an approximate 32 % increase in the AHI, a 10% weight loss predicts a 26% decrease in the AHI, and a 10% weight gain predicts a six-fold increase in the odds of developing moderate to severe OSA [20, 21]. Obesity affects OSA mainly through two mechanisms: 1) Increase in airway narrowing and collapse, as a result of excess fat in the (peri- and para) pharyngeal tissues; 2) Excess fat in the thoracic and abdominal walls increases the respiratory effort in these patients. It is estimated that BMI increment above the 50th percentile is associated with a 10% increased risk for OSAS [21]. Body Mass Index (BMI) is the most commonly used measurement of obesity. This parameter should always be considered in relation with UA anatomical characteristics [2].

UA clinical examination is an essential step in the evaluation of an OSA patient. Multilevel anatomical obstruction may play a role in OSA. Therefore, clinical examination should encompass evaluating the different UA anatomical levels which may be involved in OSA pathogenesis [12, 13].

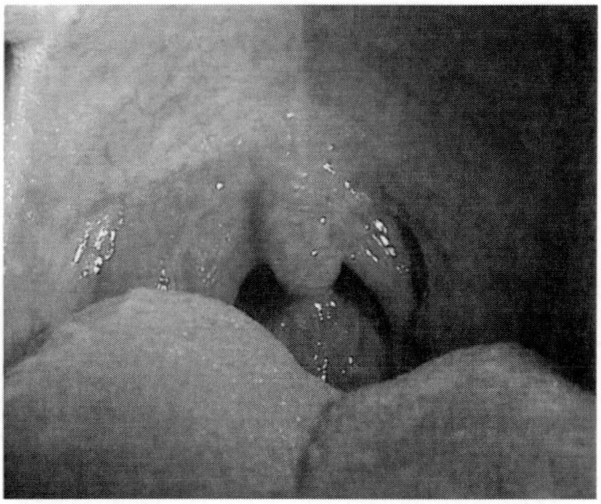

Figure 1. OSAS oropharyngeal characteristics example: soft palate ptosis, tonsillar pillars medialization.

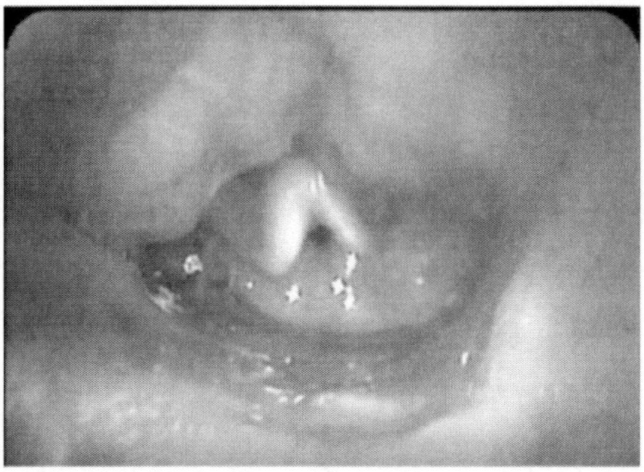

Figure 2. OSAS hypopharyngeal characteristics example: closing-book shape epiglottidis, arytenoid edema with lingual tonsil hypertrophy.

The different UA levels and associated pathological conditions that could contribute to OSA are reported as follows.

- Nose and nasopharynx: inferior turbinates hypertrophy, nasal septal deviation, nasal valve collapse, nasal polyposis, adenoid hypertrophy, signs of chronic sinusitis.
- Mouth: limited opening of the oral cavity, conformation of the hard palate, volume of the tongue and its relationship with the soft palate area, malocclusion and dental classes.
- Oropharynx: enlarged and elongated soft palate, enlarged uvula, palatine tonsils hypertrophy and narrow lateral pharyngeal wall. (Figure 1).
- Hypopharynx: lingual tonsil hypertrophy, supra-laryngeal anatomical changes (epiglottic and/or arytenoid edema) (Figure 2).

Alone or in combination, these anatomical features can contribute to airway obstruction and should always be analyzed in an OSA patient in awake state or during sedation [13, 14].

The oropharyngeal examination is the first step in the clinical evaluation of an OSA patient in the outpatient setting, taking into consideration the oral tongue volume and palatine tonsil size. According to Friedman classification, oral tongue volume allows the visualization of the following pharyngeal structures [22]:

- The whole uvula and tonsils/pillar (Friedman Tongue Position: FTP I),
- most of the uvula but not the whole tonsils/pillars (FTP IIa),
- the entire soft palate and base of uvula (FTP IIb),
- only the soft palate (FTP III)
- only the hard palate (FTP IV).

Regarding the palatine tonsil size, Friedman et al. suggests the following grading system [22, 23]:

- absence of tonsillar tissue (grade 0)
- tonsils within the pillars (grade 1)
- extending to the pillars (grade 2)
- extending past the pillars (grade 3)
- extending to the midline (grade 4).

UA fiber optic endoscopic assessment in the awake patient is considered the second step. Endoscopy must start with the evaluation of the nasal cavity and continue with all subsequent anatomical structures/levels with the patient in a supine position.

Obstructive anatomical signs in the nasal cavity such as nasal septal deviation, inferior turbinate hypertrophy, obstructive congestion of the nasal mucosa and nasal polyposis are strongly related to patients with simple snoring. Nasal obstruction is a frequent symptom reported in OSA patients [24, 25]. Various authors have supported the theory that nasal obstruction is a contributing factor in the pathogenesis of OSA despite numerous controversies. They report that nasal obstruction leads to mouth breathing, which is thought to destabilize the upper airway facilitating pharyngeal anatomical collapsibility and aggravating the OSA syndrome. Moreover, nasal breathing obstruction might represent a factor influencing the clinical history of OSA as well as the patient's compliance with CPAP [25].

The endoscopic observation of the retro-palatal area from the nasopharynx allows the description of the anatomical pattern of the soft palate. Woodson et al. have classified the relationship between the soft palate and the hard palate based on the angle that they configure, and the consequent pattern of posterior collapse that occurs. According to the analysis three patterns have been described: oblique, intermediate and vertical [26]. Below to the inferior edge of the soft palate, it is possible to examine the anatomy of the pharyngeal walls and the impact of palatine tonsils hypertrophy.

The anatomy and role of the base of the tongue (BOT) is another point that should be investigated during fiber optic examination. Moore et al. [27] classified base of tongue as high tongue base (type A), high tongue base with retro-epiglottic narrowing (type B1) or diffuse tongue base narrowing (type B2), and isolated retro-epiglottic narrowing (type C). More recently, Friedman et al. proposed a new classification system according to the degree of development of the lingual tonsil [22, 23, 28].

- no lymphoid tissue (LTH0)
- scattered lymphoid tissue (LTH1)
- lymphoid tissue covering the entire tongue base, limited vertical thickness (LTH2)
- lymphoid tissue covering the entire tongue base, significant vertical thickness of approximately 5–10 mm (LTH3)
- lymphoid tissue covering the entire tongue base, rising to or above the tip of the epiglottis, approximately 1 cm in height (LTH 4).

This is a standardized grading score proposed by Friedman et al. [22, 23] to measure LT on the BOT. It is the most widely used method due to its good cost-effective ratio, and its easy application in clinical practice. Furthermore, the systematic use of this classification avoids heterogeneous approaches to describe lingual tonsil size/volume.

Finally, epiglottis abnormalities or laryngeal obstructive conditions can be evaluated with the use of the fiber optic endoscope. During endoscopic fiber optic evaluation, it is possible to perform Müller's maneuver. It is done by forced and prolonged inspiration with the mouth and nose closed [12, 13]. Müller's maneuver helps us to assess the pharyngeal collapsibility and may predict different pharyngeal sites, and patterns of obstruction. However, the reliability of Müller's maneuver in an awake patient in identifying sites and collapse patterns is not 100%. One should keep in mind that this maneuver is carried out in an awake patient with a preserved pharyngeal muscular tone [12-14, 29].

Soares et al. [30] studied and compared fiber optic nasal endoscopy with Müller's maneuver (FNMM) versus drug-induced sleep endoscopy (DISE) in diagnosing the presence of level-specific UA collapse in OSA patients. Fifty-three patients were included in this study. Fiber-optic nasal endoscopy with Müller's maneuver and DISE did not differ significantly when assessing the presence of severe retro-palatal airway collapse. However, there was a statistically significant difference in the incidence of severe retro-lingual collapse identified by DISE (84.9% DISE vs 35.8% of FNMM).

The introduction of DISE has allowed dynamic airway evaluation in a state that closely mimics natural sleep. Different authors concord that DISE, when performed with a standardized protocol, can offer additional and pivotal information concerning sites and patterns of obstruction [31-33]. Airway evaluation obtained with sleep endoscopy have been shown to have good correlation with the respiratory disturbance index (RDI). During DISE, the following information should be considered: severity of event, sound generation (snoring vs stridor), partial/ complete obstruction/collapse of UA, sites of obstruction (e.g., tongue base, supraglottis and glottis) and pattern of collapse at different sites (antero-posterior, lateral and circumferential) [31].

DISE has been found to be useful for treatment option selection in OSA patients. DISE can also aid in identifying why some patients fail CPAP therapy. Similarly, when surgery fails, DISE assessment of the UA may shed some light on the residual problem [31-33].

Correlation between UA Clinical Examination and UA Anatomical Collapsibility

Several literature studies have reported the association between UA clinical examination and UA anatomical collapsibility [12, 13, 20, 21]. Friedman et al. [14] introduced a surgical staging system considering the relation between tongue position, palatine tonsil size and patients' BMI (Table 1).

Table 1. Friedman staging system as determined by Friedman tongue position (FTP), tonsil size, and BMI

STAGE	FTP	TONSIL SIZE	BMI
I	I, IIa, IIb	3 or 4	<40
II	I, IIa, IIb	0, 1, or 2	<40
	III or IV	3 or 4	<40
III	III or IV	0, 1, or 2	<40
IV*	I–IV	0-4	>40

* All patients with significant craniofacial or other anatomic abnormalities.

According to Friedman staging and grading systems [14], OSA patients with a grade I or II of Friedman tongue position, grade 3-4 palatine tonsils hypertrophy and low LTH represent the best candidates for palatal surgery (UPPP with tonsillectomy), achieving a success rate higher than 80% (stage I disease). OSA patients with high FTP and low palatine tonsils hypertrophy (stage III disease) should not be considered as candidates for palatal surgery alone as the success rate is reported at 8% (Table 1).

In another clinical study Friedman et al. demonstrated that patients classified with this staging system showed significant improvement in AHI after 6-months follow-up compared with a group of patients treated without the benefit of a staging system [9].

Palatine tonsil (PT) hypertrophy is one of the most important anatomical factors that correlate with oropharyngeal obstruction in OSA patients. Jara et al. [34] have showed a relationship between PT size and OSA. They report that subjective PT grade was more strongly associated with AHI compared with PT volume. These data suggest that the space that the tonsils occupy within the oropharyngeal airway, maybe more predictive of OSA severity in adult patients than the actual measured volume of the tonsils [34]. Evidence in the literature of the primary role of tonsil hypertrophy in OSA pathogenesis has been confirmed by evaluating the effect of palatine tonsillectomy in adult OSA patients [35, 36]. Senchak et al. [35] reported the effect of tonsillectomy alone in adult obstructive sleep apnea patients with significant PT hypertrophy. The authors reported that the mean AHI decreased from 18.0 to 3.2 events per hour after surgery, with a reduction of 82%. The response rate (with subjects achieving at least a 50% reduction of AHI to a value <15) was 94.7%. Following tonsillectomy, there were statistically significant reduction in median lowest saturation of oxygen level and improvement in Epworth Sleepiness Scale and Berlin scores [35]. Similar results have been reported by Holmlund et al. [36] Their study comprised of 28 OSA patients with apnea-hypopnea index of >10, large tonsils (Friedman tonsil size 3 and 4), and age between 18 to 59 years. The apnea-hypopnea index was reduced from a mean of 40 per hour to 7 per hour, $p < 0.001$, at 6 months follow-up post isolated palatine tonsillectomy [36]. This study confirmed the main role of palatine tonsil hypertrophy in OSA syndrome and that tonsillectomy is effective on obstructive sleep apnea (OSA) in adults with large tonsils [36].

Evidence suggesting the importance of hypertrophy of the base of tongue in hypopharyngeal obstruction has also been reported in the literature [19, 20, 22]. In a recent study by Iannella et al. [37], preoperative and postoperative characteristics of sixty-eight OSAS patients who underwent trans-oral robotic resection of the base of tongue were analyzed. Lymphatic hypertrophy (LTH) in the region of the BOT was endoscopically documented in the preoperative evaluation of all these patients: 26 (38.3%) patients had LTH grade 3 according to the Friedman classification, and 42 (61.7%) had a preoperative LTH grade 4. 91.2 % of the patients were noted to have an absence of lymphatic tissue on the tongue at the endoscopic follow-up. The mean preoperative value of AHI decreased from 38.2 (95% confidence interval [CI]: 33.57-42.97) to a mean of 21.6 (95% CI: 16.93-26.33) at the last follow-up. There was a statistical difference between preoperative and postoperative AHI (P = .001). These evidences suggest the importance of lymphatic hypertrophy of the base of tongue in the hypopharyngeal obstruction [37].

PEDIATRIC OSA PATIENTS

Obstructive sleep apnea is one of the most common cause of SDB in children. Symptoms and polysomnographic characteristics of OSA in children are substantially different when compared with adult patients with OSA [38, 39].

Night symptoms of pediatric OSA include loud snoring (three or more nights per week), episodes of breathing cessation, awakening, mouth breathing, dry mouth or sore throat. Daytime symptoms of OSA are very non-specific. These non-specific symptoms may present as hyperactivity, difficulty concentrating/learning difficulties, behavioural difficulties, excessive daytime sleepiness and moodiness. The presence of these symptoms together with nighttime symptoms, may alert clinicians to clinically significant obstructive SDB. In addition, children with OSA may suffer from growth disturbances and poor school achievement [38-41].

The diagnosis of pediatric OSA include a detailed clinical history, evaluating nocturnal and diurnal symptoms, investigations, followed by specific questionnaires administered to parents. The Pediatric Sleep Questionnaire (PSQ) is the most widely used questionnaire consisting of 22 close-ended questions. The current guidelines of the European Respiratory Society Task Force define PSQ as a good test for identifying children affected by OSAS with an apnea-hypopnea index (AHI) > 5 [41, 42].

Nocturnal oximetry is the most widely used screening technique for children with a strong clinical suspicion of pediatric OSA. In fact, it has a low cost and is easy to carry out and interpret. However, despite its positivity which allows the diagnosis of OSA, its negativity does not exclude the pathology [38-40]. According to Kirk et al. [43], the sensitivity and specificity of oximetry for the identification of moderate OSA (AHI > 5/h), compared to the laboratory PSG test, were 67% and 60%, respectively.

Nocturnal in-laboratory polysomnography (PSG) is considered the gold standard test for OSA diagnosis in children with a high suspicion of this pathology. It is indicated for quantifying the severity of the disease, for preoperative evaluation, for predicting post-operative complications and the persistence of sleep breathing disorders after treatment. According to the American Academy of Sleep Medicine, children with an AHI within the range of 1.5 to 5 events/hour is defined to have mild OSA, an AHI within the range of 5 to 10 events/hour defines moderate OSA, and an AHI>10 events/hour of total sleep time is considered as severe OSA [38-40, 43].

Adenoid and/or tonsil hypertrophy are the most common cause of UA obstruction in children. Adenoid hypertrophy contributes to the narrowing of the retro-palatal area, that due to the smallest cross-sectional area compared to adults, is a frequent site of obstruction. This pathology can lead to mouth breathing, nasal congestion, nasal speech, snoring, chronic sinusitis, and recurrent otitis media [38, 39].

Palatine tonsil (PT) hypertrophy is the cause of oropharyngeal obstruction in children. It is the cause of narrowing of the oropharynx contributing to collapse of the lateral walls. Some authors report an increased expression of various inflammatory mediators to be the cause of adeno-tonsillar hypertrophy in OSA children [38-40].

Clinical Investigation

UA clinical evaluation of all anatomical alterations contributing to OSA is an essential step in children with OSA [38, 39].

Friedman et al. have defined a grading scale for evaluating the degree of tonsillar hypertrophy in children. This grading system is reported in Table 2 [39, 44].

In particular, children with Grade IV tonsils (kissing tonsils) are very susceptible to developing sleep disorders, due to oropharyngeal narrowing and lateral collapse.

The close correlation between adeno-tonsillar hypertrophy and pediatric OSA, and the effect of adeno-tonsillectomy in children with OSA have been confirmed in numerous studies in the literature [45-47]. In a study by Suri et al. [46] reporting 50 children who underwent adeno-tonsillectomy, the average RDI value reduced significantly from 16.2 ± 10.7 to 6.46 ± 4.8 ($p < 0.001$) post-operatively and the AHI decreased from 8.5 (SD ± 5.7) to 1.3 (SD ± 1) post-operatively. Adenotonsillectomy showed a greater impact on resolution of apneas in OSA children. Similar conclusions were reported by Mitchell et al. [47] who studied the outcome of adenotonsillectomy in 79 children with OSA. The mean preoperative AHI for the study population was 27.5, whereas the mean postoperative AHI was 3.5. This change was highly significant ($P < .001$). His study also reported that the quality of life in OSA children improved significantly after adenotonsillectomy [47].

Table 2. Friedman palatine tonsil grading of tonsillar size

Grade	Description
0	No tonsils seen
I	In tonsillar fossa
II	Visible beyond anterior pillars
III	Extended 3/4 of way to midline
IV	Completely obstructing airway (kissing tonsils)

Functional nasal obstruction in children may contribute to sleep-disordered breathing. However, it is considered an independent risk factor in pediatric OSA patients [38-40].

Nasal congestion secondary to nasal mucosal inflammation induces increased airway resistance and may result in oral breathing, sleep disruption, and fatigue [42].

Hard palate conformation and dental occlusion is another anatomical feature not to be underestimated in children with OSA. Orthodontic treatment represents a valid alternative in patients with high-arched or narrow palates, susceptible to OSA. The use of rapid maxillary expansion, an appliance to widen the palate and flatten the palatal arch, has shown very good polysomnographic outcomes in a recent meta-analysis [38, 39, 45]. Villa et al. [48] proposed the oral appliance therapy for moderate to severe OSAS children with malocclusion (Figure 2).

Some authors have claimed that genetic causes may also play a role in the pathogenesis of pediatric OSA. However, this is currently still controversial, though it is well recognized that some clinical syndromes such as Downs, Prader–Willi and Beckwith–Wiedemann are strongly associated with OSAS risk in children [38, 39, 49]

Finally, craniofacial abnormalities can also be a cause of UA obstruction syndrome in pediatric OSA patients. Alterations of the size, position, and geometry of the mandible and tongue can lead to thickening of the retro-palatal region [38, 39]. Maxillo-mandibular advancement (MMA) is one of the most common type of surgical procedure performed in pediatric OSA patients with cranio-facial abnormalities. It provides an enlargement of the nasopharynx, oropharynx, and hypopharynx by advancing the soft palate and tongue, and shrinking the lateral pharyngeal walls [45, 50]. On the other hand, such as in the adult population, the indication for mid-face advancement should take into consideration the complication rate and cosmetic sequelae. For this reason, MMA is not considered as a first line option in children without facial abnormalities [38, 45].

Different factors such as age at time of surgery, high-arched palate, and pre-treatment severity of disease were found to be associated with poor outcome of adenotonsillectomy in these children. A large number would require postoperative polysomnographic evaluation and treatment of residual disease [41, 45]. DISE could be used in this instance to detect the anatomical site of potential collapse in children with residual OSA after adenotonsillectomy or in children after maxillofacial alterations [51].

Final Considerations

In every OSA patient, a complete medical history should be collected. This encompasses collecting nocturnal and daytime symptoms, risk factors, comorbidities, as well as measuring the quality of sleep and its impact on daily life in terms of excessive daytime sleepiness and quality of life [2, 7].

The analysis of UA anatomy during clinical examination is of pivotal importance both in adult and pediatric OSA patients. The ENT specialist should clarify the role of anatomical factors in each patient, identify the level and grade of UA obstruction before deciding on a customized surgical treatment for the OSA patient. During clinical examination, the authors suggest keeping in mind the Friedman surgical staging system, and to always perform an awake UA endoscopic examination with a Mueller maneuver [12-14].

The success rate of palatal surgery, independent of the different palatal surgical techniques employed, is strongly related to the anatomical relationship between soft palate, palatine tonsil size, oral tongue volume and position, and hypopharyngeal obstruction. If a stage I disease is detected (Table 1), soft palatal surgery could achieve a surgical success rate greater than 80% [14].

The analysis of the anatomical BOT conformation is of pivotal importance, as suggested by Moore [27]. High grade lymphatic tissue at the base of tongue according to Friedman classification system leads to high collapsibility of this region and significant improvement of AHI after trans-oral robotic surgery. Therefore, the therapeutic success rate of isolated palatal surgery is lower if a hypo-pharyngeal or larynx obstruction is present [31, 37].

In cases of suspected hypopharyngeal obstruction, we suggest performing DISE as simple awake endoscopy may not show site and pattern of obstruction at this level. During DISE, the ENT specialist should pay attention not only to the retropalatal pattern of obstruction, but also to the lateral pharyngeal wall obstruction, base of tongue and epiglottic collapse [31]. During this procedure the ENT specialist should observe whether the oral tongue contribute to the soft palate collapse. If a soft palate collapse is observed to be secondary to tongue retro-position, treatment options to the base of the tongue should be considered [52].

In children with OSA the main anatomical feature to be evaluated is the presence of adeno-tonsillar hypertrophy. Brietzke et al. [53] have reported the resolution of polysomnographic findings in 83% of children with OSAS without other co-morbidities after adenotonsillectomy. High-arched hard palate and dental malocclusion are anatomical features not to be underestimated in children with OSA [38, 39]. Oral appliance therapy should be considered in these situations as it has shown to achieve good results in children with moderate and severe OSAS with malocclusion [48].

In cases of failure after adeno-tonsillar surgery, DISE may be performed to further evaluate anatomical collapse [39].

References

[1] Berry RB, Budhiraja R, Gottlieb DJ, and American Academy of Sleep Medicine. Rules for scoring respiratory events in sleep: update of the 2007 AASM Manual for the Scoring of Sleep and Associated Events. Deliberations of the Sleep Apnea

Definitions Task Force of the American Academy of Sleep Medicine. *J Clin Sleep Med.* 2012;8:597-619.

[2] Epstein LJ, Kristo D, Strollo PJ Jr et al. Clinical guideline for the evaluation, management and long-term care of obstructive sleep apnea in adults. *J Clin Sleep Med.* 2009; 5:263–276.

[3] Shochat T, Pillar G. Sleep apnoea in the older adult: pathophysiology, epidemiology, consequences and management *Drugs Aging.* 2003;20:551-60.

[4] Yaggi HK, Concato J, Kernan WN, Lichtman JH, Brass LM, Mohsenin V. Obstructive sleep apnea as a risk factor for stroke and death. *N Engl J Med.* 2005;353:2034–2041.

[5] Pan L, Xie X Liu D, Ren D, Guo Y. Obstructive sleep apnoea and risks of all-cause mortality: preliminary evidence from prospective cohort studies. *Sleep Breath.* 2016 Mar;20:345-53.

[6] Eckert DJ, White DP, Jordan AS, Malhotra A, Wellman A. Defining phenotypic causes of obstructive sleep apnea. Identification of novel therapeutic targets. *Am J Respir Crit Care Med.* 2013;188:996-1004.

[7] Wellman A, Edwards BA, Sands SA, et al. A simplified method for determining phenotypic traits in patients with obstructive sleep apnea. *J Appl Physiol* 114: 911–922, 2013.

[8] Eckert D. Phenotypic approaches to obstructive sleep apnoea - new pathways for targeted therapy. *Sleep Medicine Reviews*, 2018-02-01, Volume 37, Pages 45-59.

[9] Bosi M, De Vito A, Gobbi R, Poletti V, Vicini C. The importance of obstructive sleep apnoea and hypopnea pathophysiology for customized therapy. *Eur Arch Otorhinolaryngol.* 2017;274:1251-1261.

[10] Bosi M, De Vito A, Kotecha B et al. Phenotyping the pathophysiology of obstructive sleep apnea using polygraphy/polysomnography: a review of the literature. *Sleep Breath.* 2018;22:579-592.

[11] Owens RL, Edwards BA, Eckert DJ, et al. An Integrative Model of Physiological Traits Can be Used to Predict Obstructive Sleep Apnea and Response to Non Positive Airway Pressure Therapy. *Sleep.* 2015 Jun 1;38(6):961-70.

[12] Virk JS, Kotecha B. Otorhinolaryngological aspects of sleep-related breathing disorders. *J Thorac Dis* 2016;8:9-17.

[13] Friedman M, Tanyeri H, La Rosa M et al. Clinical predictors of obstructive sleep apnea. *Laryngoscope.* 1999;109:1901-7.

[14] Friedman M, Ibrahim H, Bass L. Clinical staging for sleep-disordered breathing. *Otolaryngol Head Neck Surg* 2002; 127:13–21.

[15] Lin CM, Davidson TM, Ancoli-Israel S. Gender differences in obstructive sleep apnea and treatment implications. *Sleep Med Rev.* 2008;12:481-96.

[16] Iannella G, Vicini C, Colizza A, et al. Aging effect on sleepiness and apneas severity in patients with obstructive sleep apnea syndrome: a meta-analysis study. *Eur Arch Otorhinolaryngol.* 2019;276:3549-3556.

[17] Young T, Shahar E, Nieto FJ et al. Predictors of sleep-disordered breathing in community-dwelling adults: the sleep heart health study. *Arch Intern Med.* 2002; 162:893–900.

[18] Ancoli-Israel S, Kripke DF, Klauber MR, Mason WJ, Fell R, Kaplan O. Sleep-disordered breathing in communitydwelling elderly. *Sleep.* 1991; 14:486–495.

[19] Yaremchuk K Sleep disorders in the elderly. *Clin Geriatr Med.* 2018; 34:205–216.

[20] Fogel RB, Malhotra A, Dalagiorgou G, et al. Anatomic and physiologic predictors of apnea severity in morbidly obese subjects. *Sleep.* 2003. 15;26:150-5.

[21] Mannarino MR, Di Filippo F, Pirro M. Obstructive sleep apnea syndrome. *Eur J Intern Med.* 2012;23:586-93.

[22] Friedman M, Salapatas AM, Bonzelaar LB. Updated Friedman Staging System for Obstructive Sleep Apnea. *Adv Otorhinolaryngol.* 2017;80:41-48.

[23] Friedman M, Hamilton C, Samuelson CG, Lundgren ME, Pott T. Diagnostic value of the Friedman tongue position and Mallampati classification for obstructive sleep apnea: a meta-analysis. *Otolaryngol Head Neck Surg.* Apr; 148:540-7.

[24] Meen EK, Chandra RK. The role of the nose in sleep-disordered breathing. *Am J Rhinol Allergy.* 2013;27:213-20.

[25] Mickelson SA. Nasal Surgery for Obstructive Sleep Apnea Syndrome. *Otolaryngol Clin North Am.* 2016;49:1373-1381.

[26] Woodson BT. A method to describe the pharyngeal airway. *The Laryngoscope* 2015;125:1233-8.

[27] Moore KE, Phillips C. A Practical Method for Describing Patterns of Tongue-Base Narrowing (Modification of Fujita) in Awake Adult Patients with Obstructive Sleep Apnea. *J Oral Maxillofac Surg* 60:252-260, 2002.

[28] De Vito A, Carrasco Llatas M, Vanni A et al. European position paper on drug-induced sedation endoscopy (DISE). *Sleep Breath.* 2014;18:453-65.

[29] Campanini A, Canzi P, De Vito A, Dallan I, Montevecchi F, Vicini C. Awake versus sleep endoscopy: personal experience in 250 OSAHS patients. *Acta Otorhinolaryngol Ital.* 2010;30:73-7.

[30] Soares D, Folbe AJ, Yoo G, Badr MS, Rowley JA, Lin HS. Drug-induced sleep endoscopy vs awake Müller's maneuver in the diagnosis of severe upper airway obstruction. *Otolaryngol Head Neck Surg.* 2013;148:151-6.

[31] De Vito A, Carrasco Llatas M, Ravesloot MJ et al. European position paper on drug-induced sleep endoscopy: 2017 Update. *Clin Otolaryngol.* 2018;43:1541-1552.

[32] Carrasco-Llatas M, Matarredona-Quiles S, De Vito A, Chong KB, Vicini C. Drug-Induced Sleep Endoscopy: Technique, Indications, Tips and Pitfalls. *Healthcare* (Basel). 2019 24;7.

[33] De Vito A, Cammaroto G, Chong KB, Carrasco-Llatas M, Vicini C. Drug-Induced Sleep Endoscopy: Clinical Application and Surgical Outcomes. *Healthcare* (Basel). 20192. 5;7(3).

[34] Jara SM, Weaver EM. Association of palatine tonsil size and obstructive sleep apnea in adults. *Laryngoscope*. 2018;128:1002-1006.

[35] Senchak AJ, McKinlay AJ, Acevedo J, et al. The effect of tonsillectomy alone in adult obstructive sleep apnea. Otolaryngol *Head Neck Surg*. 2015;152:969-73.

[36] Holmlund T, Franklin KA, Levring Jäghagen E, et al. Tonsillectomy in adults with obstructive sleep apnea. *Laryngoscope*. 2016 Dec;126:2859-2862.

[37] Iannella G, Magliulo G, Montevecchi F, et al. Lingual tonsil lymphatic tissue regrowth in patients undergoing transoral robotic surgery. *Laryngoscope*. 2019;129:2652-2657.

[38] Savini S, Ciorba A, Bianchini C, Stomeo F, Corazzi V, Vicini C, Pelucchi S. Assessment of obstructive sleep apnoea (OSA) in children: an update. *Acta Otorhinolaryngol Ital*. 2019;39:289-297.

[39] Gulotta G, Iannella G, Vicini C, et al. Risk Factors for Obstructive Sleep Apnea Syndrome in Children: State of the Art. *Int J Environ Res Public Health*. 2019. 4;16.

[40] Horne RS, Wijayaratne P, Nixon GM, Walter LM. Sleep and sleep disordered breathing in children with down syndrome: Effects on behaviour, neurocognition and the cardiovascular system. *Sleep Med Rev*. 2019;44:1-11.

[41] Li Z, Celestin J2, Lockey RF. Pediatric Sleep Apnea Syndrome: An Update. *J Allergy Clin Immunol Pract*. 2016;4:852-61.

[42] Isaiah A, Shikara M, Pereira KD, Das G. Refining screening questionnaires for prediction of sleep apnea severity in children. *Sleep Breath*. 2019; 27.

[43] Kirk V, Baughn J, D'Andrea L, Friedman N, et al. American Academy of Sleep Medicine Position Paper for the Use of a Home Sleep Apnea Test for the Diagnosis of OSA in Children. *J Clin Sleep Med*. 201715;13:1199-1203.

[44] Esteller E. Obstructive sleep apnea-hypopnea syndrome in children: beyond adenotonsillar hypertrophy. *Acta Otorrinolaringol Esp*. 2015; 66:111-9.

[45] Bluher AE, Ishman SL, Baldassari CM. Managing the Child with Persistent Sleep Apnea. *Otolaryngol Clin North Am*. 2019;52:891-90.

[46] Suri JC, Sen MK, Venkatachalam VP, et al. Outcome of adenotonsillectomy for children with sleep apnea. *Sleep Med*. 2015;16:1181-6.

[47] Mitchell RB. Adenotonsillectomy for obstructive sleep apnea in children: outcome evaluated by pre- and postoperative polysomnography. *Laryngoscope*. 2007;117:1844-54.

[48] Villa MP, Rizzoli A, Rabasco J, Vitelli O, Pietropaoli N, Cecili M, Marino A, Malagola C. Rapid maxillary expansion outcomes in treatment of obstructive sleep apnea in children. *Sleep Med.* 2015;16:709-16.

[49] Simpson R, Oyekan AA, Ehsan Z, Ingram DG. Obstructive sleep apnea in patients with Down syndrome: current perspectives. *Nat Sci Sleep.* 2018;10:287-293.

[50] Garg RK, Afifi AM, Garland CB, Sanchez R, Mount DL. Pediatric Obstructive Sleep Apnea: Consensus, Controversy, and Craniofacial Considerations. *Plast Reconstr Surg*. 2017;140:987-997.

[51] Collu MA, Esteller E, Lipari F, Haspert R, Mulas D, Diaz MA, Dwivedi RC. A case-control study of Drug-Induced Sleep Endoscopy (DISE) in pediatric population: A proposal for indications. *Int J Pediatr Otorhinolaryngol*. 2018;108:113-119.

[52] Green KK, Kent DT, D'Agostino MA, et al. Drug-Induced Sleep Endoscopy and Surgical Outcomes: A Multicenter Cohort Study. *Laryngoscope*. 2019;129:761-770.

[53] Brietzke SE, Gallagher D. The effectiveness of tonsillectomy and adenoidectomy in the treatment of pediatric obstructive sleep apnea/hypopnea syndrome: a meta-analysis. *Otolaryngol Head Neck Surg*. 2006;134:979-84.

In: Sleep Medicine in Critical Care
Editors: Antonio M. Esquinas et al.
ISBN: 978-1-53617-768-8

Chapter 5

DEVICES FOR DIAGNOSIS OF SLEEP BREATHING DISORDERS

Adam J. Birdseye, Richard Brown and Sakina F. Dastagir*

Guy's and St Thomas' NHS Foundation Trust, Lane Fox Respiratory Unit/Sleep Disorders Centre, London, UK

ABSTRACT

Sleep related breathing disorders (SRBDs) can be diagnosed using various devices commonly categorised into Type I-IV studies. These are classified according to; the number of parameters, whether they require an attending sleep technologist and their setting. Type I and II studies combine 7 channels including respiratory parameters and electroencephalogram (EEG), to give the most accurate respiratory analysis. However, these may be impractical in a standard critical care setting. Type III and IV studies are both portable and easier to set up. Type III devices measure respiratory parameters only and can provide information on the type of SRBD. Type IV devices measure 1-2 parameters, but cannot differentiate the nature of the SRBD. Both devices may underestimate the severity of the SRBD as they do not directly measure sleep. Peripheral arterial tonometry (PAT) is easy to use and offers an indirect measure of sleep, without EEG, but has limited evidence in the critical care setting. Finally, CO_2 monitoring can be used in conjunction with these studies to help assess hypoventilation.

* Corresponding Author's E-mail: sakina.f.dastagir@gmail.com.

INTRODUCTION

Sleep related breathing disorders (SRBDs) can be identified using a number of different physiological parameters, including; oxygen saturation, pulse rate, respiratory effort, airflow and associated sleep architecture. The most frequently and easily monitored of these parameters include fluctuations in oxygen saturation and pulse rate. Analysis of this can provide the oxygen desaturation index (ODI) – how often oxygen desaturations occur per hour. An elevated ODI can be caused by the presence of respiratory events, known as apnoeas and hypopnoeas. These are identified as temporary cessations or reductions in breathing. They can be further classified by their cause, such as an obstruction in the upper airway or due to a failed drive to breathe. Devices that recognize the frequency of both apnoeas and hypopnoeas are therefore able to ascertain the apnoea-hypopnoea index (AHI). Identifying the nature of these respiratory events enables insight into which treatment is most appropriate. Electroencephalography (EEG) can be used to establish how frequently these respiratory events cause arousals, as demonstrated by the respiratory disturbance index (RDI).

There are several devices which can assist in the diagnosis of sleep related breathing disorders (SRBDs) within the critical care setting. These devices are classified using guidelines from organisations such as the American Association of Sleep Medicine (AASM), the Association for Respiratory Technology and Physiology (ARTP)/British Thoracic Society (BTS) and the National Institute for Health and Care Excellence (NICE). These bodies assign 'levels/types/classes' to sleep studies and the devices they incorporate. This categorisation is based on the number of parameters they record, the environment in which they are used and whether they require the attendance of a sleep technologist for set up and maintenance of signals. The AASM guidelines are universally recognised and accepted [1]. For this reason and to allow for consistency, the devices will be referred to as per the AASM guidelines; Type I, Type II, Type III and Type IV studies (Table 1).

Newer technologies, such as Peripheral Arterial Tonometry (PAT) cannot be categorised as Type I – IV and so an alternative classification scheme has been proposed which classifies devices based on the parameters they record and incorporates Sleep, Cardiovascular, Oximetry, Position, Effort and Respiratory parameters; the SCOPER system. However, SCOPER is deemed more complicated and has not yet been adopted by most clinicians or the task force that established the AASM guidelines. Therefore, PAT technology will be discussed separately.

Carbon Dioxide (CO_2) monitoring is often used alongside the types of studies mentioned above, particularly within the critical care setting. There is no specific mention of CO_2 monitoring in the AASM guidelines. However, the AASM manual [2] which provides the rules, terminology and technical specification for the analysis of sleep and associated events, refers to CO_2 monitoring in the context of identifying hypoventilation.

Hypoventilation is seen in a number of conditions within the critical care setting including chronic obstructive pulmonary disease (COPD), obstructive sleep apnoea (OSA), obesity hypoventilation syndrome (OHS), congenital central hypoventilation syndrome (CCHS), and neuromuscular conditions such as Duchenne-type muscular dystrophy (DMD) and spinal muscular dystrophy (SMA).

Table 1. Summary of sleep study types as per AASM guidelines

Type of Study	Description
Type I	Polysomnography study - measures 7 or more channels Attended by a sleep technologist at set up and across the duration of the study Performed in a sleep laboratory Not portable (Natus®, Embla®, SDx and Compumedics®, Grael PSG®)
Type II	Polysomnography study - measures 7 or more channels Not attended by a sleep technologist across the recording of the study (unattended study) Portable device (Natus® Embletta® MPR Sleep System, Compumedics® Somté PSG, Philips Respironics® Alice PDx®, NOX A1®)
Type III	Measures more than 4 channels Unattended study Portable device (Embletta®, Domino Light®, ApneaLink®, Alice NightOne®, NOX T3®)
Type IV	Measures 1-2 channels Unattended Study Portable Device (Konica Minolta Pulsox®300i, WristOx$_2$®, Viatom Checkme™ O2, Masimo SET®, BresoDX®, RUSleeping™ RTS, Wizard™)

Finally, within the intensive care unit (ICU) ventilators are used for the monitoring of airway pressures as well as delivering treatment. Ventilators can detect changes in flow, pressure, respiratory rate and the rate of change of a patient's respiratory cycle. Ventilators can be adjusted to various modes and settings, which can detect what ventilator support a patient requires. In patients with central hypoventilation syndromes, the spontaneous breathing rate is detected, when this falls below the minimum breath rate requirement the ventilator will deliver timed breaths.

Type IV Studies

Type IV sleep studies are classed as unattended limited diagnostic tools that record one or two channels, typically oxygen saturation, heart rate (HR) or just nasal airflow alone [1]. However, advancement in technology has resulted in the addition of further channels, such as sound and movement. Type IV studies are derived from portable and non-invasive devices and can record data continuously for multiple nights. This can minimise any potential errors from night-to-night variability of SRBDs. These devices are also considered to be self-administrated, without the need for a qualified sleep technologist.

Two-Channel Type IV Sleep Studies

Pulse oximetry is considered the most widely-used two-channel Type IV sleep study in clinical practice. It is typically recorded with a device that typically uses a finger sensor with spectrophotometry and pulsatile flow to sense oxygen saturation (SpO_2) and pulse rate, where SpO_2 is the surrogate of arterial blood oxygen saturation (SaO_2). These devices use two different wavelengths of light; red (660 nm) and infra-red (940 nm). The amount of light transmitted through human tissue alters depending on the changes in arterial blood volume which occurs during the periodic movement of arterial blood flow caused by each heart beat (pulsatile flow). As the two light wavelengths pass through the nail bed of the finger, the absorption ratio of these lights measures the amount of oxygenated and deoxygenated haemoglobin in the blood.

Most conventional pulse oximeter devices have an accuracy of SpO_2 ± 2% above 70% and they have been shown to be accurate at tracking changes in oxygen saturation, although there is a time lag. The accuracy of the pulse rate monitor in the pulse oximetry can be ± 2beats per min (bpm) whilst in the range of 30-100bpm or ± 2% of the value whilst in the range of 100-230 bpm.

The ability to record SpO_2 and pulse rate continuously means that pulse oximetry can provide insights into important physiological changes associated with SRBD (Figure 1(c)). The number of desaturations per hour, typically as a 3% or a 4% drop in SpO_2 (the ODI) is most commonly considered for the assessment of SRBD. Other important parameters include the mean SpO_2, the percentage of time spent below SpO_2 of 90% and the nadir of desaturations. These parameters are important to distinguish between nocturnal hypoxaemia, sleep apnoea and its severity along with any suggestion of presumed hypoventilation. Changes in pulse rate, in association with the oxygen desaturations, can give an indication of subsequent arousals from sleep which may indicate one of the clinical features of Obstructive Sleep Apnoea-Hypopnoea Syndrome (OSAHS). An increase in the pulse rate of more than 6 bpm occurring more than 15 times per hour can be a significant marker of OSAHS, even if no oxygen desaturations are recorded [3].

Pulse oximetry has been shown to have a sensitivity of 87.4% (±3.8) for moderate to severe OSAHS. However, it has a specificity of 64.9% (±6.7) to exclude OSAHS [4].

Therefore, this method can provide false negative as well as false positive results, where false negatives are most commonly seen in young and non-obese subjects and false positives in other SRBDs such as central sleep apnoea, Cheyne-Stokes breathing and hypoventilation disorders. As a result of its specificity and the limited channels it records, the AASM do not recommend pulse oximetry as a standalone diagnostic tool in either an unattended or attended setting [5]. However, due to its sensitivity, it is widely accepted as a screening tool for patients demonstrating a high clinical pre-test likelihood of moderate to severe OSAHS. This is usually assessed by clinical history which includes a physical examination and various symptom questionnaires such as the Snoring, Tiredness, Observed apnoeas, high blood Pressure, Body mass index, Age, Neck circumference and Gender (STOP-BANG) [3].

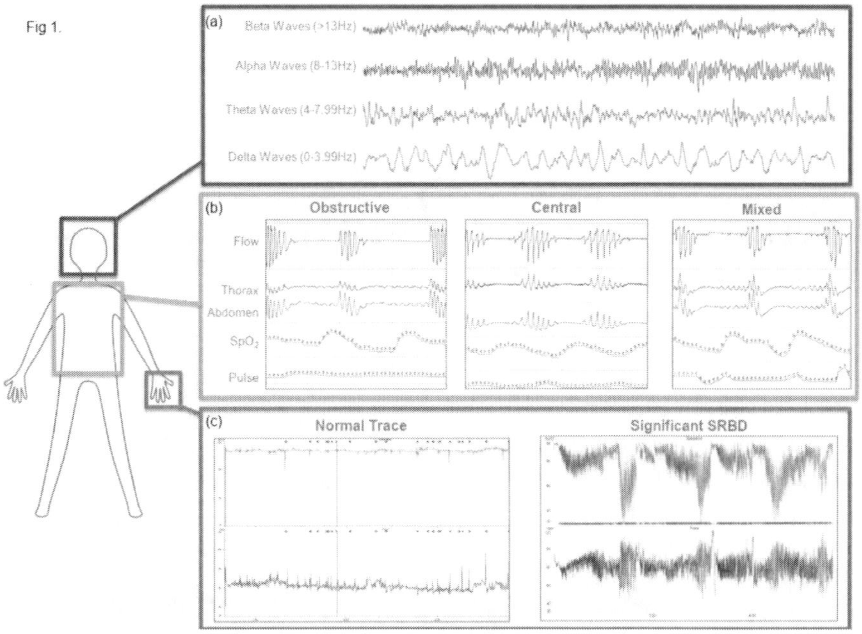

Figure 1. (a) Waveforms associated with different stages of sleep (b) Pattern of airflow, RIP belt, SpO_2 and pulse during obstructive, central and mixed apnoeas.
(c) Pulse oximetry trace with normal results and significant SRBD.

The use of pulse oximetry is clinically acceptable in the diagnosis of nocturnal hypoxemia [5]. Nocturnal hypoxemia can be seen in patients with COPD, OHS, Cystic Fibrosis, Sickle Cell and neuromuscular disorders, such as post-polio syndrome. It is defined as a nocturnal SpO2 of <90%, and in severe cases the SpO_2 is <80%. However, in cases where severe hypoxemia or low pre-test likelihood of OSAHS is clinically present, caution should be taken due to the limitations of the accuracy of pulse oximetry alone.

A common limitation of pulse oximetry includes motion artefact which can result in ambiguous measurement of SpO_2 and pulse rate. Excessive movements of the probe site location can lead to false recordings or complete loss of the channel. Additionally, ambiguous SpO_2 readings can be the result of poor perfusion, incorrect probe placement, finger nail polish, acrylic nails, and pigmentation of the skin. Other causes include; intravenous contrast dyes, ambient light, high levels of carbo-xyhaemoglobin in smokers, severe hypoxia, autonomic neuropathy and anaemia. Other factors such as poor pulse palpation, atrial fibrillation, beta blocking medication, or if a subject has a pacemaker, can render the pulse rate channel ineffective as a reliable indicator of arousal.

Other Type IV Studies

Sound and movement can also used as a two channel type IV study. This recent development in technology has been validated with a high sensitivity and specificity in the screening of OSAHS [6]. The use of a microphone to record breathing sounds and an accelerometer to record movements has been shown to be a reliable tool to indicate snoring, oronasal breathing sounds, apnoeas, and hypopnoeas whilst also estimating posture and sleep time. A recent publication has looked at using breathing sounds for the detection of central sleep apnoea (CSA) with 85.7% sensitivity and 88.9% specificity [7]. However, further validation studies are required before this method is considered in standard clinical practice.

Single-Channel Type IV Sleep Studies

There are type IV studies which record only nasal airflow via a pressure transducer or a thermistor. The devices which are currently available use a pressure transducer in the form of a nasal cannula and provide diagnostic information in relation to apnoea index only. This nasal cannula picks up pressure fluctuations and transmits them to a transducer which converts this signal into an electrical waveform. The nasal cannula detects the negative pressures seen during inhalation and positive pressures created during exhalation. The oronasal thermistor consists of two temperature sensitive sensors that monitor the temperature differences at the nose and mouth with cooler air flowing during inspiration compared to the warmer air which flows during expiration. These temperature differences are then converted into an electrical waveform.

The routine use of single-channel nasal airflow devices as a diagnostic tool in an unattended setting is minimal. This is due to a limited number of readily available devices on the market and also due to the wide-use of pulse oximetry as the first line tool. Limited data have been published on the validation of nasal airflow as a single indicator in SRDB, with most studies being carried out in an attended setting. Additionally, they are battery operated and dependent on manual start and stop which can increase the risk of human error. In an unattended setting, the displacement of the nasal cannula may cause insufficient flow data due to pressure leak and result in poor data acquisition.

Visual analysis of the overall graphical trace provided by pulse oximetry can give suggestive information about the type of SRBD: More detailed analysis, using shorter epochs of the overall trace can allow an understanding of the nature of the oxygen desaturations or 'dips' present. Both obstructive and central events have characteristic forms; both obstructive and central events have a slow initial onset and take some time to reach the nadir, but obstructive event have a faster return to baseline compared to central events (Figure 1 (b)). However, actual discrimination between an obstructive and central event cannot be reliable as no actual measurement of airflow or inspiratory effort is being recorded.

Other types of SRBD can be recognised by their pattern via visual analysis of the overall graphical traces, including Rapid Eye Movement (REM) and/or positional SRBDs. REM sleep may be identified through periodic increases in the heart rate with high variability compared to baseline, commonly known as a "REM hump." This observation combined with the knowledge of when to expect REM sleep during the night and episodic repetitive oxygen desaturations may give an indication of REM related sleep disordered breathing. Positional SRBDs can involve desaturations and associated heart rate variability occurring in distinct clusters across the night, that do not coincide with expected REM timings.

OHS may be identified alongside sleep apnoea, here repetitive oxygen desaturations are seen and after reaching a nadir there is visual evidence of oxygen saturations not returning back to baseline due to hypoventilation with low minute ventilation.

Type III Studies

Type III studies, often referred to as unattended cardio-respiratory or cardiopulmonary studies, use devices to measure at least 4 physiological parameters. These include one cardiac variable such as Electrocardiogram (ECG) or HR, two respiratory variables including airflow and/or respiratory effort and oxygen saturation.

The AASM manual provides recommended and acceptable technical specifications for all home sleep apnoea tests (HSATs). For type III tests this incorporates recommendations for detecting; oxygen saturation with pulse oximetry and airflow via the recommended nasal pressure transducer or oronasal thermal airflow sensor. The technical specifications also recommend technology for monitoring respiratory effort: the dual thoraco-abdomnial Respiratory Inductance Plethysmography (RIP) belts. Dual RIP belt technology consists of two belts, each with an insulated coiled wire positioned in a sinusoidal fashion within it. One belt is placed at the level of the thorax and the other at the level of the abdomen. An approximate measure of cross sectional area is obtained across both levels and a digital waveform is produced as the belts expand with inhalation and contract with exhalation. The amplitude of the waveform is proportional to the breath volume and when calibrated to a known volume RIP belts can provide a measure of tidal volume.

The airflow sensor and respiratory effort devices used within Type III studies allow for important details to be made available, including the nature and duration of the respiratory events. This means the airflow sensor allows the analyser to distinguish between apnoeas and hypopnoeas based on the degree of airflow reduction compared to baseline breathing seen in the flow trace. Simultaneously, the RIP belts will allow for the differentiation of apnoeas into obstructive, central or mixed events. The point at which the event starts and ends can also be clearly observed. This is useful when looking for breathing disorders such as Cheyne-Stokes respiration, which is seen in patients in critical care. This diagnosis is based in part on breathing pattern and the duration of each event which will clearly be displayed by this type of study.

The ability to see the pattern of breathing allows for more complex analysis of sleep studies. Paradoxical breathing can be identified during obstructive events; the respiratory bands do not move synchronously with each other as they do in normal breathing, instead they move in opposite directions. Central apnoeas can also be depicted by a unique pattern in the respiratory band trace. As the patient does not display any effort to breath, a horizontal flat line is seen in both the thorax and abdomen traces during a central apnoea. Mixed apnoeas can be defined by seeing the flat lines of a central followed by the paradoxical breathing of an obstructive in one event (Figure 1 (b)).

This type of study is designed to be assembled and attached by the patient themselves or a family member. This can be done after education from a sleep technologist or with an educational manual in the absence of a sleep technologist. This portable and self-assembly method means Type III devices can be used within critical care settings. In this setting they can be applied by a family member or non-sleep specialist healthcare professional. The application of these sensors may be slightly more complicated on patients in critical care. If a patient is immobile attaching the RIP belts around the patient may be more difficult. Also if a patient is on supplemental oxygen, the device will need to be able to deliver oxygen and pick up the airflow concurrently, so more specialised equipment (such as a split cannula) will need to be sourced and attached. Similarly, specialised equipment would be needed for patients on mechanical ventilation.

Studies assessing the diagnostic accuracy of Type III devices compared to Type I devices have found that Type III devices score well for their sensitivity and specificity for AHI in patients with a high pre-test probability for OSA. Often, as with Type IV devices, as disease severity increased Type III devices decreased in sensitivity. Also, the milder the OSA the lower the specificity [8]: The same degree of specificity is found in elderly patients [9] and those with coronary disease [10]. Further research needs to be conducted to test the accuracy of these devices in the critical care setting. Most studies assess these devices in patients with OSAHS and more research needs to be done for other types of SRBDs.

The Type III study does not specifically assess sleep stages; however, REM sleep has a characteristic erratic breathing pattern [11]. This is seen in the RIP bands and can be used to assess if SRBD is present during REM. Type III devices also often have a position sensor which can be useful in determining if any SRBD present is related to sleeping position.

Type III devices all have automated scoring available, but a sleep technologist is needed to review and potentially edit the data manually. Without the presence of an EEG, even for a trained sleep technologist, it can be unclear when the patient is awake or asleep during the night. In the worst case, this can result in an inaccurate AHI and ODI being generated.

These devices are designed for unattended settings but even with training there is a chance of poor sensor placement and sensor dislodgement. For instance, the RIP belts can be placed in the wrong position at the beginning of the study, or they can shift as the patient repositions overnight. The abdominal RIP belt can rise up towards the bottom of the chest which can make paradox less clear on the respiratory effort trace and this may lead to incorrect classification of the respiratory event. Studies have shown a 10% technical failure rate when compared with Type I studies [8].

Type III devices are portable which means they have a battery or need charging prior to use and so their ability to record multiple nights can vary. Some Type III studies can be adjusted to record for 2 nights. In these scenarios they need to be set to record between certain times and this may not always reflect the patient's sleep routine. Other devices will only download the longest recording when used on more than one night. With no means of choosing which data is kept, this may result in data from a more informative night being discarded.

Type II and I Studies

A Type I sleep study is defined as an attended Polysomnography (PSG) which is commonly performed in a sleep laboratory where a sleep technologist is available to help maintain high quality signals throughout the recording. This is considered the gold-standard study in the diagnosis of OSA and other forms of SRBD in healthy patients and those with significant co-morbid respiratory conditions, cardiovascular conditions, opioid use or insomnia [1]. However, the requirement for a dedicated sleep laboratory and attending overnight sleep technologist means that a Type I sleep study cannot be conducted within most standard critical care settings.

A Type II study, which is defined as an unattended portable PSG, is performed without an attending overnight sleep technologist and therefore can be conducted within the critical care setting. This must have a minimum of 7 channels and commonly combines the respiratory channels monitored by a Type III device with; 6 lead EEG, right and left electrooculogram (EOG), 3 lead submental electromyogram (EMG), bilateral 2 lead tibialis anterior EMG, and 2 lead electrocardiogram (ECG). These PSG sensors must be attached by an appropriately qualified sleep technologist using the standardised method detailed by the AASM Manual [2].

The EEG measures the postsynaptic electrical activity produced by large groups of cortical neurons. The sleep EEG monitors the synchronous activity of these neurons via bilateral frontal, central and occipital scalp electrodes which are referenced to the contralateral mastoid process. The electrical activity measured by these electrodes provides the characteristic 'brainwaves' seen during wake and sleep. These brainwaves are categorised by their frequency range as; beta waves (>13 Hz), alpha waves (8 – 13 Hz), theta waves (4 – 7.99 Hz), and delta waves (0 – 3.99 Hz) (Figure 1 (a)). The EEG data are used alongside the signals produced by the electrical activity of the eyes (EOG) and Submentalis muscle (submental EMG) in order to differentiate between sleep stages and identify cortical arousals.

The sleep technologist uses the AASM Manual to categorise 30 second epochs as either; Stage W (Wakefulness), Stage N1 (Non-Rapid Eye Movement (NREM) 1), Stage N2 (NREM 2), Stage N3 (NREM 3), or Stage R (REM). Once sleep staging and cortical arousal scoring has been completed, the sleep technologist can then assess SRBDs in relation to sleep duration and analyse its effect on sleep disruption and sleep architecture. Finally, the patient's RDI is then calculated by combining the number of obstructive apnoeas, central apnoeas, mixed apnoeas, hypopnoeas, and respiratory effort related arousals (RERAs) per hour of sleep.

The use of the PSG study as the gold standard measure of OSA and other forms of SRBD is in part because analysis of cortical arousals allows for detection of RERAs and Hypopnoeas that cause arousal without an observable ≥3% oxygen desaturation. These subtypes of respiratory events are uniquely identified by the PSG and are therefore incorporated into the RDI generated by Type II studies. Furthermore, quantification of sleep duration via an EEG allows for the Type II study to establish an RDI in relation to total sleep time opposed to total recording time. This distinction may be particularly important in the critical care setting where numerous factors are known to contribute to poor sleep efficiency [12]. This can result in an actual sleep time which is much shorter than the total recording time. This is taken into consideration by the RDI of the Type II device and avoids any under-estimation of SRBDs which may occur when using total recording time. Finally, as with Type III devices, classification of different types of SRBDs is made via automatic or manual analysis of respiratory events. With Type II devices this occurs in the presence of both sleep stage and position and can therefore help to differentiate between sleep stage or position dependent SRBDs.

The requirement for specialist Type II PSG equipment and trained sleep technologists to set-up and analyse the data may make this study difficult to perform in certain critical care settings. Additionally, questions have been raised about the feasibility of performing unattended PSGs within the critical care setting due to the increased risk of sensor dislodgement and potential poor tolerance of the equipment by severely ill patients. The acquisition of high-quality PSG data via Type II studies within critical care has been demonstrated within both mechanically ventilated and non-mechanically ventilated patients [13]. However, although demonstrated as feasible, patients with terminal illness, coma, deep sedation, head/neck related injuries, and severe agitation were excluded. Furthermore, numerous patients were excluded due to poor patient, family and caregiver equipment tolerance. Therefore, this suggests that the Level II study is only appropriate for a specific subsection of critical care patients and these patients may need to be selected carefully.

The appropriateness of the Type II study within critical care is further complicated by the presence of atypical EEG features which have been identified in medically unstable mechanically ventilated patients [14]. These atypical EEG features include; featureless Stage N2 with no observable sleep spindles of K complexes, the presence of polymorphic delta, burst suppression and isoelectric electro-encephalography. These may result from a variety of factors including; sepsis-associated encephalopathy and the effects of sedatives and analgesics. The presence of these atypically fast EEG frequencies in sleep and slow EEG frequencies in wake prevents use of the standard AASM sleep staging rules. Alternative EEG frameworks for analysing wake and sleep in critical care patients have been proposed but these are not currently in wide-use. Therefore, in critical care patients with these atypical EEG features sleep stages cannot be delineated, sleep duration cannot be quantified and cortical arousals cannot be identified. This means that the RDI generated by Type II studies in these patients will no longer be able to accurately identify hypopnoeas causing arousals, RERAs or any type of SRBD in relation to sleep duration.

PAT

PAT technology detects changes in peripheral sympathetic arterial tone to recognise respiratory events. Devices which use this technology are worn on the wrist with a probe placed on the finger. The wrist device contains an actigraph and the finger probe incorporates PAT and pulse oximetry. These devices use these channels to help identify a PAT derived substitute for total sleep time (TST) which can then be used to find an approximation of AHI and ODI. These channels are also used to identify PAT surrogates for sleep architecture, body position and snoring.

PAT technology works by assessing the blood volume in the finger. The finger has high vascular density and blood flow variability which is controlled largely by alpha adrenergic pathways [15]. At the end of a respiratory event there is increased sympathetic tone resulting in constriction of the blood vessels in the finger which causes a decrease in fingertip volume and the PAT signal.

When the PAT and pulse oximetry signals are combined, respiratory events can be identified. This is seen with an initial reduction in PAT signal alongside an oxygen desaturation, followed by an increase in both signals along with an increase in HR. The built in actigraph records motion and with the use of algorithms this can distinguish between wake and sleep. Each sleep stage shows different characteristic HR, oxygen saturation, movement and PAT signal. PAT devices estimate sleep stages by combining all these variables. This allows the AHI to be derived in relation to the PAT derived total sleep time. Studies have been conducted which have shown high correlation for the RDI ($r = 0.879$), the AHI ($r = 0.893$) and the ODI ($r = 0.942$) with type I studies [16].

The PAT device provides automated scoring of the studies but full manual scoring is available. This provides more accurate analysis, however, the detail available with the PAT device can make manual editing a time-consuming process.

These devices require signals from alpha-adrenergic receptors to function and so should not be used on patients taking alpha-blockers such as doxazosin mesylate. The PAT derived AHI is poorly correlated with PSG derived AHI in patients with increased arterial stiffness [17] which may require the exclusion of certain patients, particularly those in critical care.

Assessment of OSA in patients with myocardial infarction using the PAT device compared well to type III devices for assessing the AHI in moderate to severe OSA [18]. Smaller studies have found that in an intensive care unit PAT technology overestimated TST and REM sleep [19]. This may result in inaccurate respiratory analysis.

Monitoring of Carbon Dioxide

During sleep, changes in our central respiratory control system leads to an increase in the arterial partial pressure of carbon dioxide (P_aCO_2) when compared to wake supine values. In sleep-related hypoventilation disorders, the rise in P_aCO_2 is greater than normal which can lead to acute and chronic type 2 respiratory failure, therefore the monitoring of P_aCO_2 is an important parameter.

The gold standard to measure P_aCO_2 is by arterial blood gas (ABG) analysis, which is invasive and difficult to obtain without causing sleep disruption and a subsequent change in P_aCO_2 and therefore surrogate markers for P_aCO_2 are considered.

Transcutaneous monitoring of carbon dioxide ($TcCO_2$) is a validated and quantitative, non-invasive method where a Severinghaus electrode based sensor measures gas tension of the underlying tissue by heating the site of application, usually the earlobe, thorax or the forearm. $TcCO_2$ monitors are small, easy to use, have direct compatibility with type I-III study equipment and have built in batteries, allowing long-term monitoring. Most conventional monitors also provide transcutaneous oxygen levels (TcO_2) a surrogate for arterial pressure of oxygen (P_aO_2).

$TcCO_2$ values can lag behind changes in P_aCO_2 by up to two minutes or more. Precision and performance is limited by the presence of hypoxemia, increased skin thickness, oedema of the skin or increased capillary blood flow induced by movement [20].

End-tidal carbon dioxide ($EtCO_2$), or capnography, is an alternative non-invasive measurement. $EtCO_2$ is obtained via nasal cannula and refers to the graphical measurement of carbon dioxide partial pressure during expiration. $EtCO_2$ can provide false low values in patients who have marked nasal obstruction, profuse nasal secretions, receiving supplemental oxygen or are oral venters.

The AASM, recommend that for detection of hypoventilation during a diagnostic study either $TcCO_2$ or $EtCO_2$ can be used, however, during a sleep study with non-invasive ventilation, $TcCO_2$ is recommended [2].

CONCLUSION

Type IV sleep studies are portable and cost effective. However, they have significant limitations, including; low specificity for recognising SRBDs and an inability to distinguish between different SRBDs or between wake and sleep. Type I - III studies may be able to provide more detail, especially when there is clinical evidence of more complex SRBDs.

The AHI and nature of the SRBD can be identified using portable type III devices, allowing a more detailed diagnosis in the critical care setting. Studies have shown it has high sensitivity and specificity for detecting moderate-severe OSA.

The Type II study allows for analysis of SRBDs in relation to objectively measured sleep. However, PSG studies are not viable in all critical care patients and therefore careful patient selection is required.

PAT testing provides an alternative strategy to defining sleep and SRBDs and is comparable with type I studies for defining the RDI. The PAT derived TST does not use EEG and this needs to be taken into consideration. The method of data acquisition may exclude certain patient groups in critical care.

CO_2 monitoring can be considered an important in patients with possible complex SRBD, particularly in the critical care setting.

References

[1] Kapur VK, Auckley DH, Chowdhuri S, Kuhlmann DC, Mehra R, Ramar K, Harrod CG. 2017. "Clinical practice guideline for diagnostic testing for adult obstructive sleep apnea: an American Academy of Sleep Medicine clinical practice guideline." *J Clin Sleep Med.* 13(3):479–504. doi: 10.5664/jcsm.6506

[2] Berry RB, Albertario CL, Harding SM, Lloyd RM, Plante DT, Quan SF, Troester MM, Vaughn BV. 2018. *The AASM Manual for the Scoring of Sleep and Associated Events: Rules, Terminology and Technical Specifications.* Version 2.5. Darien, IL: American Academy of Sleep Medicine.

[3] Association for Respiratory Technology & Physiology. 2018. *ARTP Standards of Care – Sleep Apnoea Service (Diagnostics). 2018; V8.* Staffordshire: ARTP. http://www.artp.org.uk/en/sleep/sleep-standards/sleep-documents.cfm.

[4] Ross SD, Sheinhait IA, Harrison KJ, Kvasz M, Connelly JE, Shea SA, Allen IE. 2000. "Systematic review and meta-analysis of the literature regarding the diagnosis of sleep apnea." *Sleep.* Jun 15;23(4):519-532.

[5] Kushida CA; Littner MR; Morgenthaler T, Alessi CA, Bailey D, Coleman J Jr, Friedman L et al. 2005. "Practice parameters for the indications for polysomnography and related procedures: An update for 2005." *Sleep.* Apr;28(4):499-521. doi: 10.1093/sleep/28.4.499

[6] Alshaer H, Fernie GR, Tseng WH, Bradley TD. 2016. "Comparison Of In-Laboratory And Home Diagnosis Of Sleep Apnea Using A Cordless Portable Acoustic Device." *Sleep Medicine*. Jun;22:91-96. doi: 10.1016/j.sleep.2015.11.003

[7] Alshaer H, Hummel R, Bradley TD. 2017. "Distinguishing Patients with Central from Obstructive Sleep Apnea Using Overnight Breath Sound Recordings." *European Respiratory Journal.* Sep, 50 (suppl 61) OA3204; doi: 10.1183/1393003.congress-2017.OA3204

[8] El Shayeb M, Topfer LA, Stafinski T, Pawluk L, Menon D. 2014. "Diagnostic accuracy of level 3 portable sleep tests versus level 1 polysomnography for sleep-disordered breathing: a systematic review and meta-analysis." *Canadian Medical Association journal.* Jan 7; 186(1): E25-51. doi:10.1503/cmaj.130952.

[9] Polese JF, Santos-Silva R, de Oliveira Ferrari PM, Sartori DE, Tufik S, Bittencourt L. 2013. "Is portable monitoring for diagnosing obstructive sleep apnea syndrome suitable in elderly population?" *Sleep Breath.* May;17(2):679–686. doi: 10.1007/s11325-012-0742-y.

[10] Ayappa I, Norman RG, Seelall V, Rapoport DM. 2008. "Validation of a self-applied unattended monitor for sleep disordered breathing." *Journal of clinical sleep medicine:* Feb 15; 4(1):26-37.

[11] Drakatos P, Patel K, Thakrar C, Williams AJ, Kent BD, Leschziner GD. 2016. "Sleep-stage sequencing of sleep-onset REM periods in MSLT predicts treatment response in patients with narcolepsy." *J Sleep Res.* Apr;25(2):203-210. doi: 10.1111/jsr.12363.

[12] Pisani MA, Friese RS, Gehlbach BK, Schwab RJ, Weinhouse GL, Jones SF. 2015. "Sleep in the intensive care unit." *Am J Respir Crit Care Med.* Apr 1;191(7):731–738. doi: 10.1164/rccm.201411-2099CI.

[13] Knauert MP, Yaggi HK, Redeker NS, Murphy TE, Araujo KL, Pisani MA. 2014. "Feasibility study of unattended polysomnography in medical intensive care unit patients." *Heart Lung.* Sep-Oct; 43(5):445–452. doi: 10.1016/j.hrtlng.2014.06.049.

[14] Watson PL, Pandharipande P, Gehlbach BK, Thompson JL, Shintani AK, Dittus BS, Bernard GR, Malow BA, Ely EW. 2013. "Atypical sleep in ventilated patients: empirical electroencephalography findings and the path toward revised ICU sleep scoring criteria." *Crit Care Med.* Aug;41(8):1958–1967. doi: 10.1097/CCM.0b013e31828a3f75.

[15] Berry, RB. 2012. *Fundamentals of Sleep Medicine.* Elsevier. Pages 189-218. https://doi.org/10.1016/B978-1-4377-0326-9.00013-0.

[16] Yalamanchali S, Farajian V, Hamilton C, Pott TR, Samuelson CG, Friedman M. 2013. "Diagnosis of obstructive sleep apnea by peripheral arterial tonometry: meta-analysis." *JAMA Otolaryngol Head Neck Surg.* Dec;139(12):1343-1350. doi: 10.1001/jamaoto.2013.5338.

[17] Carter, JC, Auckley D. 2018. "Watch What You're Doing!" *J Clin Sleep Med.* Mar 15; 14(3):301-302. doi: 10.5664/jcsm.6962.

[18] Ting J, Tan LL, Balakrishnan ID, Chan SP, Yeo TC, Lee CH. 2018. "Watch-PAT versus level III device in diagnosing sleep disordered breathing in first myocardial infarction." *Clin Respir J.* Aug;12(8):2332-2339. doi: 10.1111/crj.12909.

[19] Namba S, Ujike Y, Ikegami T, Shimoyama I, Easton PA. 2011. "Sleep monitoring with portable devices in ICU patients." *European Respiratory Journal.* 38: p5011.

[20] Restrepo RD, Hirst KR, Wittnebel L, and Wettstein R. 2012 "AARC Clinical Practice Guideline: Transcutaneous Monitoring of Carbon Dioxide and Oxygen: 2012" *Respiratory Care.* Nov;57(11):1955-1962. doi: 10.4187/respcare.02011.

In: Sleep Medicine in Critical Care
Editors: Antonio M. Esquinas et al.
ISBN: 978-1-53617-768-8

Chapter 6

How to Diagnose Sleep-Related Breathing Disorders outside the Sleep Laboratory

Eui-Sik Suh*
Consultant in Respiratory and Ventilation Medicine,
Lane Fox Respiratory Service,
Guy's and St Thomas' NHS Foundation Trust, London, UK

Abstract

Attended in-laboratory polysomnography remains the gold standard method for diagnosing sleep-related breathing disorders. However, it is expensive, time-consuming, and requires expert technical input to assure the quality of the measurement. Therefore alternative diagnostic tests may be required in the general ward and critical care environments. Unattended polysomnography is increasingly used in the home, as well as in the hospital environment, and has a high degree of correlation with the results of attended in-laboratory polysomnography. Portable respiratory polygraphy is an alternative that allows diagnosis of both obstructive and central events during nocturnal recording, but is limited by the inability to detect sleep stage, and tends to underestimate the apnoea-hypopnoea index. Nocturnal pulse oximetry and transcutaneous capnography is useful for screening for patients in whom there is a high index of suspicion for sleep-disordered breathing and can detect response to treatment. Capnography is particularly helpful for those patients requiring ventilator support for sleep hypoventilation syndromes. Technologies such as peripheral arterial tonometry are helpful in diagnosing patients with sleep-disordered breathing. However, in cases where unattended, portable modalities used to screen patients with suspected sleep-related breathing disorders give negative or inconclusive results, then attended laboratory polysomnography should be deployed."

* Corresponding Author's E-mail: euisik.suh@gstt.nhs.uk.

INTRODUCTION

Sleep-related breathing disorders (SRBDs) are commonly encountered in the hospital setting outside the confines of the sleep laboratory, in clinical environments where both the appropriate diagnostic equipment and specialist expertise may be absent, for example in critical care units and on the general medical ward. Furthermore, a suspicion of the presence of a SRBD may be raised during a hospital stay and need to be investigated in the home environment following discharge from hospital. It is important, therefore, to ensure that well-validated, relatively simple tools are available to clinicians to enable accurate diagnosis of SRBDs and to assess the response to treatment outside the sleep department.

Obstructive sleep apnoea, central sleep apnoea and sleep hypoventilation syndromes are the most common SRBDs seen outside the sleep centre environment. With the prevalence of obesity standing at 29% in the UK and increasing [1], there is need to ensure that obesity-related respiratory failure (ORRF) and obstructive sleep apnoea (OSA) can be diagnosed by community and hospital-based non-specialists. The prevalence of OSA among hospitalised patients lies between 2% and 6% [2, 3]. Where obesity hypoventilation exists as a comorbid condition, it adversely affects the outcome of a hospital admission, with increased rates of intensive care unit admission, long-term care at discharge and mechanical ventilation, and hence diagnosing and effectively treating patients with SRBDs is clearly a priority.

Since the prevalence of ORRF and OSA is also increasing among patients undergoing surgery, and given that these conditions are associated with increased peri-operative risk, it is important that simple and effective diagnostic tools are readily available to surgical and anaesthetic teams to enable optimal risk assessment and management prior to embarking on surgical intervention [4]. Furthermore, the widespread use of sedative agents and opioid analgesics may increase the risk of respiratory compromise in patients with OSA.

Using a definition of OSA as apnoea-hypopnoea index (AHI) of ≥5/hour in the Wisconsin Sleep Cohort, the prevalence of OSA was found to be 24% in men and 9% in women aged between 30 and 60 years [5]. The prevalence of OSA with associated excessive daytime somnolence is approximately 3% to 7% in adult men and 2% to 5% in adult women [6]. Screening data suggest that large numbers of patients are undiagnosed and untreated [7-9], and therefore remain at risk of the well-established adverse associations of OSA, including poorly controlled hypertension, type 2 diabetes, glaucoma, impaired daytime vigilance, and increased risk of cardiovascular and cerebrovascular events. With increasing BMI and worsening apnoea-hypopnoea index (AHI), patients with OSA may develop hypercapnic respiratory failure, termed the obesity hypoventilation syndrome (OHS), and may require ventilatory support in the form of non-invasive ventilation (NIV). Depending on the severity and phenotype of

OHS, patients may need positive airway pressure (PAP) therapy in the form of continuous positive airway pressure (CPAP) or NIV. The optimal treatment for OHS is yet to be established [10, 11], but lies beyond the scope of this chapter. OHS confers greater risk to patients as they may present with decompensated respiratory failure, requiring acute ventilatory support; perioperative complications are also higher among patients with untreated OHS compared with patients with OSA and obese subjects without obesity [12].

Central sleep apnoea (CSA) is a less common cause of sleep-disordered breathing and is found predominantly in patients with cardiac and neurological disease, although psychotropic medications are also an important cause. 10% of SRBDs are attributable to CSA [13]. It is more common among the elderly and in men. This may be due to women having a lower apnoeic threshold which has the effect of stabilising respiration. It is characterised by recurrent apnoeas during sleep in the absence of respiratory effort. CSA can be associated with sleep fragmentation, insomnia and daytime somnolence. The International Classification of Sleep Disorders defines five CSA syndromes: 1) Primary (or idiopathic) CSA; 2) Cheyne-Stokes breathing pattern; 3) CSA due to high-altitude periodic breathing; 4) Drug-related CSA; and 5) Primary sleep apnoea of infancy. Primary CSA is a diagnosis of exclusion when all alternative causes have been explored; it is associated with a heightened hypercapnic ventilatory response, low $PaCO_2$ and sleep state instability [14].

Cheyne-Stokes respiration is common among patients with heart failure, with a prevalence of 37% among patients with heart failure and left ventricular ejection fraction <45% in one study on 100 patients [15]. Although it is predominantly seen in patients with left ventricular systolic dysfunction, it has also been observed in patients with diastolic dysfunction [16]. Sleep disturbance is common in Cheyne-Stokes respiration (CSR). There is a characteristic crescendo-decrescendo pattern of respiratory effort and airflow, with a typical cycle time of 60-90 seconds. The pathophysiology of CSR is incompletely understood and centres around instability of respiratory control in sleep, but has as its most prominent features 1) hyperventilation leading to hypocapnia below the apnoeic threshold (AT) and thus central apnoea, which in turn leads to hypercapnia; 2) elevated central hypercapnic ventilatory response; 3) hypoxaemia leading to increased peripheral chemoreceptor stimulation; 4) increased pulmonary vagal afferent traffic due to pulmonary venous congestion and C-fibre stimulation, leading to increased sympathetic activity that drives an exuberant response to hypercapnia; 5) circulatory delay leading to a prolonged time for oxygenated blood leaving the pulmonary artery to reach peripheral chemoreceptors; 6) reduced blood-buffering capacity [14].

TECHNOLOGIES TO DIAGNOSE SLEEP-DISORDERED BREATHING

Polysomnography

According to the American Association of Sleep Medicine (AASM), attended nocturnal polysomnography (PSG) remains the gold standard technique for diagnosing sleep-disordered breathing [17]. PSG enables recording of multiple data channels, including electroencephalography (EEG) to allow sleep staging, electro-oculogram (EOG) to detect rapid eye movement (REM) sleep, thoracic and abdominal efforts and transcutaneous oxygen saturations (SpO_2). The minimum parameters to be recorded during PSG according to AASM recommendations are shown in Table 1.

Disadvantages of Polysomnography

There are, however, several disadvantages to this approach. Firstly, attended PSG in a sleep laboratory is costly, with an average tariff of approximately $1800 in the USA for a PSG-based diagnosis with CPAP therapy [18]. Reimbursement for investigation of sleep disorders is variable between healthcare systems and there is understandably a desire among patients and healthcare providers to ensure a lower-cost, validated diagnostic test for sleep-disordered breathing. Secondly, polysomnography requires considerable technical expertise to set up the study and then to interpret the data robustly. Therefore, alternative strategies are available to allow clinicians to achieve a diagnosis of sleep-disordered breathing. Thirdly, while PSG can be performed in the home, or in general medical ward and critical care environments, patients typically are not attended by trained sleep technicians overnight, so the quality of data acquisition cannot be assured. Furthermore, PSG studies can be hampered in the hospital environment by additional monitoring of vital functions as well as treatment modalities; this is particularly true of the ICU environment. A recent systemic review of sleep deprivation in the ICU identified only five studies that investigated sleep quality using polysomnography in a small number of patients (range 4-21 patients) [19], underlining the challenges of performing PSG in a critical care setting. Finally, given the intensity of resources required to provide attended PSG in an accredited sleep laboratory, waiting lists for diagnostic studies can be prolonged [20, 21].

Classification of Diagnostic Devices for Sleep Disordered Breathing

The AASM has a well-established classification of diagnostic modalities to detect SRBDs [22]. Type 1 refers to attended nocturnal PSG, which is usually carried out in the sleep laboratory. Type 2 studies refer to unattended PSG studies, which may be performed in the home or hospital environment. Type 3 tests have at least four recording channels – a measure of respiratory effort, airflow, SpO_2 and either electrocardiogram (ECG) or heart rate. Such studies are often term limited respiratory polygraphy. Type 4 devices record one or two parameters such as SpO_2 and heart rate. Collectively, type 2-4 devices are referred to as home sleep apnoea tests (HSAT) or portable sleep monitoring devices.

Table 1. Minimum recommended parameters recorded for polysomnography. From reference [17]

Central monopolar recording
Occipital mono- or bipolar recording
Chin electromyogram
Left and right anterior tibial electromyogram
Left and right electro-oculogram
Electrocardiogram
Snoring microphone
Nasal/oral airflow
Thoracic and abdominal effort
Transcutaneous oximetry (SpO_2)
Body position

Polysomnography Outside the Sleep Laboratory

Unattended PSG

A large number of devices are available to perform full PSG in a patient's home, but there are relatively few studies that compare Type 2 devices with attended laboratory PSG. A recent systematic review by Bruyneel and Ninane [23] of six such studies found that home PSG was reliable in detecting obstructive sleep apnoea: in one study [24], using an AHI cut-off of ≥10/hour, home PSG diagnosed OSA with a sensitivity of 91% and specificity of 89%. Similarly, Bruyneel et al., using an AHI cut-off of ≥20/hour, reported a sensitivity of 76% and specificity of 85% for home PSG [25]. Overall, home PSG tended to over-estimate AHI for mild-to-moderate OSA, but underestimated severity for more severe cases, compared with laboratory PSG. This disparity may be due to night-to-night variability arising from differences in body posture (patients tend to sleep more in the supine position in sleep laboratory studies), differences in medications taken at home and in the sleep laboratory, alcohol consumption at home or nasal congestion [23]. Unsurprisingly, sleep quality tends to be better in the home environment; in the studies of Bruyneel et al. and Kingshott et al., sleep efficiency was 81-85% at home compared with 71-75% in the laboratory [25, 26]. Home PSG studies are however limited by failed recordings due to, for example, dislodged nasal cannulae or EEG leads. Adequate recordings are obtained in 79-100% of cases [REF Bruyneel and Ninane review], and failure rates tend to be lower when PSG hook-ups are performed in the patient's home rather in the sleep laboratory.

The 2017 AASM guideline on the diagnosis of OSA in adults reviewed data from only two studies that compared Type 2 HSAT devices against PSG [17]; in high-risk populations using a cut-off of AHI ≥ 5, diagnostic accuracy ranged from 84% to 91%. Using a cutoff of AHI ≥ 15, the accuracy of Type 2 HSAT devices was 88%. Currently there remains no direct recommendation for the use of home PSG in the diagnosis of OSA and data on cost reductions are difficult to derive, given the wide variation in reimbursements for diagnostic sleep studies across healthcare systems. However, home PSG clearly offers the opportunity to obtain a definitive diagnosis of OSA in a large proportion of patients without the inconvenience and cost of an overnight stay in hospital.

Portable Respiratory Polygraphy (Type 3 Devices)

For patients in whom a history and examination raise the suspicion of moderate-to-severe OSA, portable respiratory polygraphy (RPG) offers the opportunity for diagnosis with high sensitivity and specificity, with the additional benefits of portability, lower cost and convenience to the patient. Recent AASM guidelines for the diagnosis of OSA cite seven studies that evaluated type 3 devices against PSG [27-33]; the accuracy of diagnosis depended on the AHI cut-off. For AHI ≥5/hour, the diagnostic accuracy ranged from 94-91 in a high-risk population assuming a prevalence of 87%, and 70-78% in a low-risk population with a prevalence of 55%. For AHI ≥15/hour, diagnostic accuracy ran at 65-91% in a high-risk population, while for AHI ≥30, with 88% in a high-risk population. These data indicate that in patients with high pre-test probability of OSA, RPG is both accurate and convenient. As there are fewer data channels, there is less chance of test failure compared with PSG, and type 3 devices can be fitted relatively easily by patients themselves in their own home. Furthermore, diagnostic protocols that include automated scoring systems are cost-effective [33], although manual scoring remains more accurate and should be performed. Most studies have focused on comparing PRG-based treatment protocol against PSG in patients with AHI ≥15, thus excluding patients with potentially treated mild OSA who may or may not need CPAP. In a broad population of patients requiring a sleep study for intermediate-to-high suspicion of OSA, Corral et al. found that home RPG was non-inferior to PSG-based diagnosis and treatment in terms of improvements in Epworth Sleepiness Score, quality of life and blood pressure [34]. Importantly, a cost analysis demonstrated that RPG-based diagnosis and treatment was €416 cheaper than PSG at €320 per patient.

There are however limitations to the use of RPG. It does not detect sleep stage; therefore, RPG tends to underestimate AHI, as the denominator for calculating the AHI is total recording time, which is longer than PSG-detected total sleep time. RPG is also unable to detect hypopnoeas associated with arousals that do not involve oxygen desaturation, which can be picked up on PSG. The average difference between PSG-derived respiratory event index (REI) and RPG-derived AHI is 10/hour [28].

Nocturnal Pulse-Oximetry and Type 4 Devices

Nocturnal pulse-oximetry is frequently used as a screening tool to identify patients who may require treatment for OSA and other SRBDs. It is convenient, easy for the patient to use at home or in hospital, and can yield important data regarding nocturnal oxygen saturations. Transcutaneous arterial oxygen saturation can be continuously monitored using a probe on the finger or on the ear-lobe. It must be borne in mind however that, like respiratory polygraphy, sleep stage cannot be identified by nocturnal oximetry. Similarly, nocturnal pulse-oximetry does not identify apnoeas or hypopnoeas per se. However, since these events are usually associated with oxygen desaturations, the hourly frequency of desaturations by 2%, 3% or 4% are often taken as surrogates for the AHI. A wealth of other data may be derived from nocturnal pulse oximetry. Percentage of the total recording time spent below, for example, and SpO_2 of 90% may give an indication of the severity of SRBD and is an independent predictor in obese patients of daytime hypercapnia [35]. Prolonged desaturations over several minutes may occur in patients with alveolar hypoventilation syndrome during presumed REM sleep. The rapidity with which SpO_2 falls and then recovers during a presumed apnoeic or hypopnoeic event may allow the clinician to distinguish between obstructive (rapid, repetitive desaturations from baseline) and central (lower frequency of desaturations, re-saturation to above the baseline in keeping with hyperventilation) events.

Technical considerations are important for sleep oximetry. Typically, the cyclical drops in SpO_2 in apnoeas and hypopnoeas lag 45-60 seconds behind the respiratory event. It is important that the SpO_2 sampling frequency at a level that will detect these events as discrete episodes. SpO_2 measurements can be significantly affected by changes in peripheral perfusion due for example to ambient temperature, hypotension and use of vasopressor drugs. Darker skin tone can lead to a falsely elevated measurements at low levels of SpO_2 [36]. Patient movement during nocturnal recording can introduce artefact. Since pulse oximetry depends on the detection of differential absorption of infra-red frequencies by oxygenated and deoxygenated haemoglobin, SpO_2 measurements are affected by met- and carboxy-haemoglobinaemia, both of which lead to an overestimation of SpO_2. Conversely, anaemia leads to an overestimation of SpO_2. Tissue optics can be affected to an important degree by severe obesity. Finally, oximetry is limited by its inability to detect SRBDs which are not associated with oxygen desaturations, for example, pure CSA in Ondine's curse and upper airway resistance syndrome.

Agreement of Pulse Oximetry Parameters with PSG-Derived AHI

Several studies have investigated the utility of pulse oximetry in the screening and diagnosis of OSA, but interpretation of the data is hampered by the heterogeneity of the oximetry parameters that were compared with PSG-derived AHI. Deegan and McNicholas showed that overnight pulse oximetry combined with clinical features could only make the diagnosis of OSA (confirmed by PSG) in one third of cases in a large population of patients attending a sleep clinic [37]. By contrast, Williams et al. found in a smaller cohort of 40 patients that visual assessment of a pattern of repetitive desaturation on overnight pulse oximetry could reliably detect OSA as defined on PSG by AHI ≥10/hour [38]. All 15 patients with a consistent pattern for OSA on oximetry had OSA; five of the 18 patients with a negative oximetry had OSA on PSG, i.e., false negatives, but had substantially milder disease. 10% of tracings were inadequate for interpretation. Cooper et al. established that the accuracy of qualitative inspection of overnight oximetry traces in detecting OSA was dependent on the AHI threshold [39], with diagnostic sensitivity increasing with worsening disease severity of OSA. At AHI ≥25/hour, visual inspection of oximetry traces had 100% sensitivity and 95% specificity in diagnosing OSA, while at AHI ≥5/hour the sensitivity was just 60% with specificity at 80%.

Olson et al. compared the cumulative percentage time at $SaO_2 < 90\%$ (CT_{90}) and a saturation variability index (ΔIndex, the sum of the differences between successive readings divided by the number of readings – 1) in a population of 793 patients with suspected OSA. CT_{90} was only weakly correlated with AHI (Spearman $\rho = 0.36$, $p < 0.0001$), with ΔIndex having only a slightly better correlation with AHI (Spearman $\rho = 0.59$ $p < 0.0001$). Magalung et al. compared the relative utility of the different indices derived from pulse oximetry in a total of 516 patients investigated for OSA, and found that the ΔIndex was the best predictor of AHI on PSG with a c index of 0.881 [40]. However, the 2%, 3% and 4% oxygen desaturation indices (ODI) has similar levels of accuracy (c indices 0.868, 0.873 and 0.852, respectively). There was further validation of the ΔIndex in a study 301 patients undergoing PSG for suspected OSA [41]. Using an AHI cut-off of ≥15/hour as the diagnostic criterion for OSA and a ΔIndex threshold of 0.6, nocturnal oximetry was able to detect OSA with a sensitivity of 98% and a specificity of 46%. The positive predictive value was 77% and the negative predictive value 94%. Schäfer et al. compared 4% ODI with PSG in 114 patients with suspected OSA and found a significant correlation between ODI and PSG-derived respiratory disturbance index (RDI) ($r = 0.7$, $p < 0.001$). ODI had a high sensitivity (94%) but low specificity (41%) for diagnosing OSA. Similar results were obtained in the study of Golpe et al., with only a weak correlation found between AHI and 4% ODI ($r = 0.60$) and an area under the receiver-operator curve of less than 0.8 for the diagnosis of OSA as defined by AHI ≥10/hour [42]. Half of patients in this study could not have been diagnosed with nocturnal oximetry alone.

It appears that while pulse oximetry can yield important information regarding nocturnal desaturations, it is insufficiently accurate to diagnose SRBD compared with PSG. The performance of nocturnal oximetry as a diagnostic improves as the severity of OSA increases, i.e., at higher AHI cut-offs, and in patients with a higher pre-test probability of OSA. It is therefore more helpful as a rule-in test in higher-risk populations than as a rule-out test. However, all the studies validating nocturnal oximetry as a diagnostic tool have used PSG as the gold standard, and it is widely acknowledged that there can be significant night-to-night variability in both PSG and home sleep apnoea tests (HSATs) [43]. Furthermore, the AHI in itself has limited clinical significance in that it is poorly correlated with symptoms or with treatment outcomes. The population distribution of AHI is unimodal, so an AHI cut-off is essentially arbitrary. The utility of PSG and nocturnal oximetry arises from their ability to identify patients whose quality of life is likely to improve with treatment. In a randomised controlled trial reported by Whitelaw et al., PSG-directed management of patients with suspected OSA was no better than oximetry-based management in identifying patients who were likely to improve their quality of life with CPAP therapy [44]. Automated algorithms for analysing nocturnal oximetry are now commonplace and accurate – Vazquez et al. established in a study of 246 patients with suspected OSA that automatically calculated ODI from nocturnal oximetry were highly correlated with PSG-derived AHI (r=0.97), with a sensitivity of 98% and specificity of 88% [45]. Nonetheless, nocturnal oximetry is not currently recommended by the AASM as a diagnostic tool for OSA [17], as the evidence points towards its use as a "rule-in" test rather than a "rule-out" test.

As briefly alluded to above, nocturnal pulse oximetry can yield important qualitative information about the nature of sleep disturbance in SRBDs.

The Oximetry Trace

The frequency of desaturations of 2%, 3% and 4% below the baseline are routinely analysed in an automated manner to yield the ODI. The duration of desaturations and the speed of resaturation (i.e., recovery of the SpO_2 to the baseline level) can also produce useful information. In OSA, the frequency of desaturations tends to be higher than in CSA and importantly, resaturation occurs rapidly, giving a characteristic saw-tooth morphology of the SpO2 waveform [Figure 1]. In Cheyne-Stokes respiration, the frequency of desaturations may be lower due to the inherent duration of the apnoea-hyperventilation cycle, which is typically 60-90 seconds. Resaturation tends not only to be slower in CSA, but also occurs to a higher level of SpO2 than might be expected in OSA, due to the hyperventilation that characterises CSA. Automated algorithms have been developed to differentiate OSA from CSA utilising the photoplethysmographic properties of the oximetry trace, which give an indication of intrathoracic pressure changes during respiration [46-48], and therefore of respiratory effort.

Patients with OSA are expected to have lower mean SpO_2 values over the recording period than healthy subjects; accordingly, the percentage of recording time with SpO_2 below 90% increases with severity of OSA. Furthermore, patients with OSA have greater variability of SpO_2. Although oximetry does not give a reliable measure of alveolar ventilation during sleep, periods of prolonged desaturation over several minutes with or without repetitive desaturations associated with upper airway obstruction, for example during presumed REM sleep, can suggest the presence of REM-related hypoventilation in the obese or neuromuscular patient. Mandal et al. reported that, in a cohort of 245 obese patients referred to a tertiary home mechanical ventilation centre for assessment of sleep-disordered breathing, the percentage of analysis time with SpO_2 below 90% on baseline nocturnal oximetry was higher in the group with daytime hypercapnia than in the eucapnic group [35].

These features of nocturnal oximetry allow the clinician to identify different phenotypes of obesity-related sleep-disordered breathing:

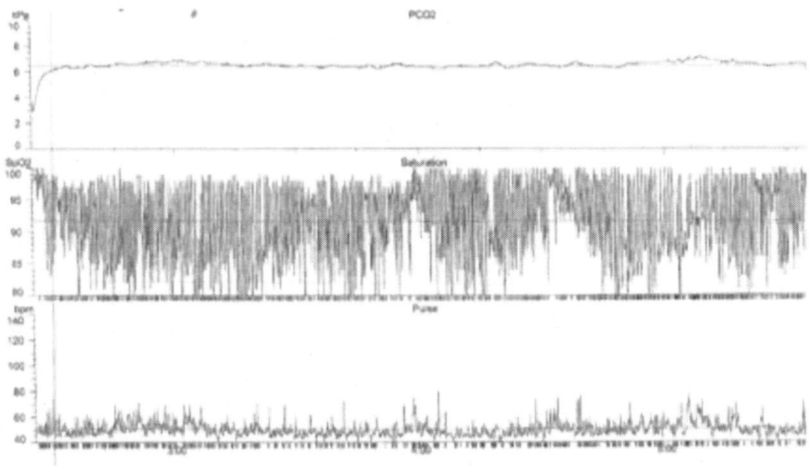

Figure 1. Nocturnal oximetry and transcutaneous capnography in a patient with hypercapnic obstructive sleep apnoea. PCO2: transcutaneous partial pressure of carbon dioxide; SpO2: transcutaneous oxygen saturations.

1. OSA – rapid repetitive desaturations without prolonged periods of hypoxaemia; the patient may be eucapnic or hypercapnic [Figure 1].
2. OSA with OHS – rapid repetitive desaturations with prolonged periods of hypoxaemia in presumed REM sleep, which may be associated with hypercapnic respiratory failure [Figure 2].

3. Lone OHS – prolonged periods of hypoxaemia in presumed REM sleep with associated daytime hypercapnia, in the absence of rapid repetitive desaturations [Figure 3].

The Heart Rate Trace

It is often easy for the clinician to neglect the heart rate trace on nocturnal pulse oximetry, when there is in fact a great deal of information to be gleaned. Increased heart rate variability is a sensitive indicator of arousal during a desaturation event [49, 50] [Figure 2]. The heart rate trace may indicate the presence of atrial fibrillation or other hitherto undiagnosed rhythm disorders, which may be an important contributing factor in their SRBD, particularly CSA.

A fall in heart rate can give an indication, although not always reliably, of sleep onset. Similarly, REM sleep is heralded by an increase in heart rate, arising from increased sympathetic drive [51], and may be accompanied by a period of prolonged hypoxaemia as minute ventilation decreases during REM sleep as a result of reduced central respiratory drive and respiratory muscle activity [Figures 2 and 3].

Recently, a characteristic pattern of heart rate variability has been identified that is associated with a diagnosis of periodic limb movement disorder (PLMD). Krishnaswamy et al. explored an observation that patients with PLMD had increased heart rate variability in the absence of oxygen desaturations on nocturnal oximetry. 70 patients with daytime somnolence and a PSG diagnosis of PLMD were studied, and 81% of these were found to have increased heart rate variability on their oximetry trace in the absence of significant desaturations [52].

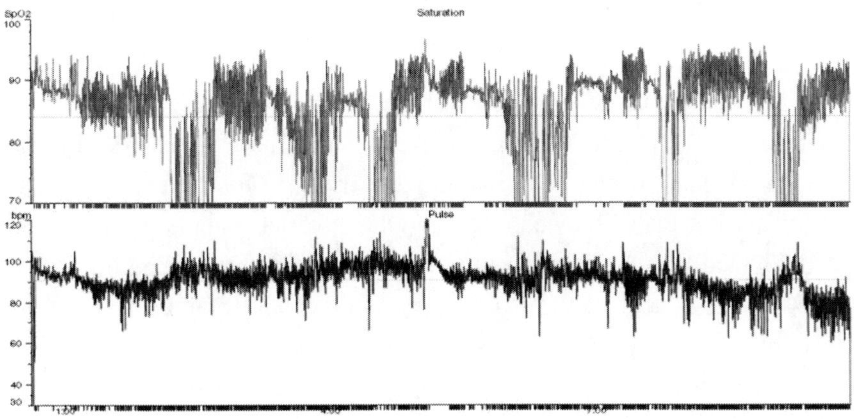

Figure 2. Nocturnal oximetry in a patient with obstructive sleep apnoea and obesity hypoventilation syndrome. Note the prolonged oxygen desaturations in presumed rapid eye movement sleep in conjunction with rapid, repetitive desaturations. SpO2: transcutaneous oxygen saturations.

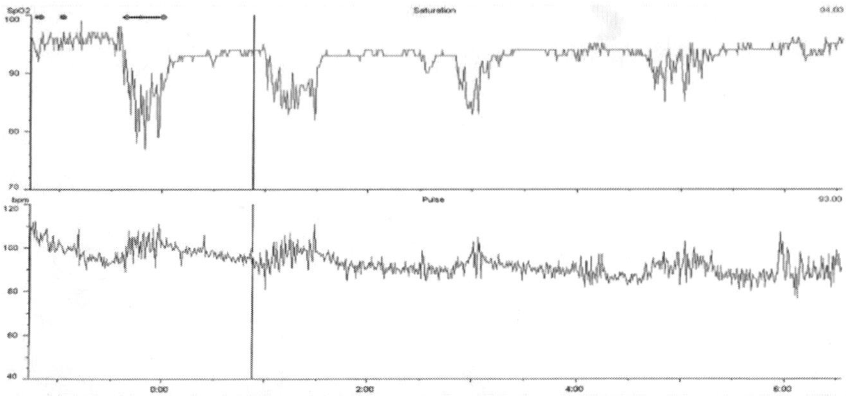

Figure 3. Nocturnal oximetry in a patient with lone obesity hypoventilation syndrome. Note the prolonged oxygen desaturations in presumed rapid eye movement sleep in the absence of rapid repetitive desaturations. SpO2: transcutaneous oxygen saturations.

Pulse Oximetry in Patients with Underlying Lung Disease

Patients with significant airways or parenchymal lung disease may also have concomitant OSA or other SRBD. The prevalence of obesity in COPD patients ranges from 15% in European cohorts [53, 54] to 54% in the United States [55]. The prevalence of OSA in patients with mild airflow obstruction is similar to that found in the general population, but coexistent OSA in COPD further degrades sleep quality [56-58]. Some features of COPD increase the risk of OSA, in particular, patients with chronic bronchitis and cor pulmonale are more likely to develop OSA due to a tendency to higher BMI and a rostral shift of fluid in the supine position [59]. By contrast, those with predominant emphysema are likely to have a lower body mass index (BMI) and more pronounced lung hyperinflation. The latter increases upper airway closing pressure and may protect against airways collapse and OSA. Importantly, the prognosis for COPD-OSA overlap syndrome patients is worse than for those with COPD alone; in one study, all-cause mortality over a nine-year period was 42% for COPD-OSA overlap patients not treated with continuous positive airways pressure (CPAP), compared with just 24% for patients with COPD only [60]; mortality did not differ between COPD-OSA overlap patients treated with CPAP and patients with COPD only. It is therefore of vital importance to diagnose such patients with accuracy. However, the diagnosis of OSA and other SRBD in COPD is hampered in many patients by underlying persistent hypoxaemia, which can have a marked effect on ODI. In fact, the current AASM guidelines on the diagnosis of SRBD does not recommend the use of any HSAT in patients with significant underlying cardiopulmonary condition, on the basis that validation studies for HSAT explicitly excluded these patients [17]. Robust diagnosis therefore depends on attended PSG, which may be challenging to obtain in hospital environments where the suspicion of SRBD in patients with cardiopulmonary disease are often raised, i.e., on the general medical ward or in critical care units. A reasonable compromise is often reached, with limited nocturnal respiratory polygraphy being used to identify the presence of obstructive or central sleep apnoea.

Nocturnal Transcutaneous Capnography

An important, often overlooked element in the investigation of SRBDs is the presence or absence of hypoventilation and eucapnia. Daytime hypercapnia is present in 10-38% of patients with OSA and its prevalence increases with worsening frequency of desaturations, increasing restrictive ventilatory defect and with rising body mass index (BMI) [35, 61-66]. Arterial blood gas sampling should be performed if there is a suspicion of daytime hypercapnia, based on the severity of symptoms and on the appearance of the oximetry trace. As noted above, the percentage of the recording time spent with $SpO_2 < 90\%$ is associated with the presence of nocturnal hypoventilation. Furthermore, clinic $SpO_2 < 95\%$ and vital capacity <3L should prompt arterial blood gas sampling [35]. Although OHS is defined by daytime hypercapnia, there is an increasing recognition that this definition may miss those patients who hypoventilate overnight but maintain daytime eucapnia; hence, a definition of OHS that includes patients with elevated bicarbonate >27mmol/L and arterial base excess >3mmol/L would allow earlier diagnosis and consideration of bi-level positive pressure ventilation rather than CPAP [67].

The detection of nocturnal hypercapnia can be achieved in the critical care environment by frequent intermittent arterial blood sampling via an arterial catheter. However, this can be unnecessarily invasive in stable patients who are undergoing inpatient assessment of SBRD. While end tidal carbon dioxide tensions ($ETCO_2$) may be helpful in assessing ventilatory adequacy in patients undergoing invasive mechanical ventilation, it is less useful in self-ventilating patients or those receiving non-invasive ventilation. Furthermore, $ETCO_2$ may not give an accurate measure of arterial CO_2 in patients with obstructive airways disease [68]. Transcutaneous capnography (TCO_2) has been available for many years and allows estimation of arterial CO_2 tensions in non-invasively in real-time. It depends on the diffusion of capillary CO_2 to a cutaneous electrode and is facilitated by heating of the skin. There are limitations to this technique due to a relatively long stabilization time (5-10 minutes) and reaction time (5-10s). The sensor requires periodic repositioning, particularly to prevent skin damage from the heater element of the electrode. Technical drift of the transcutaneous CO_2 measurement over time can be corrected retrospectively. As for transcutaneous SpO_2 monitoring, TCO_2 measurements can be confounded by hypoperfusion and low cardiac output states, oedema or increased skin thickness. Nonetheless, TCO_2 enables recognition of hypoventilation in real-time nocturnally in a non-invasive manner, as well as assessment of response to ventilation. TCO_2 correlates well with $PaCO_2$ [69], although high $PaCO_2$

levels may increase the $PaCO_2/TCO_2$ bias. It is important to anchor TCO_2 readings with an arterial blood gas sample for $PaCO_2$ when the TCO_2 electrode is applied at the at the beginning off a recording period, to ensure that the two values are comparable. The close agreement between TCO_2 and $PaCO_2$ is preserved when patients are undergoing NIV, and thus nocturnal transcutaneous capnography enable assessment of ventilatory sufficient in patients during both the diagnostic and treatment phases of SRBD [70].

Peripheral Arterial Tonometry to Diagnose Sleep-Related Breathing Disorders

Sympathetic activation increases between slow-wave and REM sleep, and between quiet wakefulness and REM sleep. Furthermore, sympathetic activation increases in response to apnoeic episodes of 10-60s duration, with greatest activity occurring at the end of each apnoea, leading to sharp elevations in blood pressure and heart rate [51, 71, 72]. Peripheral arterial tonometry (PAT) has been developed method to assess autonomic activation non-invasively during sleep [73] and relies on the pulsatile plethysmographic signal measured from the finger as a surrogate for sympathetic activity. In combination with wrist-worn actigraphy and pulse oximetry (as in the Watch-PAT device), PAT can be used to detect apnoea and hypopnoea by measuring peripheral arterial volume changes. The algorithm incorporated into the Watch-PAT devices correlates arousals detected from PAT with oxygen desaturations to determine respiratory effort-related arousals. Several studies have found high levels of agreement between the respiratory disturbance index (RDI) and AHI generated by the Watch-PAT and PSG. In a recent meta-analysis of 14 studies comparing Watch-PAT with PSG, a correlation coefficient of $r = 0.89$ was found between Watch-PAT RDI and PSG RDI, and a correlation coefficient of $r = 0.89$ between Watch-PAT AHI and PSG AHI [74]. However, most of these studies compared Watch-PAT with PSG performed in the sleep laboratory, rather than in the home environment. Zou et al. compared Watch-PAT with unattended home PSG in 98 patients in Sweden, and found Watch-PAT-derived RDI, AHI, and ODI correlated closely (0.88, 0.90, and 0.92; $p < 0.0001$, respectively) with the same indices obtained from PSG [75]. A further study from O'Brien et al. found a good level of agreement between home Watch-PAT measurements and unattended PSG in 31 pregnant women (AHI, $r = 0.76$, $p < 0.001$; RDI, $r = 0.68$, $p < 0.001$) [76]. Garg et al. evaluated the performance of home Watch-PAT against laboratory PSG using a cut-off of AHI $\geq$ 5/hour and reported a low specificity of 0.43 [77]. At an AHI cut-off of $\geq$30, they reported a higher specificity of 0.82 and sensitivity of 0.92. In light of the risks of false-negative results using Watch-PAT, PSG continues to be recommended in patients with negative or non-diagnostic results [17].

CONCLUSION

Although PSG remains the gold standard for the diagnosis of patients with sleep-related breathing disorders, this is not a pragmatic solution for many patients in the hospital inpatient or home environments. For patients in whom the index of suspicion of SRBD is moderate or high, limited respiratory polygraphy and nocturnal oximetry are useful tools to both screen for SRBD and to assess response to treatment. Nocturnal oximetry, in particular, may provide a wealth of useful physiological data to guide the clinician at relatively low cost and without great inconvenience to the patient, not only in suggesting a diagnosis but also in assessing response to treatment. The proviso however remains that clinicians proceed to PSG for such patients whose initial investigations are either negative or inconclusive.

REFERENCES

[1] Lifestyles Team ND. *Statistics on Obesity, Physical Activity and Diet*, England, 2019. Health and Social Care Information Centre; 2019.

[2] Nowbar, S; Burkart, KM; Gonzales, R; Fedorowicz, A; Gozansky, WS; Gaudio, JC; et al. Obesity-associated hypoventilation in hospitalized patients: prevalence, effects, and outcome. *Am J Med.*, 2004, 116(1), 1-7.

[3] Spurr, KF; Graven, MA; Gilbert, RW. Prevalence of unspecified sleep apnea and the use of continuous positive airway pressure in hospitalized patients, 2004 national hospital discharge survey. *Sleep and Breathing.*, 2008, 12(3), 229-34.

[4] Hillman, DR; Chung, F. Anaesthetic management of sleep-disordered breathing in adults. *Respirology.*, 2017, 22(2), 230-9.

[5] Young, T; Palta, M; Dempsey, J; Skatrud, J; Weber, S; Badr, S. The occurrence of sleep-disordered breathing among middle-aged adults. *N Engl J Med.*, 1993, 328(17), 1230-5.

[6] Punjabi, NM. The epidemiology of adult obstructive sleep apnea. *Proc Am Thorac Soc.*, 2008, 5(2), 136-43.

[7] Appleton, SL; Vakulin, A; McEvoy, RD; Vincent, A; Martin, SA; Grant, JF; et al. Undiagnosed obstructive sleep apnea is independently associated with reductions in quality of life in middle-aged, but not elderly men of a population cohort. *Sleep Breath.*, 2015, 19(4), 1309-16.

[8] Simpson, L; Hillman, DR; Cooper, MN; Ward, KL; Hunter, M; Cullen, S; et al. High prevalence of undiagnosed obstructive sleep apnoea in the general population and methods for screening for representative controls. *Sleep Breath.*, 2013, 17(3), 967-73.

[9] Kapur, V; Strohl, KP; Redline, S; Iber, C; O'Connor, G; Nieto, J. Underdiagnosis of sleep apnea syndrome in U.S. communities. *Sleep Breath.*, 2002, 6(2), 49-54.

[10] Masa, JF; Mokhlesi, B; Benítez, I; Gomez de Terreros, FJ; Sánchez-Quiroga, MÁ; Romero, A; et al. Long-term clinical effectiveness of continuous positive airway pressure therapy versus non-invasive ventilation therapy in patients with obesity hypoventilation syndrome: a multicentre, open-label, randomised controlled trial. *The Lancet.*, 2019, 393(10182), 1721-32.

[11] Murphy, PB; Piper, AJ; Hart, N. Obesity hypoventilation syndrome: is less really more? *The Lancet.* 2019, 393(10182), 1674-6.

[12] Raveendran, R; Wong, J; Singh, M; Wong, DT; Chung, F. Obesity hypoventilation syndrome, sleep apnea, overlap syndrome: perioperative management to prevent complications. *Current Opinion in Anaesthesiology.*, 2017, 30(1), 146-55.

[13] Sateia, MJ. International classification of sleep disorders-third edition: highlights and modifications. *Chest.*, 2014, 146(5), 1387-94.

[14] Eckert, DJ; Jordan, AS; Merchia, P; Malhotra, A. Central sleep apnea: Pathophysiology and treatment. *Chest.*, 2007, 131(2), 595-607.

[15] Javaheri, S. Sleep disorders in systolic heart failure: a prospective study of 100 male patients. The final report. *Int J Cardiol.*, 2006, 106(1), 21-8.

[16] Bitter, T; Faber, L; Hering, D; Langer, C; Horstkotte, D; Oldenburg, O. Sleep-disordered breathing in heart failure with normal left ventricular ejection fraction. *Eur J Heart Fail.*, 2009, 11(6), 602-8.

[17] Kapur, VK; Auckley, DH; Chowdhuri, S; Kuhlmann, DC; Mehra, R; Ramar, K; et al. Clinical Practice Guideline for Diagnostic Testing for Adult Obstructive Sleep Apnea: An American Academy of Sleep Medicine Clinical Practice Guideline. *J Clin Sleep Med.*, 2017, 13(3), 479-504.

[18] Kim, RD; Kapur, VK; Redline-Bruch, J; Rueschman, M; Auckley, DH; Benca, RM; et al. An Economic Evaluation of Home Versus Laboratory-Based Diagnosis of Obstructive Sleep Apnea. *Sleep.*, 2015, 38(7), 1027-37.

[19] Medrzycka-Dabrowska, W; Lewandowska, K; Kwiecień-Jaguś, K; Czyż-Szypenbajl, K. Sleep Deprivation in Intensive Care Unit - Systematic Review. *Open Med (Wars).*, 2018, 13, 384-93.

[20] Masa, Jimenez, JF; Barbe, Illa, F; Capote, Gil, F; Chiner Vives, E; Diaz de Atauri, J; Duran Cantolla, J; et al. [Resources and delays in the diagnosis of sleep apnea-hypopnea syndrome]. *Arch Bronconeumol.*, 2007, 43(4), 188-98.

[21] Flemons, WW; Douglas, NJ; Kuna, ST; Rodenstein, DO; Wheatley, J. Access to diagnosis and treatment of patients with suspected sleep apnea. *Am J Respir Crit Care Med.*, 2004, 169(6), 668-72.

[22] Collop, NA; Anderson, WM; Boehlecke, B; Claman, D; Goldberg, R; Gottlieb, DJ; et al. Clinical guidelines for the use of unattended portable monitors in the diagnosis of obstructive sleep apnea in adult patients. Portable Monitoring Task

Force of the American Academy of Sleep Medicine. *Journal of clinical sleep medicine: JCSM: official publication of the American Academy of Sleep Medicine.*, 2007, 3(7), 737-47.

[23] Bruyneel, M; Ninane, V. Unattended home-based polysomnography for sleep disordered breathing: current concepts and perspectives. *Sleep Med Rev.*, 2014, 18(4), 341-7.

[24] Campbell, AJ; Neill, AM. Home set-up polysomnography in the assessment of suspected obstructive sleep apnea. *J Sleep Res.*, 2011, 20(1 Pt 2), 207-13.

[25] Bruyneel, M; Sanida, C; Art, G; Libert, W; Cuvelier, L; Paesmans, M; et al. Sleep efficiency during sleep studies: results of a prospective study comparing home-based and in-hospital polysomnography. *J Sleep Res.*, 2011, 20(1 Pt 2), 201-6.

[26] Kingshott, RN; Douglas, NJ. The effect of in-laboratory polysomnography on sleep and objective daytime sleepiness. *Sleep.*, 2000, 23(8), 1109-13.

[27] Gjevre, JA; Taylor-Gjevre, RM; Skomro, R; Reid, J; Fenton, M; Cotton, D. Comparison of polysomnographic and portable home monitoring assessments of obstructive sleep apnea in Saskatchewan women. *Can Respir J.*, 2011, 18(5), 271-4.

[28] Masa, JF; Corral, J; Pereira, R; Duran-Cantolla, J; Cabello, M; Hernandez-Blasco, L; et al. Effectiveness of home respiratory polygraphy for the diagnosis of sleep apnoea and hypopnoea syndrome. *Thorax.*, 2011, 66(7), 567-73.

[29] Polese, JF; Santos-Silva, R; de Oliveira Ferrari, PM; Sartori, DE; Tufik, S; Bittencourt, L. Is portable monitoring for diagnosing obstructive sleep apnea syndrome suitable in elderly population? *Sleep Breath.*, 2013, 17(2), 679-86.

[30] Santos-Silva, R; Sartori, DE; Truksinas, V; Truksinas, E; Alonso, FF; Tufik, S; et al. Validation of a portable monitoring system for the diagnosis of obstructive sleep apnea syndrome. *Sleep.*, 2009, 32(5), 629-36.

[31] Yin, M; Miyazaki, S; Ishikawa, K. Evaluation of type 3 portable monitoring in unattended home setting for suspected sleep apnea: factors that may affect its accuracy. *Otolaryngol Head Neck Surg.*, 2006, 134(2), 204-9.

[32] Planes, C; Leroy, M; Bouach Khalil, N; El Mahmoud, R; Digne, F; de Roquefeuil, F; et al. Home diagnosis of obstructive sleep apnoea in coronary patients: validity of a simplified device automated analysis. *Sleep Breath.*, 2010, 14(1), 25-32.

[33] Masa, JF; Corral, J; Pereira, R; Duran-Cantolla, J; Cabello, M; Hernandez-Blasco, L; et al. Effectiveness of sequential automatic-manual home respiratory polygraphy scoring. *Eur Respir J.*, 2013, 41(4), 879-87.

[34] Corral, J; Sanchez-Quiroga, MA; Carmona-Bernal, C; Sanchez-Armengol, A; de, la, Torre, AS; Duran-Cantolla, J; et al. Conventional Polysomnography Is Not Necessary for the Management of Most Patients with Suspected Obstructive Sleep Apnea. Noninferiority, Randomized Controlled Trial. *Am J Respir Crit Care Med.*, 2017, 196(9), 1181-90.

[35] Mandal, S; Suh, ES; Boleat, E; Asher, W; Kamalanathan, M; Lee, K; et al. A cohort study to identify simple clinical tests for chronic respiratory failure in obese patients with sleep-disordered breathing. *BMJ open respiratory research.*, 2014, 1(1), e000022.

[36] Bickler Philip, E; M.D. Ph.D. Feiner John, R; M.D. Severinghaus John, W. M.D. Effects of Skin Pigmentation on Pulse Oximeter Accuracy at Low Saturation. *Anesthesiology: The Journal of the American Society of Anesthesiologists.*, 2005, 102(4), 715-9.

[37] Deegan, PC; McNicholas, WT. Predictive value of clinical features for the obstructive sleep apnoea syndrome. *Eur Respir J.*, 1996, 9(1), 117-24.

[38] Williams, AJ; Yu, G; Santiago, S; Stein, M. Screening for sleep apnea using pulse oximetry and a clinical score. *Chest.*, 1991, 100(3), 631-5.

[39] Cooper, BG; Veale, D; Griffiths, CJ; Gibson, GJ. Value of nocturnal oxygen saturation as a screening test for sleep apnoea. *Thorax.*, 1991, 46(8), 586-8.

[40] Magalang, UJ; Dmochowski, J; Veeramachaneni, S; Draw, A; Mador, MJ; El-Solh, A; et al. Prediction of the Apnea-Hypopnea Index From Overnight Pulse Oximetry. *Chest.*, 2003, 124(5), 1694-701.

[41] Levy, P; Pepin, JL; Deschaux-Blanc, C; Paramelle, B; Brambilla, C. Accuracy of oximetry for detection of respiratory disturbances in sleep apnea syndrome. *Chest.*, 1996, 109(2), 395-9.

[42] Golpe, R; Jimenez, A; Carpizo, R; Cifrian, JM. Utility of home oximetry as a screening test for patients with moderate to severe symptoms of obstructive sleep apnea. *Sleep.*, 1999, 22(7), 932-7.

[43] Aarab, G; Lobbezoo, F; Hamburger, HL; Naeije, M. Variability in the apnea-hypopnea index and its consequences for diagnosis and therapy evaluation. *Respiration.*, 2009, 77(1), 32-7.

[44] Whitelaw, WA; Brant, RF; Flemons, WW. Clinical Usefulness of Home Oximetry Compared with Polysomnography for Assessment of Sleep Apnea. *American Journal of Respiratory and Critical Care Medicine.*, 2005, 171(2), 188-93.

[45] Vazquez, JC; Tsai, WH; Flemons, WW; Masuda, A; Brant, R; Hajduk, E; et al. Automated analysis of digital oximetry in the diagnosis of obstructive sleep apnoea. *Thorax.*, 2000, 55(4), 302-7.

[46] Sommermeyer, D; Zou, D; Grote, L; Hedner, J. Detection of sleep disordered breathing and its central/obstructive character using nasal cannula and finger pulse oximeter. *Journal of clinical sleep medicine: JCSM: official publication of the American Academy of Sleep Medicine.*, 2012, 8(5), 527-33.

[47] Barak-Shinar, D; Amos, Y; Bogan, RK. Sleep disordered breathing analysis in a general population using standard pulse oximeter signals. *Sleep Breath.*, 2013, 17(3), 1109-15.

[48] Romem, A; Romem, A; Koldobskiy, D; Scharf, SM. Diagnosis of obstructive sleep apnea using pulse oximeter derived photoplethysmographic signals. *J Clin Sleep Med.*, 2014, 10(3), 285-90.

[49] Zamarron, C; Gude, F; Barcala, J; Rodriguez, JR; Romero, PV. Utility of oxygen saturation and heart rate spectral analysis obtained from pulse oximetric recordings in the diagnosis of sleep apnea syndrome. *Chest.*, 2003, 123(5), 1567-76.

[50] Zamarron, C; Romero, PV; Gude, F; Amaro, A; Rodriguez, JR. Screening of obstructive sleep apnoea: heart rate spectral analysis of nocturnal pulse oximetric recording. *Respir Med.*, 2001, 95(9), 759-65.

[51] Somers, VK; Dyken, ME; Mark, AL; Abboud, FM. Sympathetic-nerve activity during sleep in normal subjects. *N Engl J Med.*, 1993, 328(5), 303-7.

[52] Krishnaswamy, UM; Higgins, SE; Kosky, CA; Delacy, S; Williams, AJ. Diagnosis of PLMD from increased pulse rate variability on overnight oximetry. *Nature and science of Sleep.*, 2010, 2, 107-14.

[53] van den Bemt, L; van, Wayenburg, CAM; Smeele, IJM; Schermer, TRJ. Obesity in patients with COPD, an undervalued problem? *Thorax.*, 2009, 64(7), 640-.

[54] Steuten, LM; Creutzberg, EC; Vrijhoef, HJ; Wouters, EF. COPD as a multicomponent disease: inventory of dyspnoea, underweight, obesity and fat free mass depletion in primary care. *Prim Care Respir J.*, 2006, 15(2), 84-91.

[55] Eisner, MD; Blanc, PD; Sidney, S; Yelin, EH; Lathon, PV; Katz, PP; et al. Body composition and functional limitation in COPD. *Respir Res.*, 2007, 8, 7.

[56] McNicholas, WT. COPD-OSA Overlap Syndrome. *CHEST.*, 2017, 152(6), 1318-26.

[57] Bednarek, M; Plywaczewski, R; Jonczak, L; Zielinski, J. There is no relationship between chronic obstructive pulmonary disease and obstructive sleep apnea syndrome: a population study. *Respiration.*, 2005, 72(2), 142-9.

[58] Sanders, MH; Newman, AB; Haggerty, CL; Redline, S; Lebowitz, M; Samet, J; et al. Sleep and sleep-disordered breathing in adults with predominantly mild obstructive airway disease. *Am J Respir Crit Care Med.*, 2003, 167(1), 7-14.

[59] White, LH; Bradley, TD. Role of nocturnal rostral fluid shift in the pathogenesis of obstructive and central sleep apnoea. *J Physiol.*, 2013, 591(5), 1179-93.

[60] Marin, JM; Soriano, JB; Carrizo, SJ; Boldova, A; Celli, BR. Outcomes in patients with chronic obstructive pulmonary disease and obstructive sleep apnea: the overlap syndrome. *Am J Respir Crit Care Med.*, 2010, 182(3), 325-31.

[61] Kaw, R; Hernandez, AV; Walker, E; Aboussouan, L; Mokhlesi, B. Determinants of hypercapnia in obese patients with obstructive sleep apnea: a systematic review and meta analysis of cohort studies. *Chest.*, 2009, 136(3), 787-96.

[62] Akashiba, T; Kawahara, S; Kosaka, N; Ito, D; Saito, O; Majima, T; et al. Determinants of chronic hypercapnia in Japanese men with obstructive sleep apnea syndrome. *Chest.*, 2002, 121(2), 415-21.

[63] Resta, O; Foschino-Barbaro, MP; Bonfitto, P; Talamo, S; Legari, G; De Pergola, G; et al. Prevalence and mechanisms of diurnal hypercapnia in a sample of morbidly obese subjects with obstructive sleep apnoea. *Respir Med.*, 2000, 94(3), 240-6.

[64] Mokhlesi, B; Tulaimat, A; Faibussowitsch, I; Wang, Y; Evans, AT. Obesity hypoventilation syndrome: prevalence and predictors in patients with obstructive sleep apnea. *Sleep Breath.*, 2007, 11(2), 117-24.

[65] Golpe, R; Jiménez, A; Carpizo, R. Diurnal Hypercapnia in Patients With Obstructive Sleep Apnea Syndrome. *Chest.*, 2002, 122(3), 1100-1.

[66] Leech, JA; Onal, E; Baer, P; Lopata, M. Determinants of hypercapnia in occlusive sleep apnea syndrome. *Chest.*, 1987, 92(5), 807-13.

[67] Hart, N; Mandal, S; Manuel, A; Mokhlesi, B; Pepin, JL; Piper, A; et al. Obesity hypoventilation syndrome: does the current definition need revisiting? *Thorax.*, 2014, 69(1), 83-4.

[68] Nickol, AH; Dunroy, H; Polkey, MI; Simonds, A; Cordingley, J; Corfield, DR; et al. A quick and easy method of measuring the hypercapnic ventilatory response in patients with COPD. *Respir Med.*, 2009, 103(2), 258-67.

[69] Cuvelier, A; Grigoriu, B; Molano, LC; Muir, JF. Limitations of transcutaneous carbon dioxide measurements for assessing long-term mechanical ventilation. *Chest.*, 2005, 127(5), 1744-8.

[70] Janssens, J-P; Borel, J-C; Pépin, J-L. Nocturnal monitoring of home non-invasive ventilation: the contribution of simple tools such as pulse oximetry, capnography, built-in ventilator software and autonomic markers of sleep fragmentation. *Thorax.*, 2011, 66(5), 438-45.

[71] Somers, VK; Dyken, ME; Clary, MP; Abboud, FM. Sympathetic neural mechanisms in obstructive sleep apnea. *J Clin Invest.*, 1995, 96(4), 1897-904.

[72] Narkiewicz, K; Somers, VK. Sympathetic nerve activity in obstructive sleep apnoea. *Acta Physiol Scand.*, 2003, 177(3), 385-90.

[73] Schnall, RP; Shlitner, A; Sheffy, J; Kedar, R; Lavie, P. Periodic, profound peripheral vasoconstriction--a new marker of obstructive sleep apnea. *Sleep.*, 1999, 22(7), 939-46.

[74] Yalamanchali, S; Farajian, V; Hamilton, C; Pott, TR; Samuelson, CG; Friedman, M. Diagnosis of Obstructive Sleep Apnea by Peripheral Arterial Tonometry: Meta-analysis. *JAMA Otolaryngology–Head & Neck Surgery.*, 2013, 139(12), 1343-50.

[75] Zou, D; Grote, L; Peker, Y; Lindblad, U; Hedner, J. Validation a portable monitoring device for sleep apnea diagnosis in a population based cohort using synchronized home polysomnography. *Sleep.*, 2006, 29(3), 367-74.

[76] O'Brien, LM; Bullough, AS; Shelgikar, AV; Chames, MC; Armitage, R; Chervin, RD. Validation of Watch-PAT-200 against polysomnography during pregnancy. *J Clin Sleep Med.*, 2012, 8(3), 287-94.

[77] Garg, N; Rolle, AJ; Lee, TA; Prasad, B. Home-based diagnosis of obstructive sleep apnea in an urban population. *J Clin Sleep Med.*, 2014, 10(8), 879-85.

In: Sleep Medicine in Critical Care
Editors: Antonio M. Esquinas et al.
ISBN: 978-1-53617-768-8

Chapter 7

HYPOXIC AND HYPERCAPNIC RESPIRATORY FAILURE: IMPLICATIONS FOR SLEEP MEDICINE, DIAGNOSIS AND PRACTICAL APPROACH

*Gül Gürsel**, *MD*
Department of Pulmonary Critical Care Medicine,
Gazi University, Ankara, Turkey

ABSTRACT

Chronic hypoventilation affects patients with disorders on any level of the respiratory system.

Obesity hypoventilation syndrome (OHS), COPD, neuromuscular diseases and congestive heart failure are most frequent causes of respiratory failure and hypoventilation worsens during sleep in these diseases. Optimal treatment of patients with chronic hypoventilation with NIV crucially depends on the underlying pathophysiological mechanisms. Treatment of chronic hypercapnic respiratory failure with noninvasive ventilation improves daytime dyspnea, PaCO2, hypersomnolence, exacerbations, readmissions and survival.

Keywords: respiratory failure, intensive care unit, hypoventilation, obesity hypoventilation, COPD, neuromuscular disease, noninvasive mechanical ventilation, home ventilation

* Corresponding Author's E-mail: gurselgl@gmail.com.

INTRODUCTION

Respiratory failure occurs when the body is unable to carry out oxygenation, ventilation or both.

Hypoxemic respiratory failure is defined by partial pressure of oxygen in arterial blood (PaO_2) <60 mm Hg on room air and hypercapnic (or hypercarbic) respiratory failure is defined by partial pressure of carbon dioxide in arterial blood ($PaCO_2$) >45 mm Hg.

The most recent revision of the American Academy of Sleep Medicine (AASM) scoring criteria suggest to score sleep relate hypoventilation (SRH) in case of: PaCO2 > 55 mm Hg for ≥10 minutes during sleep or; increases of the PaCO2 ≥ 10 mm Hg as compared to awake supine value up to a level of >50 mm Hg for ≥10 minutes [1].

Chronic hypoventilation affects patients with disorders on any level of the respiratory system.

Obesity hypoventilation syndrome (OHS), COPD, neuromuscular diseases and congestive heart failure are most frequent causes of respiratory failure and hypoventilation worsens during sleep in these diseases. The cornerstone of managing chronic hypercapnic respiratory failure is ventilatory support. Depending on the aetiology of chronic respiratory failure, criteria for patient selection for home noninvasive mechanical ventilation (HNIV) differ. In patients with COPD, chronic nocturnal ventilatory support with HNIV may improve daytime dyspnea, PaCO2, hypersomnolence, exacerbations, and readmissions. In chronic hypercapnic respiratory failure related to neuromuscular disease, HNIV has been shown to slow the progression of chronic respiratory failure and improve survival in patients with amyotrophic lateral sclerosis (ALS).

OBESITY HYPOVENTILATION SYNDROME

Obesity is an increasing global epidemic that adversely affects respiratory system. Sleep-disordered breathing and obesity hypoventilation syndrome (OHS) are among the most common pulmonary complications related to obesity. The prevalence of obesity among patients admitted to the ICU have reported between 9% and 26% for patients with BMI >30 kg/m [2]. Patients with OHS may present with acute hypercapnic respiratory failure that necessitates immediate noninvasive ventilation (NIV) or invasive ventilation and intensive care unit (ICU) monitoring. OHS is defined by the combination of obesity (body mass index [BMI] >30 kg/m2), sleep-disordered breathing (SDB), and awake daytime hypercapnia (awake resting PaCO2 > 45 mm Hg at sea level), after excluding other causes for hypoventilation [2]. Approximately 90% of patients with OHS have coexistent obstructive sleep apnea (OSA), with nearly 70% having severe OSA. The remaining 10% of patients with OHS without OSA have non-obstructive, sleep-dependent hypoventilation [3].

Patients with OHS have decreased lung compliance, reduction in functional residual capacity and chest wall compliance, and increased pulmonary resistance. Decreased chest wall compliance because of obesity causes an excessive increase in the work of breathing. Individuals with OHS tend to have lower tidal volume and higher respiratory rate, which increases the dead space effect. Another possible mechanism of hypoxaemia is ventilation-perfusion mismatching at the base of the lungs, where microatelectasis is likely to occur. Chemosensitivity is progressively impaired by increased CO2 levels. Chronic hypercapnia is also believed to result from the inability to eliminate CO2, which accumulates at night during apnea and hypopnea episodes, during the day. A secondary mechanism that also impairs chemosensitivity is elevated serum and cerebrospinal fluid levels of bicarbonate.

If increased compensatory respiratory drive cannot be maintained, hypoventilation, initially occurs during rapid eye movement (REM) sleep. The repetitive occurrence of hypoventilation, initially limited to REM sleep, induces a secondary depression of respiratory centers leading to daytime hypercapnia and obesity hypoventilation syndrome.

OHS, is the most common indication for HMV in many countries. Positive pressure ventilation is indicated in patients with OHS at the time of diagnosis to improve respiratory mechanics, adjust neural respiratory drive, and keep the upper airway patent during sleep.

HMV can usually be applied non-invasively. However, HMV is commonly initiated within the course of emergency hospitalisations due to acute on chronic respiratory failure in OHS. Although both continous positive airway pressure (CPAP) and NIV have been shown to correct respiratory failure, NIV is superior to CPAP in improving exercise capacity and pulmonary hypertension. The degree of sleep hypoventilation and apnoeas or hypopnoeas contributing to hypercapnia differs across the spectrum of OHS/OSAS, and the dominating underlying sleep-disordered breathing may guide the choice of initial positive pressure ventilation. CPAP is easier to implement and less expensive, and both CPAP and NIV have been shown to improve gas exchange. OHS patients often need relatively high expiratory positive airway pressure (EPAP, 8-14 cm H2O) to guarantee upper airway patency, and additional pressure support or target volume to overcome the restrictive respiratory system physiology and to correct hypoventilation: the back-up rate can be set around 14-18/min. In these patients, opening and stabilization of the upper airways is crucial to deliver effective ventilation. CPAP is generally considered the initial therapy in patients with OHS and compensated hypercapnic respiratory failure with a predominant OSA component [4]. If persistent sleep hypoventilation or sustained desaturations remain after elimination of upper airway obstruction by CPAP, a trial of

BPAP-S is indicated. In those patients with a predominant lack of respiratory drive despite BPAP-S therapy, a trial of BPAP-ST or VAPS is recommended [5]. Additional supplementary oxygen is sometimes needed in the initial phase of ventilation, but usually unnecessary with an effective ventilator setting and in the absence of pulmonary comorbidity.

Recent American Thoracic Society guideline recommends CPAP mode as first line treatment for stable ambulatory patients diagnosed with OHS and concomitant severe OSA (apnea-hypopnea index >30 events/h), rather than NIV. However, panel members lacked certainty on the clinical benefits of initiating treatment with CPAP, rather than NIV, in patients with OHS who have sleep hypoventilation without severe OSA. They suggest that hospitalized patients with respiratory failure suspected of having OHS be started on NIV therapy before being discharged from the hospital, until they undergo outpatient workup and titration of positive airway pressure therapy in the sleep laboratory, ideally within the first 3 month after hospital discharge [3].

Chronic Obstructive Pulmonary Disease (COPD)

Chronic hypercapnia in patients with COPD is associated with a high mortality and frequent hospitalisations therefore patient selection and the correct ventilation strategy is crucial. Once the COPD exacerbation is resolved, noninvasive positive pressure ventilation for the treatment of severe stable chronic COPD may be considered. According to recent European Respiratory Society guideline NIV is the primary therapeutic option for home mechanical ventilation of COPD patients with chronic respiratory failure, it must be initiated when the patient presents with chronic hypercapnia in combination with the typical symptoms of respiratory failure and if hypercapnia persists for more than 2 weeks after completing acute ventilation therapy for acute respiratory acidosis [6].The aim of the ventilation therapy should be to normalise PaCO2; this may require sufficiently high ventilation intensity with effective ventilation pressures as well as the use of controlled ventilation modes.

In the non-ICU hospital setting/sleep laboratory, nocturnal NIV for chronic severe COPD is commonly titrated under PSG and guided by oximetry, transcutan CO2 measurements (TcCO 2), ABG analysis, or a combination. Patients with COPD with an OSA comorbidity (overlap syndrome) may benefit from the use of CPAP or BPAP-S, with adjustment of EPAP pressure to eliminate apneic events. In overlap syndrome, CPAP has proved to improve survival and decrease first-time hospitalization from COPD exacerbation. Conversely, in those patients with severe COPD in compensated hypercapnic respiratory failure without OSA, the usual BPAP therapy (low PS) has proved ineffective (low-intensity BPAP). In this population, emerging literature supports benefits from high-intensity therapy, with high IPAP/PS adjusted to achieve total control of the patient's spontaneous breathing. A rapid rise in inspiratory pressure (within 0.1-0.2 s) is best tolerated by patients. The use of PEEP/EPAP in assisted or assisted-controlled ventilation prevents upper airway collapse during sleep, which is especially useful in comorbid obstructive sleep apnoea syndrome (OSAS). In addition, EPAP has to be titrated high enough to overcome intrinsic positive airway pressure and its inspiratory threshold load, but a too high EPAP may aggravate hyperinflation. The most important criterion for long-term NIV is either symptomatic chronic respiratory insufficiency or persistent hypercapnia following an acute NIV-dependent exacerbation requiring hospitalisation. HNIV indication criteria are given in Table 1 [7].

Patients with mild daytime hypercapnia (PaCO2 45-50 mm Hg) require nocturnal diagnostic tests. Patient-ventilator asynchronies are common in COPD and should be considered during set-up. COPD patients usually need a much higher pressure support than NMD or obesity related respiratory failure. HMV is typically applied non-invasively during sleep and extended into the daytime as needed. Overall, titrating NIV in COPD needs time and monitoring. Patient selection criteria for HMV in COPD have recently been established: clinicians should reassess post-acute NIV in COPD patients 2-4 weeks after clinical recovery; if the PaCO2 remains >53 mm Hg, NIV should be considered. If transcutaneous PCO2 measurements are not available, a morning blood gas analysis directly after completion of the nightly sleep can be useful for evaluating the indication for mechanical ventilation. Moreover, elevated bicarbonate values can be suggestive of nocturnal hypercapnia and hence serve as an indication for further clarification. An indication for NIV exists when mild diurnal hypercapnia is accompanied by a rise in PtcCO2 to ≥10 mm Hg during nocturnal sleep.

Table 1. Long term home mechanical ventilation criteria for patients with COPD and NMD

LTHMV criteria for COPD
Chronic diurnal hypercapnia with a PaCO2 ≥ 50 mm Hg.
- Nocturnal hypercapnia with a PaCO2 ≥ 55 mm Hg.
- Mild diurnal hypercapnia with 46-50 mm Hg and an increase in PtcCO 2 ≥ 10 mm Hg during sleep.
- When persistent hypercapnia (PaCO2 > 53 mm Hg) is present at least 14 days after finishing acute ventilation therapy for acute respiratory acidosis.
LTHMV criteria for NMD
Diurnal PaCO2 ≥ 45 mm Hg
- Nocturnal PaCO2 ≥ 45 mm Hg
- Nocturnal PtcCO2 ≥ 50 mm Hg for over 30 min
- Diurnal normocapnia with a nocturnal rise in PtcCO2 of ≥10 mm Hg
- For ALS or other fast-progressing NMDs, a rapid reduction in FVC of >10% of the initial value within 3 months.

NEUROMUSCULAR DISORDERS

Sleep-disordered breathing is common in neuromuscular and chest wall diseases and treatment with noninvasive ventilation (NIV) is associated with improved outcomes. Sleep-disordered breathing patterns include sleep hypoventilation, obstructive sleep apnea, central sleep apnea, and overlapping syndromes and are commonly associated with hypercapnic respiratory failure in this patient population [8, 9]. Respiratory failure in patients with progressive NMD is due to respiratory muscle weakness with increased respiratory load, leading to ineffective ventilation.

NIV decreases respiratory system load, increases in minute ventilation, and decreases in physiological dead space. In some patients severe bulbar disease may limit the ability to use NIV given the increased risk for aspiration. Diagnostic studies to evaluate sleep-disordered breathing include nocturnal SpO2 monitoring, nocturnal capnometry PtcCO2, respiratory polygraphy, or polysomnography. Although BPAP-ST is considered the initial therapy when it is inadequate or failed volume targeted pressure support modes in ST or pressure control modes may be considered. A target tidal volume can be set around 8 cc/kg and should be closely monitored and adjusted based on ABG or TcCO2 results, or both. In the event of mild hypercapnia (PaCO2 $\geq$45 mm Hg or diurnal normocapnia with a nocturnal rise in PtcCO2 of $\geq$10 mm Hg), non-invasive ventilation should be implemented as the primary therapy option for home mechanical ventilation in neuromuscular disease patients with chronic respiratory failure, if diurnal symptoms persist (Table 1). In amyotrophic lateral sclerosis (ALS), NIV has been proved to improve quality of life as well as survival in this population.

Criteria for starting home noninvasive mechanical ventilation changes depending on the defining institution [7]. Based on CMS/National Institute for Health and Care Excellence guidelines, there are four objective criteria that can be used to guide the initiation of noninvasive ventilation If a patient meets any of these criteria, it is appropriate to initiate noninvasive ventilation: (1) forced vital capacity <50% of predicted, (2) maximal inspiratory pressure <60 cm H2O or sniff nasal pressure <40 cm H2 O, (3) PaCO2 > 45 mm Hg, and (4) overnight nocturnal desaturation <88% for 5 min. Criteria of the German national guideline are listed in Table 1. As recommended modes BPAP with backup rate (BPAP-ST or VAPS) and home based ventilation are commonly used.

Lastly recently developed auto-titrating modes trying to titrate inspiratory and expiratory pressures according to preset tidal volume or to stabilize the upper airway have been showing promising results in patients with COPD, OHS and NMD but further studies are necessary to find out their exact role in these patient population [10].

CONCLUSION

Appropriate selection of mode and settings according to underlying mechanisms of respiratory failure are very important to improve prognosis. Patients' requirements may change during awakeness and sleep. To find out the place and role of polysomnography and autotitrating modes in determining optimal pressure combinations need more trials.

KEY POINTS

Optimal treatment of patients with chronic hypoventilation with NIV depends on the underlying pathophysiological mechanisms.

In addition to underlying respiratory pathology increased upper airway resistance and blunted respiratory drive may increase hypoventilation during sleep in patients with OHS, COPD and neuromuscular disease.

Treatment of hypoventilation with NIV decreases morbidity and mortality.

In principle the expiratory positive airway pressure (EPAP) is titrated according to the level of upper airway obstruction and when EPAP has been titrated, the level of pressure support and respiratory rate can be adjusted aiming at normalization of PaCO2.

REFERENCES

[1] Berry R. B., Budhiraja R., Gottlieb D. J., et al., 2012 Rules for scoring respiratory events in sleep: update of the 2007 AASM Manual for the Scoring of Sleep and Associated Events. Deliberations of the Sleep Apnea Definitions Task Force of the American Academy of Sleep Medicine. *J Clin Sleep Med*; 8:597-619.

[2] Sequeira T. C. A., BaHammam A. S., Esquinas A. M. 2017. Noninvasive Ventilation in the Critically Ill Patient with Obesity Hypoventilation Syndrome: A Review *Journal of Intensive Care Medicine*, Vol. 32(7) 421-428.

[3] American Thoracic Society Assembly on Sleep and Respiratory Neurobiology Evaluation and Management of Obesity Hypoventilation Syndrome (2019). An Official American Thoracic Society Clinical Practice Guideline *Am J Respir Crit Care Med*; 3:6-24.

[4] Gursel G., Aydogdu M., Gulbas G., Ozkaya S., Tasyurek S., Yildirim F. 2011. The influence of severe obesity on non-invasive ventilation (NIV) strategies and responses in patients with acute hypercapnic respiratory failure attacks in the ICU. *Minerva Anestesiol.* Jan; 77 (1):17-25.

[5] Selim B. J. Selim, Lisa Wolfe, John M. Coleman III, and Naresh A. Dewan, 2018 Initiation of Noninvasive Ventilation for Sleep Related Hypoventilation Disorders Advanced Modes and Devices *CHEST*; 153(1):251-265.

[6] Ergan B., Oczkowski S., Rochwerg B., et al., 2019. European Respiratory Society guidelines on long-term home non-invasive ventilation for management of COPD. *Eur Respir J*; 54: 1901003 https://doi.org/10.1183/13993003.01003-2019.

[7] Windisch W., Jens Geiseler, Karsten Simon, Stephan Walterspacher, Michael Dreher, on behalf of the Guideline Commission German National Guideline for Treating Chronic Respiratory Failure with Invasive and Non-Invasive Ventilation 2018 – Revised Edition: Part 2 *Respiration* 96:171-203.

[8] Hilbert J., (2018) Sleep-Disordered Breathing in Neuromuscular and Chest Wall Diseases *Clin Chest Med* 39 309-324.

[9] Crimi C., Pierucci P., Carlucci A., Cortegiani A., Gregoretti C.: Long-term ventilation in neuromuscular patients: review of concerns, beliefs, and ethical dilemmas. *Respiration* 2019;97:185-196.

[10] Gursel G., Zerman A., Basarik B., Gonderen K., Aydogdu M., Memmedova S. 2018. Noninvasive auto-titrating ventilation (AVAPS-AE) versus average volume-assured pressure support (AVAPS) ventilation in hypercapnic respiratory failure patients. *Intern Emerg Med.* Apr;13(3):359-365.

In: Sleep Medicine in Critical Care
Editors: Antonio M. Esquinas et al.
ISBN: 978-1-53617-768-8

Chapter 8

INTERMITTENT HYPOXIA, SYMPATHETIC ACTIVITY AND OXIDATIVE STRESS IN OSA AND CPAP EFFECTS

Esther I. Schwarz*[*]*, MD
Department of Pulmonology and Sleep Disorders Centre,
University Hospital of Zurich, Zurich, Switzerland

ABSTRACT

Intermittent hypoxia is the key pathophysiological feature linking obstructive sleep apnoea (OSA) with vascular damage. Severe intermittent hypoxia results in sympathetic overdrive and oxidative stress which promote systemic hypertension and endothelial dysfunction. Continuous positive airway pressure (CPAP) improves endothelial function and can reduce blood pressure in OSA. OSA and other types of sleep-disordered breathing might be aggravated in the critically ill patient in the intensive care unit, e.g., due to hypervolemia or impaired vigilance. The cardiovascular consequences of OSA, e.g., blood pressure surges or disturbed cardiac repolarisation, might be particularly disadvantageous in the critically ill patient. However, there is no data to support either diagnostic approaches nor treatment with CPAP in suspected OSA in critically ill patients to reduce the length of stay in the intensive care unit or improve the short-term outcome.

Keywords: obstructive sleep apnoea, intermittent hypoxia, sympathetic activity, oxidative stress

---

[*] Corresponding Author's E-mail: estherirene.schwarz@usz.ch.

INTRODUCTION

Obstructive sleep apnoea (OSA) is the most common sleep-related breathing disorder and its prevalence might be even higher in patients in the intensive care unit (ICU) compared to the general population. Some of the risk factors for OSA are also risk factors for ICU admission, e.g., obesity or breathing at low lung volumes such as in chronic obstructive pulmonary disease. In addition, several factors commonly seen in ICU patients, e.g., impaired vigilance, anal gosedation, myopathy and neuropathy, or fluid overload predispose to upper airway collapse and may worsen OSA severity.

OSA is characterised by repetitive upper airway collapse during sleep. Multiple factors of upper airway and respiratory mechanics as well as respiratory control play a role in OSA. Risk factors for OSA are a narrow and collapsible upper airway such as in obesity, a large neck circumference, a narrow oropharyngeal space or a higher Mallampati classification (e.g., macroglossia, low soft palate), retrognathia, or an impaired neuromechanical control of the upper airway. The upper airway muscles are hypotonic during sleep and this makes patients more susceptible to upper airway narrowing that results in an increase in upper airway resistance. The excitatory increase in motor neurone output in response to an increased resistance is reduced during sleep. Ventilation during sleep is reduced as a consequence of the inhibited output from the respiratory control centre, the lower muscle tone, the reduced chemosensitivity and thus reduced ventilatory response to hypercapnia and hypoxia, and mechanical disadvantages of the diaphragm when lying. The repetitive collapse of the pharynx during sleep results in apnoeas or hypopnoeas associated with oxygen desaturations and arousals from sleep. Intermittent hypoxia is the key pathophysiological feature of OSA. In addition, intrathoracic pressure swings during upper airway occlusion and arousals from sleep are direct consequences of obstructive sleep apnoea. These direct pathophysiological consequences of recurrent upper airway collapse during sleep result in a sequel of pathophysiological consequences such as increased sympathetic activity and eventually oxidative stress that have cardiovascular and metabolic consequences. Therefore, it has been postulated that untreated OSA contributes to adverse outcome in critically-ill patients. However, it has never been systematically analysed how effective treatment of OSA by continuous positive airway pressure (CPAP) – in the non-mechanically ventilated patient in the ICU – affects outcomes, sleep-quality and duration of ICU stay.

In case of unknown OSA that is first suspected during an ICU stay, a thorough diagnosis is difficult to establish. Sleep is disturbed in an ICU setting and the critically-ill patient might be on drugs (e.g., opioids, sedatives) and in conditions (e.g., hypervolemia, heart failure) that affect upper airway collapse and that result in other types of sleep-disordered breathing such as hypoventilation, central sleep apnoea or Cheyne Stoke's Breathing. These other types of sleep-disordered breathing imply either no treatment or a different treatment modality compared to OSA. In addition, a sleep-related breathing disorder in a critically-ill patient might only represent a transient condition. However, if snoring, witnessed apnoeas associated with cyclic oxygen desaturations, and a history in accordance with OSA are present in a patient in the ICU, pneumologists are often asked to initiate CPAP in these patients. The evidence-base for initiating CPAP in a critically-ill patient with suspected OSA, however, is missing.

The consequences of intermittent hypoxia – the key player in terms of cardiovascular and metabolic consequences of OSA –, particularly sympathetic overdrive and oxidative stress, will be discussed in this chapter. Furthermore, the effects of CPAP on the pathophysiological consequences of OSA will be looked at using data from both conventional randomised controlled CPAP trials as well as randomised controlled CPAP withdrawal trials. In addition, the potential role of OSA-induced intermittent hypoxia in the critically-ill patient will be discussed.

Intermittent Hypoxia in OSA

The direct mechanisms that link OSA to adverse cardiovascular outcome are intermittent hypoxia leading to sympathetic overdrive and oxidative stress, abrupt intrathoracic pressure changes leading to mechanical stress on the heart and intrathoracic vessels, and arousal-induced reflex sympathetic activation associated with blood pressure surges [1]. These acute pathophysiological consequences of OSA promote endothelial dysfunction, the early and potentially reversible stage of vascular damage preceding atherosclerosis also seen in OSA [2]. Intermittent hypoxia is considered the most important factor linking OSA with vascular damage.

However, from rodent models of intermittent hypoxia it is known that the extent, the duration and the frequency of intermittent hypoxia play a role in the balance between maladaptive harmful and adaptive beneficial mechanisms (e.g., hypoxic preconditioning effects). In addition, the exact pattern of deoxygenation-reoxygenation (comparable to ischemia-reperfusion) might determine the harmful vs beneficial effects of intermittent hypoxia that might also differ between target organs [3].

Intermittent Hypoxia and Sympathetic Activity and Hypertension

There is clear evidence from cell culture, animal and human studies that intermittent hypoxia is the key factor leading to a sympathetic overdrive and systemic hypertension in OSA. Sympathetic nerve activity increases during apnoeas and hypopnoeas peaking at the termination of the event [4]. Intermittent hypoxia acts mainly via increased carotid chemoreceptor stimulation of the sympathetic nervous system [5]. Nocturnal intermittent hypoxia results not only in elevation of sympathetic activity and blood pressure during sleep, but this effect is carried over into daytime resulting in persisting elevated catecholamine levels and daytime hypertension [6]. However, nocturnal blood pressure is particularly influenced by OSA and daytime measurements or screening for hypertension might underestimate the elevated blood pressure (masked hypertension) and the increased left ventricular afterload in OSA [7].

In summary, primarily explained by intermittent hypoxia-induced chemoreflex sympathetic activation and persisting sympathetic overactivation, OSA is associated with repetitive nocturnal blood pressure surges at the end of apnoeic events, a nocturnal non-dipping pattern, masked hypertension, sustained daytime hypertension (secondary hypertension), and treatment-resistant hypertension.

CPAP Effects on Sympathetic Activity and Blood Pressure in OSA

The most effective treatment for OSA is CPAP. Whereas evidence on the effect of CPAP in primary and secondary prevention of hard cardiovascular outcomes is limited and inconclusive, respectively, there is robust evidence on CPAP effects on sympathetic activity, endothelial function and hypertension.

It has been demonstrated that abolishing OSA with CPAP results in a reduction of levels of catecholamines and muscle nerve sympathetic activity [8]. It has also been shown that CPAP results in a clinically relevant improvement of endothelial function in a diverse population with OSA [2, 9].

The overall CPAP treatment effect on cardiovascular outcomes is generally underestimated in randomised controlled trials due to insufficient treatment adherence in previously treatment-naïve patients with newly diagnosed OSA. The CPAP therapy withdrawal model was introduced to allow studying the pathophysiological consequences of OSA and treatment effects of CPAP in an effective and controlled way [10]. Optimally treated patients previously diagnosed with OSA, established on CPAP therapy and using their CPAP device every night and all night are included. A therapy withdrawal results in recurrence of OSA and allows studying pathophysiological changes that can be attributed to OSA in a controlled model. The randomised controlled CPAP withdrawal trials have provided robust evidence on diverse cardiovascular and metabolic consequences of OSA and also CPAP effects [10]. Recurrence of OSA during a short-term CPAP therapy withdrawal was associated with a significant increase in urinary catecholamines as marker of increased sympathetic activity and a progressive decrease in peripheral endothelial function compared to the control group continuing CPAP [6]. Along with these changes, a clinically relevant increase in morning systolic and diastolic blood pressure was found [11]. The observed change in blood pressure in untreated OSA in this group of patients with an optimal CPAP adherence was considerably larger than in conventional CPAP trials, in which CPAP usage is usually suboptimal and the treatment effect underestimated. A higher apnoea-hypopnoea-index, the use of more antihypertensive drugs, a lower blood pressure at baseline and the absence of statin usage were independent predictors of a pronounced increase in blood pressure in response to CPAP withdrawal. This highlights the role of OSA as a secondary cause of hypertension and the need for a combined treatment by antihypertensive drugs and CPAP in hypertensive patients with OSA.

CPAP has been shown to reduce blood pressure in moderate to severe symptomatic OSA in several randomised controlled trials and meta-analyses. Meta-analyses have shown that CPAP results in a significant but modest reduction of blood pressure of 2-3 mmHg in unselected patients with varying baseline blood pressure, antihypertensive treatment, severity of OSA and CPAP adherence [12, 13]. Meta-analyses only including RCTs on OSA and resistant hypertension have found a larger blood pressure lowering effect of CPAP of 4-7 mmHg [14].

The Effects of Intermittent Hypoxia and CPAP on the Cardio- and Cerebrovascular System

The heart and the brain are important target organs potentially being affected by the detrimental pathophysiological sequelae of OSA. In a randomised controlled CPAP withdrawal trial powered to detect a minimal clinically important difference in myocardial perfusion as assessed by the gold standard technique N^{13}-ammonia-positron emission tomography, OSA recurrence had no effect on myocardial perfusion and coronary endothelial function during daytime in patients with moderate or severe OSA despite a relevant increase in blood pressure and heart rate and the previously found peripheral endothelial dysfunction [15]. In line with the findings on myocardial perfusion, an additional randomised controlled trial studying cerebrovascular reactivity using functional magnetic resonance imaging measuring blood oxygen level-dependent response to breathing stimuli during daytime found no effect of OSA on cerebrovascular reactivity or cerebral blood flow [16]. However, despite preserved vascular function during daytime, the brain is exposed to OSA-induced changes during sleep that might explain the observed increased risk of stroke in OSA and neurocognitive dysfunction. Near infrared spectroscopy was used to monitor cerebral tissue oxygenation and haemoglobin concentration during in-hospital sleep studies in patients with moderate to severe OSA who were allocated to either withdraw CPAP or continue therapeutic CPAP [17]. OSA recurrence was associated with intermittent and sustained falls in cerebral tissue oxygenation during sleep of a clinically relevant degree, in some patients sufficient to cause cerebral ischemia associated with functional impairment. Cerebral autoregulation was insufficient to protect the brain from relevant nocturnal cerebral tissue deoxygenation in patients with OSA.

It is plausible that intermittent hypoxia and its consequences like endothelial dysfunction and elevated blood pressure might influence the outcome in case of an acute coronary syndrome. OSA might influence the extent of ischemic myocardial damage in case of an acute coronary syndrome. Obstructive apnoeas and hypopneas increase myocardial metabolic and oxygen demand during sleep by several mechanisms. In a prospective cohort study, a lower nadir oxygen saturation in moderate-to-severe OSA was associated with a poorer outcome after myocardial infarction [18]. Another cohort study suggested that OSA results in a larger myocardial damage and longer stay in the coronary care unit after myocardial infarction [19]. However, there are data suggesting a protective role of OSA on infarct size via hypoxemic preconditioning [20]. The hypothesis of beneficial hypoxic preconditioning of the myocardium in mild intermittent hypoxia comes from animal models [21, 22]. The largest prospective cohort study in patients with OSA undergoing a coronary intervention has shown that OSA is a risk factor for subsequent major adverse cerebro- and cardiovascular events and there is a body of literature indicating that OSA negatively affects prognosis after an acute coronary syndrome in the long-term [23, 24].

Obstructive respiratory events promote cardiac arrhythmia by intrathoracic pressure swings and by intermittent hypoxia and sympatho-vagal imbalance. Prolonged repolarization and increased dispersion of transmural cardiac repolarisation provide a mechanistic link between OSA and cardiac arrhythmias. untreated OSA has been recognised as a risk for recurrence of atrial fibrillation after catheter ablation or cardioversion. A meta-analysis of observational studies and randomised controlled trials has found a significant risk reduction of recurrence of atrial fibrillation after catheter ablation in patients with OSA by the use of CPAP [25].

Intermittent Hypoxia and Oxidative Stress

It has been postulated that cyclic intermittent hypoxia in OSA promotes the production of reactive oxygen species and results in oxidative stress that could activate pathways of systemic inflammation. Hypoxia-activated inflammatory pathways might play a role in the presence of concomitant pro-inflammatory conditions such as obesity. The increased production of reactive oxygen species has been interpreted as a result of the inhibition of oxidases and decreased levels of antioxidants induced by hypoxia and reoxygenation [26]. Oxidation of proteins, nucleic acids, and lipids, as well as decreased antioxidant activity have been described in animal models of intermittent hypoxia [27]. Reactive oxygen species generate peroxynitrite from endothelial nitric oxide that produces nitrotyrosine, which is associated with endothelial dysfunction [28]. Compared to controls, cellular expression of nitrotyrosine and NF-κB was enhanced in endothelial cells of patients with OSA and endothelial nitric oxide synthase was reduced [29]. These findings link oxidative stress in intermittent hypoxia with endothelial dysfunction.

CPAP Effects on Oxidative Stress in OSA

In an uncontrolled interventional study in patients with OSA undergoing a four week CPAP treatment, it was observed that markers of endothelial cell function improved and markers of oxidative stress (e.g., nitrotyrosine) decreased in parallel in those that used CPAP sufficiently [30]. Shortly after these data were published, a randomised controlled CPAP trial confirmed that CPAP increases markers of endothelial function (nitric oxide) and reduces plasma levels of markers of oxidative stress (8-isoprostane) [31]. Another link on oxidative processes in OSA comes from a CPAP withdrawal study using this study model to study exhalomics in OSA. Untargeted exhaled breath analysis was used to define the effect of OSA on the breath profile, which contains a wealth of metabolic information as volatile exhaled compounds that are released along the blood gas barrier. OSA recurrence resulted in an increase in exhaled molecules associated with stress, altered lipid peroxidation and the gut flora metabolism [32].

Using the randomised controlled CPAP withdrawal model as human model of intermittent hypoxia, better validated markers of oxidative stress were assessed in moderate or severe OSA. Reactivation of intermittent hypoxia during CPAP withdrawal did not result in increased levels of markers of oxidative stress, e.g., early morning blood malondialdehyde [33]. OSA recurrence led to a significant reduction in urinary F2-isoprostane suggesting a reduction in oxidative stress. A possible explanation was a significant increase in the antioxidant superoxide dismutase, a marker of hypoxic pre-conditioning, that might prevent the damage of hypoxia-reoxygenation in intermittent hypoxia. In another analysis, hypoxia-induced and endothelial-derived inflammatory markers previously described to be altered in cell cultures were analysed in morning blood samples of more than 100 patients with OSA participating in CPAP withdrawal trials. Except from a small but significant decrease in the vasoactive peptide adrenomedullin, OSA recurrence as real-life model of intermittent hypoxia had no effect on other vascular inflammatory markers linked to hypoxia [34]. The short exposure time to intermittent hypoxia of two weeks might be relevant for the unexpected finding and highlights that extent and duration of intermittent hypoxia might determine between harmful and beneficial effects.

In contrast to the evidence on sympathetic activity as a consequence of intermittent hypoxia and sleep fragmentation, data on oxidative stress and systemic inflammation in association with intermittent hypoxia are less conclusive.

In summary, intermittent hypoxia results in increased sympathetic activity and blood pressure [35, 36] and in endothelial dysfunction [37], however its role in oxidative might depend on the degree and duration of exposure to intermittent hypoxia [21, 22].

Role of Intermittent Hypoxia in the Critically-Ill Patient

The potential role of OSA for different target-organs in the critically-ill patient is discussed in the following.

Hypertension - particularly nocturnal hypertension – is a strong predictor for cardiovascular morbidity and mortality. In addition, OSA results in repetitive nocturnal blood pressure surges at the end of apnoeas and intrathoracic pressure swings that affect the transmural pressure over the heart and the intrathoracic vessels. For a critically ill-patient with an acute cardio- or cerebrovascular problem (e.g., cardiogenic shock, decompensated heart failure, aortic dissection, heart rhythm instability, ischemic or haemorrhagic stroke), these pathophysiological consequences of severe OSA are particularly disadvantageous in the acute setting. In addition, OSA is associated with disturbances in cardiac repolarisation that increase the risk for arrhythmias. This might be of importance for a haemodynamically instable ICU patient or in patients post electrical or drug-induced cardioversion. The risk of recurrence of e.g., atrial fibrillation is higher in patients with OSA.

Cerebral blood flow changes during apnoeic events; it increases during apnoeas and abruptly decreases after apnoea termination due to changes in p_aCO2 and changes in systemic blood pressure. However, cerebral autoregulation cannot counteract intermittent hypoxia-associated cerebral hypoxaemia. A randomised controlled CPAP withdrawal trial has provided evidence for severe nocturnal cerebral hypoxaemia to a degree that might result in cerebral tissue damage in severe OSA [17]. Apnoea/hypopnoea-related cyclic dips in cerebral tissue oxygenation were measured by near-infrared spectroscopy and were a bit less pronounced than corresponding peripheral arterial oxygen dips. In addition to cyclic oxygen drops in association with apnoeas and hypopnoeas resulting in intermittent cerebral hypoxemia, mean cerebral oxygen saturation significantly decreased as a result of recurrence of OSA by 3.8% [17].

Reductions in cerebral tissue oxygenation of more than 13% previously described as threshold for severe cerebral ischemia resulting in cerebral dysfunction [38] were observed in patients with severe OSA. Using the randomised controlled CPAP withdrawal protocol, it was demonstrated that OSA is associated with intermittent and sustained nocturnal cerebral tissue hypoxia of a clinically relevant degree, in some patients enough to cause cerebral ischemia associated with functional impairment. During sleep, the brain as sensitive target-organ is exposed to relevant hypoxaemia during sleep in case of severe OSA (Figure). Again, this might be particularly unfavourable in a critically-ill patient with e.g., a high metabolic demand, a failing systemic circulation, a severe acid-base-disturbance, or an encephalopathy. CPAP could prevent cerebral hypoxaemia in OSA.

However, in stroke patients, a transient ventilation disturbance and other types of sleep-disordered breathing are commonly seen in the acute post-stroke phase and there is no evidence to support treatment of acute post-stroke sleep-disordered breathing with positive airway pressure therapy.

The data on the role of intermittent hypoxia in OSA on the outcome post myocardial infarction is controversial. Whereas there is some data indicating a worse outcome after myocardial infarction in OSA, other studies suggested a beneficial effect of hypoxic preconditioning on the myocardial damage.

In conclusion, OSA is associated with a sequel of pathophysiological consequences that result in a higher risk of cardiovascular complications and end-organ damage that might be particularly disadvantageous for the critically-ill patient. However, most of the evidence on these pathophysiological consequences and associations of OSA with adverse outcome in the general population are only true for severe OSA and there is no data in critically ill patients in the ICU. Therefore, the level of OSA severity or severity of sleep-disordered breathing that is associated with pathophysiology needs to be defined to decide on early intervention by CPAP in the ICU. This is difficult, since a comprehensive sleep evaluation including a sleep study as is standard to assess severity and symptom-burden of OSA in a sleep clinic population as basis for treatment recommendation is not possible in the ICU. In addition, the condition of a critically-ill patient in the ICU is transient and influences control of breathing and severity of sleep-disordered breathing. Overall, the likelihood of severe OSA and the hypoxic burden associated with OSA need to be considered together with comorbidities and the cardiovascular condition of an ICU-patient with suspicion of OSA. Initiation of CPAP in the ICU might be considered if OSA is suspected to be severe and if the pathophysiological consequences of OSA are considered unfavourable for the ICU outcome, e.g., in uncontrolled hypertension, heart failure or arrhythmias, and if application of CPAP via an interface is feasible.

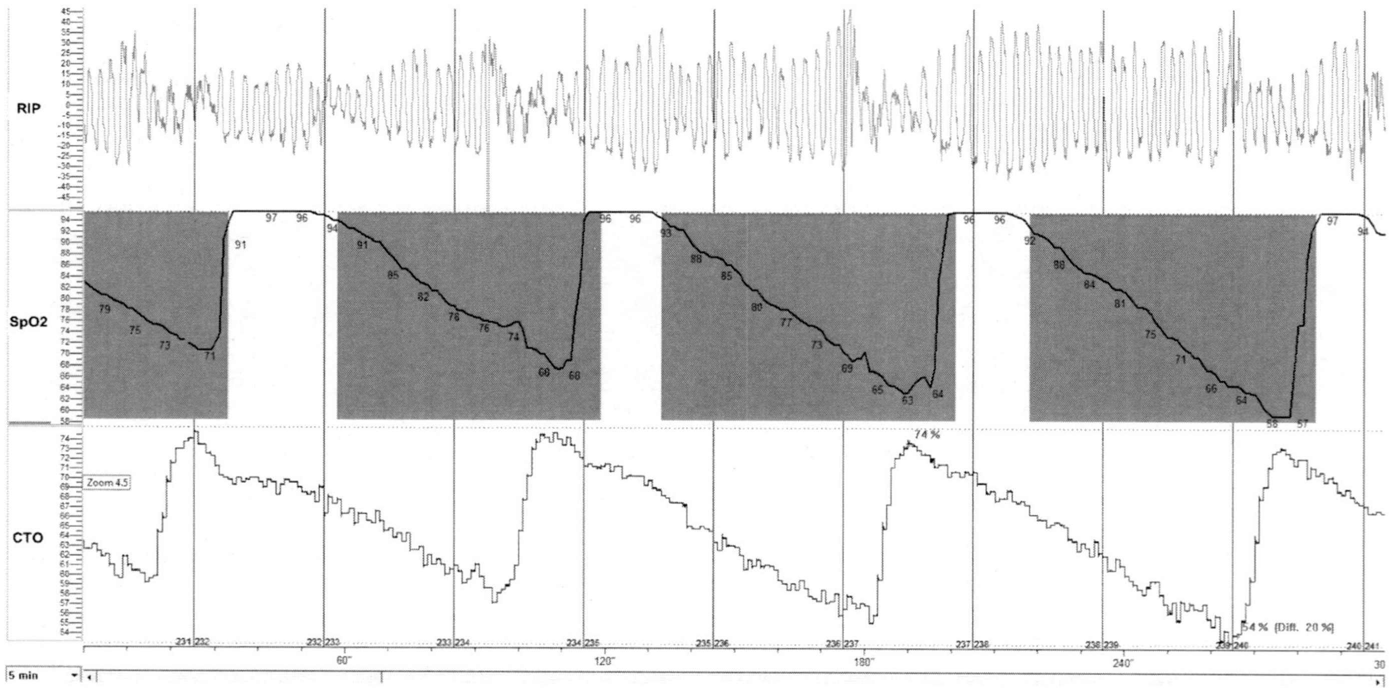

Figure 1. Five-minute window of a polygraphic and cerebral near infra-red spectroscopy recording of a patient with severe obstructive sleep apnoea. Respiratory inductance plethysmography (RIP), peripheral oxygen saturation (SpO2) and cerebral tissue oxygenation (CTO) are shown.

REFERENCES

[1] Kohler M, Stradling JR. Mechanisms of vascular damage in obstructive sleep apnea. *Nat Rev Cardiol* 2010; 7: 677-685.

[2] Schwarz EI, Puhan MA, Schlatzer C, Stradling JR, Kohler M. Effect of CPAP therapy on endothelial function in obstructive sleep apnoea: A systematic review and meta-analysis. *Respirology* 2015; 20: 889-895.

[3] Almendros I, Wang Y, Gozal D. The polymorphic and contradictory aspects of intermittent hypoxia. *Am J Physiol Lung Cell Mol Physiol* 2014; 307: L129-140.

[4] Somers VK, Dyken ME, Clary MP, Abboud FM. Sympathetic neural mechanisms in obstructive sleep apnea. *J Clin Invest* 1995; 96: 1897-1904.

[5] Dempsey JA, Veasey SC, Morgan BJ, O'Donnell CP. Pathophysiology of sleep apnea. *Physiol Rev* 2010; 90: 47-112.

[6] Kohler M, Stoewhas AC, Ayers L, Senn O, Bloch KE, Russi EW, Stradling JR. Effects of continuous positive airway pressure therapy withdrawal in patients with obstructive sleep apnea: a randomized controlled trial. *Am J Respir Crit Care Med* 2011; 184: 1192-1199.

[7] Lombardi C, Pengo MF, Parati G. Systemic hypertension in obstructive sleep apnea. *J Thorac Dis* 2018; 10: S4231-S4243.

[8] Narkiewicz K, Kato M, Phillips BG, Pesek CA, Davison DE, Somers VK. Nocturnal continuous positive airway pressure decreases daytime sympathetic traffic in obstructive sleep apnea. *Circulation* 1999; 100: 2332-2335.

[9] Kohler M, Pepperell JC, Casadei B, Craig S, Crosthwaite N, Stradling JR, Davies RJ. CPAP and measures of cardiovascular risk in males with OSAS. *Eur Respir J* 2008; 32: 1488-1496.

[10] Schwarz EI, Stradling JR, Kohler M. Physiological consequences of CPAP therapy withdrawal in patients with obstructive sleep apnoea-an opportunity for an efficient experimental model. *J Thorac Dis* 2018; 10: S24-S32.

[11] Schwarz EI, Schlatzer C, Rossi VA, Stradling JR, Kohler M. Effect of CPAP Withdrawal on BP in OSA: Data from Three Randomized Controlled Trials. *Chest* 2016; 150: 1202-1210.

[12] Pengo M, Soranna D, Giontella A, Perger E, Schwarz EI, Lombardi C, Bilo G, Zambon A, Steier J, Minuz P, Parati G, Fava C. Blood Pressure Effects of Obstructive Sleep Apnea Treatment by Continuous Positive Airway Pressure: Systematic Review, Metaanalysis and Evaluation of Phenotypes Predicting Response. *Journal of Hypertension* 2019; 37: e40-e41.

[13] Schein AS, Kerkhoff AC, Coronel CC, Plentz RD, Sbruzzi G. Continuous positive airway pressure reduces blood pressure in patients with obstructive sleep apnea; a systematic review and meta-analysis with 1000 patients. *J Hypertens* 2014; 32: 1762-1773.

[14] Iftikhar IH, Valentine CW, Bittencourt LR, Cohen DL, Fedson AC, Gislason T, Penzel T, Phillips CL, Yu-sheng L, Pack AI, Magalang UJ. Effects of continuous positive airway pressure on blood pressure in patients with resistant hypertension and obstructive sleep apnea: a meta-analysis. *J Hypertens* 2014; 32: 2341-2350; discussion 2350.

[15] Schwarz EI, Schlatzer C, Stehli J, Kaufmann PA, Bloch KE, Stradling JR, Kohler M. Effect of CPAP Withdrawal on myocardial perfusion in OSA: A randomized controlled trial. *Respirology* 2016; 21: 1126-1133.

[16] Thiel S, Lettau F, Rejmer P, Rossi C, Haile SR, Schwarz EI, Stoberl AS, Sievi NA, Boss A, Becker AS, Winklhofer S, Stradling JR, Kohler M. Effects of short-term continuous positive airway pressure withdrawal on cerebral vascular reactivity measured by blood oxygen level-dependent magnetic resonance imaging in obstructive sleep apnoea: a randomised controlled trial. *Eur Respir J* 2019; 53.

[17] Schwarz EI, Furian M, Schlatzer C, Stradling JR, Kohler M, Bloch KE. Nocturnal cerebral hypoxia in obstructive sleep apnoea: a randomised controlled trial. *Eur Respir J* 2018; 51.

[18] Xie J, Sert Kuniyoshi FH, Covassin N, Singh P, Gami AS, Wang S, Chahal CA, Wei Y, Somers VK. Nocturnal Hypoxemia Due to Obstructive Sleep Apnea Is an Independent Predictor of Poor Prognosis After Myocardial Infarction. *J Am Heart Assoc* 2016; 5.

[19] Barbe F, Sanchez-de-la-Torre A, Abad J, Duran-Cantolla J, Mediano O, Amilibia J, Masdeu MJ, Flores M, Barcelo A, de la Pena M, Aldoma A, Worner F, Valls J, Castella G, Sanchez-de-la-Torre M, Spanish Sleep N. Effect of obstructive sleep apnoea on severity and short-term prognosis of acute coronary syndrome. *Eur Respir J* 2015; 45: 419-427.

[20] Shah N, Redline S, Yaggi HK, Wu R, Zhao CG, Ostfeld R, Menegus M, Tracy D, Brush E, Appel WD, Kaplan RC. Obstructive sleep apnea and acute myocardial infarction severity: ischemic preconditioning? *Sleep Breath* 2013; 17: 819-826.

[21] Beguin PC, Joyeux-Faure M, Godin-Ribuot D, Levy P, Ribuot C. Acute intermittent hypoxia improves rat myocardium tolerance to ischemia. *J Appl Physiol (1985)* 2005; 99: 1064-1069.

[22] Cai Z, Manalo DJ, Wei G, Rodriguez ER, Fox-Talbot K, Lu H, Zweier JL, Semenza GL. Hearts from rodents exposed to intermittent hypoxia or erythropoietin are protected against ischemia-reperfusion injury. *Circulation* 2003; 108: 79-85.

[23] Lee CH, Sethi R, Li R, Ho HH, Hein T, Jim MH, Loo G, Koo CY, Gao XF, Chandra S, Yang XX, Furlan SF, Ge Z, Mundhekar A, Zhang WW, Uchoa CH, Kharwar RB, Chan PF, Chen SL, Chan MY, Richards AM, Tan HC, Ong TH, Roldan G, Tai BC, Drager LF, Zhang JJ. Obstructive Sleep Apnea and Cardiovascular Events after Percutaneous Coronary Intervention. *Circulation* 2016; 133: 2008-2017.

[24] Qu H, Guo M, Zhang Y, Shi DZ. Obstructive sleep apnea increases the risk of cardiac events after percutaneous coronary intervention: a meta-analysis of prospective cohort studies. *Sleep Breath* 2018; 22: 33-40.

[25] Deng F, Raza A, Guo J. Treating obstructive sleep apnea with continuous positive airway pressure reduces risk of recurrent atrial fibrillation after catheter ablation: a meta-analysis. *Sleep Med* 2018; 46: 5-11.

[26] Peng Y, Yuan G, Overholt JL, Kumar GK, Prabhakar NR. Systemic and cellular responses to intermittent hypoxia: evidence for oxidative stress and mitochondrial dysfunction. *Adv Exp Med Biol* 2003; 536: 559-564.

[27] Xu W, Chi L, Row BW, Xu R, Ke Y, Xu B, Luo C, Kheirandish L, Gozal D, Liu R. Increased oxidative stress is associated with chronic intermittent hypoxia-mediated brain cortical neuronal cell apoptosis in a mouse model of sleep apnea. *Neuroscience* 2004, 126: 313-323.

[28] Knepler JL, Jr., Taher LN, Gupta MP, Patterson C, Pavalko F, Ober MD, Hart CM. Peroxynitrite causes endothelial cell monolayer barrier dysfunction. *Am J Physiol Cell Physiol* 2001; 281: C1064-1075.

[29] Jelic S, Le Jemtel TH. Inflammation, oxidative stress, and the vascular endothelium in obstructive sleep apnea. *Trends Cardiovasc Med* 2008; 18: 253-260.

[30] Jelic S, Padeletti M, Kawut SM, Higgins C, Canfield SM, Onat D, Colombo PC, Basner RC, Factor P, LeJemtel TH. Inflammation, oxidative stress, and repair capacity of the vascular endothelium in obstructive sleep apnea. *Circulation* 2008; 117: 2270-2278.

[31] Alonso-Fernandez A, Garcia-Rio F, Arias MA, Hernanz A, de la Pena M, Pierola J, Barcelo A, Lopez-Collazo E, Agusti A. Effects of CPAP on oxidative stress and nitrate efficiency in sleep apnoea: a randomised trial. *Thorax* 2009; 64: 581-586.

[32] Schwarz EI, Martinez-Lozano Sinues P, Bregy L, Gaisl T, Garcia Gomez D, Gaugg MT, Suter Y, Stebler N, Nussbaumer-Ochsner Y, Bloch KE, Stradling JR, Zenobi R, Kohler M. Effects of CPAP therapy withdrawal on exhaled breath pattern in obstructive sleep apnoea. *Thorax* 2016; 71: 110-117.

[33] Stradling JR, Schwarz EI, Schlatzer C, Manuel AR, Lee R, Antoniades C, Kohler M. Biomarkers of oxidative stress following continuous positive airway pressure withdrawal: data from two randomised trials. *Eur Respir J* 2015; 46: 1065-1071.

[34] Turnbull CD, Rossi VA, Santer P, Schwarz EI, Stradling JR, Petousi N, Kohler M. Effect of OSA on hypoxic and inflammatory markers during CPAP withdrawal: Further evidence from three randomized control trials. *Respirology* 2017; 22: 793-799.

[35] Fletcher EC, Lesske J, Culman J, Miller CC, Unger T. Sympathetic denervation blocks blood pressure elevation in episodic hypoxia. *Hypertension* 1992; 20: 612-619.

[36] Fletcher EC, Lesske J, Qian W, Miller CC, 3rd, Unger T. Repetitive, episodic hypoxia causes diurnal elevation of blood pressure in rats. *Hypertension* 1992; 19: 555-561.

[37] Phillips SA, Olson EB, Morgan BJ, Lombard JH. Chronic intermittent hypoxia impairs endothelium-dependent dilation in rat cerebral and skeletal muscle resistance arteries. *Am J Physiol Heart Circ Physiol* 2004; 286: H388-393.

[38] Al-Rawi PG, Kirkpatrick PJ. Tissue oxygen index: thresholds for cerebral ischemia using near-infrared spectroscopy. *Stroke* 2006; 37: 2720-2725.

In: Sleep Medicine in Critical Care
Editors: Antonio M. Esquinas et al.
ISBN: 978-1-53617-768-8

Chapter 9

EFFECT OF CPAP ON COGNITION AND BRAIN FUNCTION

Valentina Gnoni, MD and
Ivana Rosenzweig[1,*], MD, PhD
[1]Sleep and Brain Plasticity Centre, Department of neuroimaging, King's College London & Sleep Disorders Centre, Guy's and St Thomas' Hospital, London, UK

ABSTRACT

Patients with obstructive sleep apnea (OSA) suffer from increased risk of developing cognitive and functional deficits. Significant links between OSA and several major neuropsychiatric and neurologic disorders have been proposed, and the treatment with continuous positive airway pressure (CPAP) appears to ameliorate some of these risks. Future studies will determine which cognitive domains and the associated illness-driven pathomechanisms are best targeted with various combinations of CPAP treatments.

INTRODUCTION

Obstructive sleep apnoea (OSA) is characterized by repetitive brief closures (apnea) or narrowing (hypopnea) of the pharyngeal airway during sleep [1-3]. The resulting cessation or reduction of air flow leads to reduced oxygen saturation, including commonly post-apneic arousals from sleep, increased sympathetic activity, and the resumption of airflow [1, 14, 15]. It has long been recognised that the combination of

* Corresponding Author's E-mail: ivana.1.rosenzweig@kcl.ac.uk.

frequent respiratory events and arousals from sleep throughout the night may severely fragment sleep architecture, lead to perceptions of chronically unrefreshing sleep, reduced quality of life, excessive daytime somnolence, increased risk of motor-vehicle and work accidents, and to significant changes in cognitive and brain functions of affected patients [3, 4]. The development of structural and functional changes in the brains of patients with OSA has been regularly [5, 6], if not consistently [2], described in a number of neuroimaging and cognitive studies over the years, whilst several pertinent questions still remain unanswered [2, 3, 7-9]. A wider network of structures has been shown to be affected, comprising fronto-thalamic-cerebellar regions, with significant involvement of the hippocampal formation, basal ganglia and insular cortex [2, 10-12], however, it is not yet clear whether temporal evolution of these damages occurs in a consistent matter. Similarly, it is not yet clear what pathomechanisms might dictate its severity, and in which way [2]. Additionally, the major pathomechanisms behind the cognitive changes are far from clear, and its links with dementia and other neuropsychiatric disorders is still argued, if it is no longer considered controversial [2, 13].

The role of neuroinflammation has recently been implied by the findings of a preclinical study where, in a rodent model of OSA, acute neuroinflammatory response was demonstrated following three days of exposure to intermittent hypoxia in the basal forebrain of mice, and more chronically in other parts of the frontal cortex [14]. In this study adaptive changes in specific neurocircuitry were demonstrated, with significant links to agitated (mal)adaptive behaviour under episodes of stress, and an increased ability to gain weight, with authors arguing that an innate immune response might be the missing link underlying the pathogenesis of majority of well-known structural, psychologic and metabolic changes experienced by some patients with OSA [14].

On balance, all reported neuroanatomical correlations to date have arguably shown close correlations with the clinical symptomatology observed in patients with OSA [15]. For example, patients with OSA have been noted to show deficits in information processing and psychomotor speed, difficulty in shifting between tasks, updating and monitoring working memory representations, and inhibiting predominant responses [3]. Also, in keeping with this, the involvement of the cerebellum and the subcortical areas supports the deficiency of motor skills and fine motor coordination movements demonstrated by some OSA patients [16]. Although a clearer picture of the variety of cognitive deficits triggered by OSA is emerging, reversibility of the impairments is not yet clearly established, and neither is the myriad of protective and confounding factors (e.g., genetics, ischemic preconditioning, cognitive reserve) which all might play a significant role (for a more in-depth review, see [3]).

Currently, the most effective treatment for OSA is continuous positive airway pressure (CPAP), a prosthetic non-invasive intervention [17] which has over years been reported to decrease cardiovascular morbidity and mortality, somnolence and cognitive impairments in patients with OSA [2, 16, 18-20]. Pharmacotherapy has also been used as an adjunct to CPAP for treatment of residual excessive somnolence in patients with a diagnosis of OSA [21]. Nonetheless, the findings of a recent meta-analysis have suggested that, whilst pharmacotherapy with modafinil and armodafinil, alerting psychotropics commonly used in sleep clinics, led to improvement of somnolence and attention, no significant improvements in the quality of life or other cognitive domains (including memory, executive function, and language) could be confirmed [21]. The authors, however, noted that the heterogeneity of tests and absence of standardization significantly reduced certainty as to whether actual improvement occurred in these outcomes, and to what extent additional therapy has played role in noted improvements [21]. Similarly, a recent randomised controlled trial of OSA patients with co-occurring insomnia has demonstrated a positive impact of initial treatment with cognitive and behavioral therapy for insomnia (CBT-i), on subsequent acceptance and use of CPAP therapy, and improvements in disease severity [1, 4]. In this study, participants who initially received CBT-i showed greater insomnia improvements, and greater acceptance and long-term use of CPAP compared to participants treated only with CPAP [1], leading authors to argue for an increased awareness of benefits of concomitant talking therapy in this patient sub-group.

Several major neuropsychiatric and neurologic disorders have been argued to have close bidirectional links with OSA: from stroke, epilepsy, Alzheimer's disorder to depression and posttraumatic stress disorder (also please see more in depth reviews [2, 13]). In that background, the findings of the ADIPOSA study are of particular interest [22]. In this study, which sought to elucidate the presence of non-overlapping symptoms of depression and anxiety in patients with moderate to severe OSA before and after CPAP treatment, some amelioration of depression and anxiety symptoms has been reported [22]. Moreover, the authors argued that CPAP may be effective at reducing the lack of positive affect in patient with OSA, a well-established health-protective factor [22]. The significant positive impact of CPAP treatment in patients with co-morbid OSA and stroke has also been argued recently, and benefits for patients' cognitive function, sleep quality, and daytime somnolence shown [23]. Moreover, it has been suggested that CPAP treatment should be considered as part of the rehabilitation program for patients with stroke [23]. Similarly, the positive effects of CPAP treatment for patients with co-morbid OSA and epilepsy have long been argued [2].

Notwithstanding all the positive findings and a growing body of the literature supporting the role for CPAP treatment in addressing the cognitive deficits associated with OSA, it has also been widely accepted that some accrued deficits in certain patients might be irreversible, leading to permanent cognitive decline [2, 15, 19, 24]. A close link between OSA and an early onset of cognitive impairment has been described [24, 25], while growing clinical evidence support notion that OSA should be acknowledged as one of the atypical modifiable risk factors of Alzheimer's dementia [2, 13, 24]. Of particular note is that CPAP treatment has been shown to delay cognitive decline in patients with OSA [24].

CPAP Therapy

Arguably, CPAP has proved its status as one of the most effective treatment for cognitive performance in patients with OSA [2, 3, 9, 10, 13]. The consensus in the field is that its positive therapeutic effects are reflection of its impact on the underlying causes for the pathological changes seen in patients with OSA, including hypoxia, hypercapnia, and poor sleep quality [15]. Over the last three decades numerous studies have demonstrated its role in neuroplasticity and neuroanatomical and physiologic changes in the brain (for in depth review see [2]). Some of the examples include the role of CPAP treatment in addressing the deficits in the connectivity of the default mode network and cortical thinning [10]. More specifically, an increase in the connectivity was seen in the right middle frontal gyrus after three months of CPAP treatment [10]. Further, in another study CPAP treatment almost completely reversed white matter abnormalities following a year of treatment [11]. More interestingly, significant improvements involving attention, executive function, and memory paralleled white matter changes for the therapeutic effects of CPAP [11].

Over the years, CPAP treatment has been shown to be effective in amelioration of deficits in executive functions, intelligence and memory in several studies [2, 3]. Its effects have been particularly noted in the domains of working memory, long-term verbal memory, and short-term visuospatial memory [26]. Professional well-being and job productivity have also been reported to improve in patients with severe OSA who were successfully treated with CPAP [15, 27]. Nonetheless, as already discussed, limitations of treatments with CPAP have also been well recognised [2]. Cognitive domains that have been proven more resistant to treatment with CPAP somewhat controversially similarly include those that in certain patients show significant improvement, such as working memory, attention, executive function, and psychomotor speed [28]. However, there has been consistent evidence for improvements in immediate memory [29] and following a longer duration of treatment (e.g., 12 months) have also been reported improvements in executive function, memory and reactive time [30].

Given the polymorphic findings of various studies, the importance of addressing questions such as the length of treatment required, delineation of more or less susceptible phenotypes of patients with OSA, and similarly important question, at which point in the illness progression the intervention will be at its most effective, are still far from clear [3]. These crucial questions will require future consideration through a major concerted international effort where all phenotypes of OSA will be included and investigations standardised to yield more meaningful and comparable findings [3]. Presently, however, the body of literature suggests that the length of treatment does play a major role, and it has been argued that artificial cut of point of six months of CPAP therapy might be required to address cognitive deficits in patients with OSA [31, 32].

However, shorter durations, such as three months of therapy, have also been shown to lead to significant improvement in cognition [33], especially in domains of episodic and short-term memory, as well as in the domain of the executive function [10]. In keeping with this, in patients with Alzheimer's dementia with severe OSA, CPAP treatment for three months has similarly been associated with a slower cognitive decline [34]. Much shorter duration, such as one month of CPAP treatment, has also been shown to have some beneficial effects, and to lead to improved verbal episodic memory and somnolence [9].

Nonetheless, despite ongoing neuroplasticity, it would appear that shorter durations of treatment with CPAP might not always lead to testable and perceivable effects in all patients. For example, two weeks of CPAP or oxygen-supplementation treatment have in one study failed to demonstrate significant impact on any of the cognitive domains [35]. Similarly, a comparison of patients randomized to three weeks of therapeutic versus placebo CPAP also had no significant improvements in cognition for patients with AD and OSA [36]. These findings have led some clinicians to argue that the duration of CPAP therapy is not only a crucial factor, but the main factor determining whether improvement of the cognitive performance in patients with OSA will occur [15]. Nonetheless, a more complex picture is now emerging, and it has also been recognised that the effects of treatment might be cognitive domain-specific, meaning that some domains of cognitive function might not be as sensitive to CPAP treatment as others, and or might need longer periods of treatment [37]. For example, in a prospective study, one year of the use of CPAP improved significantly the levels of somnolence and vigilance, but failed to modify neuropsychiatric symptoms of anxiety and depression [37].

In conclusion, it is no longer debatable that patients with OSA are more likely to develop cognitive impairments [3, 15]. Whilst the effected cognitive domains, associated neuropsychiatric traits, individual genetic and other protective mechanisms and the underlying illness-driven pathomechanisms are yet to be fully clarified [3], the current consensus is that a minimal therapeutic duration of four weeks, of sufficient compliance, might be needed for notifiable therapeutic effects to take place [15]. Finally, there is also some growing evidence to support the additive positive effects of pharmacotherapy and talking therapy, however, the real breakthrough will likely come about by delineating the underlying mechanism for specific cognitive impairments [13].

REFERENCES

[1] Sweetman A, Lack L, Bastien C. Co-Morbid Insomnia and Sleep Apnea (COMISA): Prevalence, Consequences, Methodological Considerations, and Recent Randomized Controlled Trials. *Brain Sci.* 2019;9(12).

[2] Rosenzweig I, Glasser M, Polsek D, Leschziner GD, Williams SC, Morrell MJ. Sleep apnoea and the brain: a complex relationship. *Lancet Respir. Med.* 2015;3(5):404-14.

[3] Bucks RS, Olaithe M, Rosenzweig I, Morrell MJ. Reviewing the relationship between OSA and cognition: Where do we go from here? *Respirology.* 2017;22(7):1253-61.

[4] Sweetman A, Lack L, Catcheside PG, Antic NA, Smith S, Chai-Coetzer CL, et al. Cognitive and behavioral therapy for insomnia increases the use of continuous positive airway pressure therapy in obstructive sleep apnea participants with co-morbid insomnia: A randomized clinical trial. *Sleep.* 2019.

[5] Tahmasian M, Rosenzweig I, Eickhoff SB, Sepehry AA, Laird AR, Fox PT, et al. Structural and functional neural adaptations in obstructive sleep apnea: An activation likelihood estimation meta-analysis. *Neurosci. Biobehav. Rev.* 2016;65:142-56.

[6] Khazaie H, Veronese M, Noori K, Emamian F, Zarei M, Ashkan K, et al. Functional reorganization in obstructive sleep apnoea and insomnia: A systematic review of the resting-state fMRI. *Neurosci. Biobehav. Rev.* 2017;77:219-31.

[7] Rosenzweig I, Morrell MJ. Hypotrophy versus Hypertrophy: It's Not Black or White with Gray Matter. *Am. J. Respir. Crit. Care Med.* 2017;195(11):1416-8.

[8] Javaheipour N, Shahdipour N, Noori K, Zarei M, Camilleri JA, Laird AR, et al. Functional brain alterations in acute sleep deprivation: An activation likelihood estimation meta-analysis. *Sleep Med. Rev.* 2019;46:64-73.

[9] Rosenzweig I, Glasser M, Crum WR, Kempton MJ, Milosevic M, McMillan A, et al. Changes in Neurocognitive Architecture in Patients with Obstructive Sleep Apnea Treated with Continuous Positive Airway Pressure. *EBioMedicine.* 2016;7:221-9.

[10] Dalmases M, Sole-Padulles C, Torres M, Embid C, Nunez MD, Martinez-Garcia MA, et al. Effect of CPAP on Cognition, Brain Function, and Structure Among Elderly Patients With OSA: A Randomized Pilot Study. *Chest.* 2015;148(5):1214-23.

[11] Castronovo V, Scifo P, Castellano A, Aloia MS, Iadanza A, Marelli S, et al. White matter integrity in obstructive sleep apnea before and after treatment. *Sleep.* 2014;37(9):1465-75.

[12] Joo EY, Tae WS, Lee MJ, Kang JW, Park HS, Lee JY, et al. Reduced brain gray matter concentration in patients with obstructive sleep apnea syndrome. *Sleep*. 2010;33(2):235-41.

[13] Polsek D, Gildeh N, Cash D, Winsky-Sommerer R, Williams SCR, Turkheimer F, et al. Obstructive sleep apnoea and Alzheimer's disease: In search of shared pathomechanisms. *Neurosci. Biobehav. Rev.* 2018;86:142-9.

[14] Polsek D, Cash D, Veronese M, Ilic K, Wood TC, Milosevic M, et al. The Innate Immune Toll-Like Receptor-2 modulates the Depressogenic and Anorexiolytic Neuroinflammatory Response in Obstructive Sleep Apnoea. 2019.

[15] Wang G, Goebel JR, Li C, Hallman HG, Gilford TM, Li W. Therapeutic effects of CPAP on cognitive impairments associated with OSA. *J. Neurol.* 2019.

[16] Devita M, Zangrossi A, Marvisi M, Merlo P, Rusconi ML, Mondini S. Global cognitive profile and different components of reaction times in obstructive sleep apnea syndrome: Effects of continuous positive airway pressure over time. *Int. J. Psychophysiol.* 2018;123:121-6.

[17] Stuck BA, Leitzbach S, Maurer JT. Effects of continuous positive airway pressure on apnea-hypopnea index in obstructive sleep apnea based on long-term compliance. *Sleep Breath.* 2012;16(2):467-71.

[18] Gildeh N, Rosenzweig I, Kent BD. Lessons from randomised controlled trials of continuous positive airways pressure therapy in the prevention of cardiovascular morbidity and mortality. *J. Thorac. Dis.* 2017;9(2):244-6.

[19] Bubu OM, Pirraglia E, Andrade AG, Sharma RA, Gimenez-Badia S, Umasabor-Bubu OQ, et al. Obstructive sleep apnea and longitudinal Alzheimer's disease biomarker changes. *Sleep*. 2019;42(6).

[20] Gildeh N, Drakatos P, Higgins S, Rosenzweig I, Kent BD. Emerging co-morbidities of obstructive sleep apnea: cognition, kidney disease, and cancer. *J. Thorac. Dis.* 2016;8(9):E901-E17.

[21] Avellar AB, Carvalho LB, Prado GF, Prado LB. Pharmacotherapy for residual excessive sleepiness and cognition in CPAP-treated patients with obstructive sleep apnea syndrome: A systematic review and meta-analysis. *Sleep Med. Rev.* 2016;30:97-107.

[22] Carneiro-Barrera A, Amaro-Gahete FJ, Saez-Roca G, Martin-Carrasco C, Ruiz JR, Buela-Casal G. Anxiety and Depression in Patients with Obstructive Sleep Apnoea before and after Continuous Positive Airway Pressure: The ADIPOSA Study. *J. Clin. Med.* 2019;8(12).

[23] Kim H, Im S, Park JI, Kim Y, Sohn MK, Jee S. Improvement of Cognitive Function after Continuous Positive Airway Pressure Treatment for Subacute Stroke Patients with Obstructive Sleep Apnea: A Randomized Controlled Trial. *Brain Sci.* 2019;9(10).

[24] Osorio RS, Gumb T, Pirraglia E, Varga AW, Lu SE, Lim J, et al. Sleep-disordered breathing advances cognitive decline in the elderly. *Neurology*. 2015;84(19):1964-71.

[25] Emamian F, Khazaie H, Tahmasian M, Leschziner GD, Morrell MJ, Hsiung GY, et al. The Association between Obstructive Sleep Apnea and Alzheimer's Disease: A Meta-Analysis Perspective. *Front. Aging Neurosci.* 2016;8:78.

[26] Turner K, Zambrelli E, Lavolpe S, Baldi C, Furia F, Canevini MP. Obstructive sleep apnea: neurocognitive and behavioral functions before and after treatment. *Funct. Neurol.* 2019;34(2):71-8.

[27] Jurado-Gamez B, Guglielmi O, Gude-Sampedro F, Buela-Casal G. Effect of CPAP therapy on job productivity and psychosocial occupational health in patients with moderate to severe sleep apnea. *Sleep Breath.* 2015;19(4):1293-9.

[28] Lau EY, Eskes GA, Morrison DL, Rajda M, Spurr KF. Executive function in patients with obstructive sleep apnea treated with continuous positive airway pressure. *J. Int. Neuropsychol. Soc.* 2010;16(6):1077-88.

[29] Jurado-Gamez B, Guglielmi O, Gude F, Buela-Casal G. Effects of continuous positive airway pressure treatment on cognitive functions in patients with severe obstructive sleep apnoea. *Neurologia*. 2016;31(5):311-8.

[30] Ng SS, Chan TO, To KW, Chan KK, Ngai J, Tung A, et al. Prevalence of obstructive sleep apnea syndrome and CPAP adherence in the elderly Chinese population. *PLoS One*. 2015;10(3):e0119829.

[31] Wu SQ, Liao QC, Xu XX, Sun L, Wang J, Chen R. Effect of CPAP therapy on C-reactive protein and cognitive impairment in patients with obstructive sleep apnea hypopnea syndrome. *Sleep Breath.* 2016;20(4):1185-92.

[32] Kotterba S, Rasche K, Widdig W, Duscha C, Blombach S, Schultze-Werninghaus G, et al. Neuropsychological investigations and event-related potentials in obstructive sleep apnea syndrome before and during CPAP-therapy. *J. Neurol. Sci.* 1998;159(1):45-50.

[33] Safiri S, Ayubi E. The effect of CPAP therapy on insulin-like growth factor and cognitive functions in obstructive sleep apnea patients: Methodological issues. *Clin. Respir. J.* 2018;12(4):1776.

[34] Troussiere AC, Charley CM, Salleron J, Richard F, Delbeuck X, Derambure P, et al. Treatment of sleep apnoea syndrome decreases cognitive decline in patients with Alzheimer's disease. *J. Neurol. Neurosurg. Psychiatry.* 2014;85(12):1405-8.

[35] Lim W, Bardwell WA, Loredo JS, Kim EJ, Ancoli-Israel S, Morgan EE, et al. Neuropsychological effects of 2-week continuous positive airway pressure treatment and supplemental oxygen in patients with obstructive sleep apnea: a randomized placebo-controlled study. *J. Clin. Sleep Med.* 2007;3(4):380-6.

[36] Ancoli-Israel S, Palmer BW, Cooke JR, Corey-Bloom J, Fiorentino L, Natarajan L, et al. Cognitive effects of treating obstructive sleep apnea in Alzheimer's disease: a randomized controlled study. *J. Am. Geriatr. Soc.* 2008;56(11):2076-81.

[37] Munoz A, Mayoralas LR, Barbe F, Pericas J, Agusti AG. Long-term effects of CPAP on daytime functioning in patients with sleep apnoea syndrome. *Eur. Respir. J.* 2000;15(4):676-81.

In: Sleep Medicine in Critical Care
Editors: Antonio M. Esquinas et al.
ISBN: 978-1-53617-768-8

Chapter 10

EFFECT OF CPAP ON CO-MORBIDITIES (CARDIAC, RENAL AND LIVER)

Martino F. Pengo*, MD, PhD, Elisa Perger, MD and Carolina Lombardi, MD, PhD
Department of Cardiovascular, Neural and Metabolic Sciences, IRCCS Istituto Auxologico Italiano, Milan, Italy

ABSTRACT

The effects of obstructive sleep apnea (OSA) treatment by means of continuous positive airway pressure (CPAP) are numerous and diverse. In fact restoring the normal breathing pattern and oxygen saturation throughout the night by treating apneas and hypopneas can resolve multiple OSA-related consequences involving different human organ systems. Some of these effects are well known such as those on the cardiovascular system: treating intermittent hypoxia allows to reduce the sympathetic nervous activation that triggers renin-angiotensin-aldosterone system, responsible of the development of arterial hypertension and, ultimately, of chronic kidney disease. Others are less studied such as the effect of CPAP on the progression of non-alcoholic fatty liver disease (NAFLD). In the present chapter we will discuss in depth the consequences of CPAP treatment in patients with OSA and cardiac, renal and hepatic co-morbidities.

CARDIAC CO-MORBIDITIES

The potential detrimental effects of sleep disordered breathing on the cardiovascular system have been extensively studied even prior to the invention of CPAP: the group of

* Corresponding Author's E-mail: m.pengo@auxologico.it.

Prof. Lugaresi, from the University of Bologna, reported for the first time the association between snoring and elevated blood pressure (BP) [1]. When CPAP was eventually introduced in clinical practice, several research groups worldwide demonstrated that indeed CPAP was able to modify, and in some cases reverse, some of the most frequent cardiac co-morbidities.

Arterial Hypertension

The pathophysiological mechanisms that link OSA and hypertension are deeply intertwined together; the most relevant ones being intermittent hypoxia and sympathetic activation, with the accompanying reduction in arterial baroreflex sensitivity. In fact, intermittent hypoxia, caused by repetitive airway obstructions, on one side promotes the peripheral chemoreceptor stimulation which causes an enhanced sympathetic activation, and on the other side, contributes to the production of reactive oxygen species, activates systemic inflammation, and ultimately impairs endothelial function.

The activation of the sympathetic branch of the autonomic nervous system is the consequence not only of intermittent hypoxia but also of arousals from sleep and increased pleural pressure swings which stimulate pulmonary stretch receptors. Such increased sympathetic discharge results in the intermittent release of dopamine, norepinephrine (noradrenaline), and epinephrine (adrenaline) which have positive inotropic, chronotropic, and dromotropic effects. Furthermore, sympathetic activation stimulates the renin-angiotensin-aldosterone system resulting in an increased production of angiotensin II which promotes vasoconstriction in venous and arterial walls smooth muscles [2].

CPAP treatment can reverse OSA and therefore restore normoxia, physiological autonomous nervous system function and a normal arterial baroreflex sensitivity therefore reducing BP values.

Since the 1990s, several randomized controlled studies (RCTs) have been trying to address the effect of CPAP on blood pressure and the results have consistently shown that CPAP use, when compared with passive control, determines a significant although modest drop in BP (systolic 2.6 ± 0.6 mmHg, diastolic 2.0 ± 0.4 mmHg) which is even more pronounced when nocturnal BP is considered [3].

Although a net BP change of a few millimeters of mercury does not seem much from a clinical perspective, it nevertheless corresponds to a considerable reduction in cardiovascular mortality over the long term.

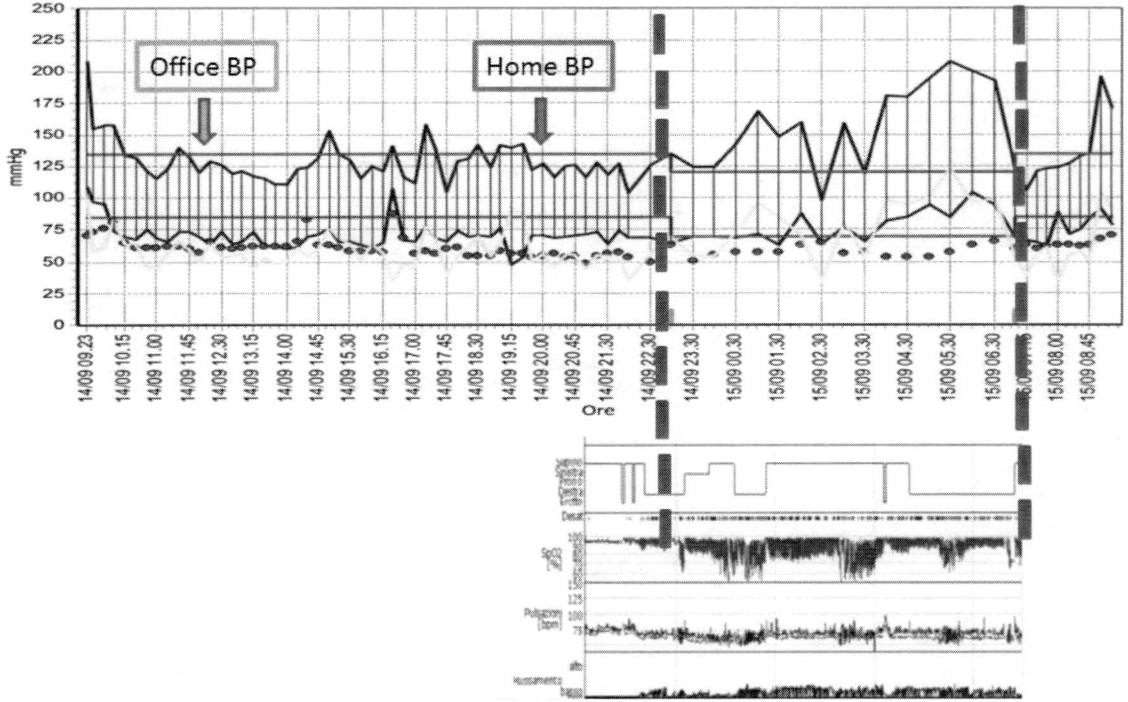

Figure 1. Ambulatory blood pressure monitoring trace (above) showing the variability of BP when measured at home or in office. Nocturnal hypertension in this patient was associated with severe obstructive sleep apnea as represented by the nocturnal oximetry trace (below).

It is important to mention that, in many RCTs, BP was measured only during clinical consultations, the so called office blood pressure, whilst only few studies have assessed ambulatory blood pressure. This methodological aspect is crucial given that OSA patients exhibit increased BP variability when compared to non-OSA subjects, making office BP less reliable and possibly not representative of the real OSA patient's BP profile. Such variability is evident when dipping BP profile is assessed: OSA is more frequent in non-dippers and particularly in reverse dippers (Figure 1).

In addition, it is well known that ambulatory BP (nocturnal BP in particular) better predicts cardiovascular outcomes in hypertensive patients as compared with office BP; its assessment thus represents a preferable approach particularly in patients with sleep disordered breathing.

Despite such limitations, The Task Force of the American Academy of Sleep Medicine Clinical Practice Guidelines suggested clinicians to use positive airway pressure (PAP) therapy to treat OSA in adults with co-morbid hypertension, without defining specific BP cut-offs or whether office or out of office BP should be considered.

Thus, understanding which are the determinants of such favorable effect of CPAP on BP could inform clinicians to implement more personalized treatment choices.

Studies on CPAP withdrawal [4] pointed out that severity of OSA was associated with a higher BP rise in response to CPAP withdrawal and with a greater net BP decrease in patients treated with CPAP, respectively. Among CPAP-related factors, patients' compliance and adherence remain the main predictors of CPAP BP-lowering effects, as confirmed in large randomized controlled trials [5]. However, studies focusing on the determinants of CPAP effect on BP are lacking thus more research is needed to understand which OSA patients might benefit the most from CPAP in terms of BP control and cardiovascular prevention.

Heart Failure

Sleep apnea is frequent in patients with heart failure (HF) who present often central respiratory events in addition to obstructive apneas. Studies investigating the potential benefits of CPAP therapy with respect to underlying heart failure have shown conflicting results. Several studies looking at surrogate end points suggested beneficial effects associated with CPAP therapy particularly in OSA patients with HF: in a pilot study 24 OSA patients with HF treated with CPAP exhibited a reduction in sympathetic nervous system signaling and a favorable hemodynamic effect, including improved left ventricular systolic and diastolic function [6].

Similarly, other trials confirmed that treatment of OSA with CPAP in HF patients improved left ventricular ejection fraction (LVEF), New York Heart Association functional class, reduced daytime blood pressure and heart rate. On hard cardiovascular endpoints some observational studies showed that patients with OSA and HF treated with CPAP had greater hospitalization-free survival and a trend to a lower mortality rate compared to untreated patients.

However, when studies focused the treatment on central other than obstructive sleep apnea, results have been disappointing: the CANPAP (Canadian Continuous Positive Airway Pressure for Patients with Central Sleep Apnea and Heart Failure) trial investigated the effect of CPAP treatment in patients with HF and central sleep apnea (CSA). No benefit was seen in the patients treated with CPAP; however, a post hoc analysis suggested a reduction in mortality among patients for whom CPAP therapy resulted in a significant improvement in AHI (to <15 events/h) [7].

Giving that many patients with heart failure present central events which do not benefit from CPAP treatment, an alternative form of bi-level positive airway pressure therapy has tested in the SAVIOR-C (Study of the Effects of Adaptive Servo ventilation Therapy on Cardiac Function and Remodeling in Patients with Chronic Heart Failure) trial which failed to show an improvement in ejection fraction or brain natriuretic peptide (BNP) levels after 24 weeks of adaptive servo-ventilation (ASV) therapy in patients with heart failure and CSA [8].

Eventually, the SERVE-HF (Treatment of Sleep-Disordered Breathing with Predominant Central Sleep Apnea by Adaptive Servo Ventilation in Patients with Heart Failure) trial was designed to test the effect of ASV on mortality in patients with left ventricular ejection fraction ≤45% and predominantly central sleep apnea. Despite effectively reducing the AHI, ASV failed to confer a survival benefit, and actually was associated with an increase in cardiovascular mortality (29.9% versus 24%) [9].

Thus, at present, ASV is not recommended in patients with heart failure, reduced ejection fraction and predominant central sleep apnea until other trials are published. One of these ongoing studies, the ADVENT-HF (Effect of Adaptive Servo Ventilation on Survival and Hospital Admissions in Heart Failure) trial, is currently investigating the effect of ASV therapy on mortality and morbidity in HF patients (left ventricular ejection fraction ≤45%) with SDB using a different algorithm than the one of SERVE-HF. Therefore in the years to come some new evidence could shed some light on the role of PAP therapy in patients with heart failure.

Atrial Fibrillation

Intermittent hypoxia, breathing efforts and autonomic derangement are also a potential promoting factor for arrhythmogenesis. OSA is associated with important hemodynamic alterations, in particular an increased right atrial and ventricular preload as well as an increased afterload related to the hypoxic pulmonary vasoconstriction have been described. Consequently, during diastole, a leftward septal displacement impairing left ventricular filling increasing also left atrial volume loading can be observed. Furthermore, long-term repeated episodes of apneas are associated with structural remodeling and changes in cardiac electrical conduction system, in particular in the atrium, which together with intermittent hypoxia and autonomic alterations could predispose to cardiac arrhythmias such as atrial fibrillation but also sudden cardiac death. Additionally, such cardiac alteration can predispose to the development of cardio embolic stroke: recently, our group showed that in patients with recent stroke the presence of OSA was associated with more pronounced cardiac structural alterations as compared with stroke patients without OSA [10]. From an epidemiological point of view, mounting evidence is now available confirming the high prevalence of cardiac arrhythmias in patients with OSA and vice versa. Atrial fibrillation (AF), the most common cardiac arrhythmia worldwide, is frequently found in OSA patients with a prevalence ranging between 3% and 5%, significantly higher than in the general population (0,4-1%) [11]. Conversely, the prevalence of OSA in patients with AF has been reported between 21% and 85%, significantly higher than in the general population. Beyond this epidemiologic association between the two conditions, there is a growing body of evidence suggesting a significant role of OSA in recurrent and/or treatment-refractory AF. Furthermore, treatment of OSA may modify these risks: in the ORBIT-AF study, OSA patients treated with CPAP were significantly less likely to develop permanent AF as compared with OSA patients not receiving CPAP [12]. Furthermore, several observational studies have demonstrated a reduction in the risk of recurrent AF following electrical cardioversion and catheter ablation among OSA patients treated with CPAP as compared with OSA patients not receiving treatment.

In conclusion, there is strong evidence supporting the screening, diagnosis and treatment of sleep disordered breathing in patients with AF. However, there is still controversy about the OSA severity to be considered as a threshold to provide treatment for such patients.

Myocardial Infarction

Prospective and cross-sectional studies report an association between OSA and coronary artery disease: the prevalence of moderate to severe OSA in patients with acute coronary syndrome is 73% and patients with severe OSA exhibit a more pronounced cardiac impairment, higher levels of Troponin-I and NT-proBNP, lower left ventricle ejection fraction and are at higher risk of ST elevation myocardial infarction. In the Sleep Heart Health study OSA was a significant predictor of incident coronary artery disease (CAD), quantified by myocardial infarction, revascularization procedures, or coronary heart disease death, in males up to 70 years of age (adjusted HR 1.10, 95% CI 1.00-1.21; per 10-unit increase in AHI) but not in older males or in females of any age.

On top of the known mechanisms linking OSA and hypertension already discussed, additional mechanisms supporting the association between OSA and CAD include endothelial dysfunction, promotion of a procoagulable state and metabolic dysregulation characterized by insulin resistance. Treatment of OSA with CPAP has been shown to mitigate these processes, offering a plausible mechanism by which treating OSA could influence cardiovascular outcomes.

However the SAVE (Sleep Apnea Cardiovascular Endpoints) trial, the largest RCT designed to investigate the question of whether treating OSA with CPAP may improve cardiovascular outcomes in patients with established CVD [5], failed to demonstrate a significant reduction in the primary end point (a composite of cardiovascular death, myocardial infarction, stroke, hospitalization for unstable angina, HF, or transient ischemic attack) among patients treated with CPAP in addition to usual care.

A recent meta-analysis aimed to assess the effects of CPAP in survival and secondary prevention of major cardiovascular events in patients with OSA and cardiovascular disease (CVD) confirmed that CPAP therapy does not significantly improve such outcomes [13].

Barbé and co-authors enrolled 725 non-sleepy patients with moderate-to-severe OSA but no prior history of CVD and randomized them to CPAP versus no therapy. After a median of 4 years, there was no difference in the incidence of systemic hypertension or cardiovascular events including cardiovascular death, nonfatal MI or stroke, TIA, or HF [14].

To conclude, current evidence showed conflicting results on the effect of OSA treatment on cardiovascular prognosis. Several potential confounding factors have been advocated with compliance to treatment being one of the most relevant. In fact, a recent meta-analysis on the effect of CPAP on major adverse cardiovascular events (MACE) in patients with moderate-to-severe OSA showed that CPAP therapy might reduce MACE and stroke among subjects with CPAP daily use exceeding 4 h/night. More randomized controlled trials ensuring adequate CPAP compliance are needed to confirm these findings.

RENAL CO-MORBIDITIES

Whilst the association of OSA with cardiovascular diseases is well recognized and described, the potential role of sleep disordered breathing in kidney disease has only recently gained attention. Sleep complaints are frequent among patients with end-stage renal disease (ESRD) and polysomnographic studies confirmed a high prevalence of sleep disorders such as OSA. OSA plays an important role in the development and progression of kidney disease. Sleep disordered breathing has been found in 54% of non-dialysis chronic kidney disease (CKD) patients, with higher prevalence of sleep apnea as the renal function deteriorates. On the other hand ESRD has itself an impact on sleep apnea severity: kidneys and lungs work closely regulating acid-base balance, maintaining fluid status and blood pressure through renin-angiotensin-aldosterone system. Metabolic factors might destabilize respiratory control by altering chemoreceptor sensitivity and reducing airway muscle tone predisposing to OSA or central sleep apnea. Another deleterious effect of ESRD which might have an impact on OSA is fluid overload: recent evidence has pointed out that fluid volume is a crucial contributory factor in sleep apnea patients with kidney diseases and that fluid removal by ultrafiltration can reduce OSA severity [15].

Furthermore, mounting evidence suggests that the treatment of moderate to severe OSA by CPAP can minimize glomerular hyperfiltration. Kinebuchi and co-authors compared the filtration fractions of 27 patients with moderate-to-severe OSA before and after one week of CPAP treatment with 32 healthy donors for renal transplantation. Considering filtration fractions and renal plasma flows as indicators of glomerular hyperfiltration, CPAP therapy significantly reduced hyperfiltration by increasing renal plasma flow and reducing the filtration fraction [16].

Analyzing the effects of CPAP treatment on kidney function in 38 men with OSA, it has been shown that 3 months of CPAP therapy were able to reduce average serum creatinine levels (0.87 to 0.82 mg/dL), and to increase average glomerular filtration rate (GFR) levels from 72.9 to 79.3 mg/dL [17]. CPAP compliance might play an important role in preserving kidney function giving that evidence suggests that a CPAP usage >4 h\night during >70% of nights was associated with a less marked decline in GFR compared to not compliant patients. Concerning the effects of CPAP on proteinuria it has been reported that CPAP use can determine a decrease in urinary albumin excretion, with the effect remaining stable for up to 3 months after commencing CPAP treatment.

Despite the literature presented above, positive impact of CPAP on kidney function has not been consistently confirmed in further studies. In a prospective, non-randomized study of the effects of fixed positive airway pressure (PAP) and auto-PAP on kidney function decline in 1807 subjects with OSA, fixed CPAP had an attenuating effect on the rate of kidney function decline whereas auto-PAP did not. In the multivariate analyses the treatment with a fixed PAP resulted also as the independent predictor of GFR amelioration at follow up [18]. The authors postulated that CPAP may have had a more significant beneficial effect on blood pressure control and sympathetic nervous system activation compared to APAP, as has previously been suggested.

A sub-study of the SAVE (Sleep Apnea Cardiovascular Endpoints) randomized control trial (RCT) offers the largest sample size to investigate the effect of CPAP on renal function: Loffler et al. aimed to assess the effects of CPAP on renal function in 200 individuals with coexisting moderate to severe OSA and cardiovascular disease [19]. The median changes in GFR or urinary albumin-to-creatinine ratio in end-of-study between the 102 CPAP users and the 98 subjects with usual care alone did not differ after a median of 4.4 years of follow-up. Although the results of this study do not support the use of CPAP for renal protection in patients with sleep apnea, the study presented several limitations: the majority of patients did not have CKD at baseline, patients with severe nocturnal hypoxia were excluded, and based on comorbidities, patients included were unlikely to be at high risk for loss of kidney function.

In conclusion, given that chronic renal hypoxia and glomerular hyperfiltration through activation of RAS are the two major pathways that lead to kidney diseases in patients with OSA and given the well-known impact of CPAP on hypoxia and RAS amelioration, more unidirectional evidences would be expected in literature about CPAP contribution to the reduction of renal function's decline. The design of future studies should focus on recruitment of OSA patients at risk for kidney disease development or of those with already established kidney failure, to better clarify the role of PAP therapy in kidney function protection among patients with sleep disordered breathing.

Liver Co-Morbidities

Liver disease represents a broad spectrum of disorders that include both alcoholic liver disease (ALD) and nonalcoholic fatty liver disease (NAFLD). Whilst the former is associated with cirrhosis and has been less investigated in the field of sleep disordered breathing, the latter includes different liver diseases such as fatty liver (liver steatosis) and nonalcoholic steato-hepatitis (NASH) and has been linked with sleep apnea through the repetitive cycles of nocturnal hypoxia which are capable of induce liver injury and steatosis. Furthermore, NAFLD has been associated with metabolic syndrome and cardiovascular co-morbidities.

However, the effect of OSA treatment, mainly by means of CPAP, on liver disease in subjects with OSA is controversial. When the main outcome was liver function, expressed with liver enzyme levels, observational studies showed that CPAP treatment allowed to obtain a significant reduction of liver enzymes with a more pronounced effect in patients compliant to CPAP treatment.

However, randomized controlled trials (RCTs) did not confirm such findings: Kohler and colleagues showed that 4 weeks of CPAP treatment did not determine a significant reduction of liver enzymes compared to sham treatment in patients with moderate to severe OSA who received either therapeutic or sub-therapeutic CPAP [20].

Observational studies assessing liver fat with computed tomography scan showed that long term CPAP treatment was associated with improvement of fatty liver in OSA patients independently of confounding factors such as body mass index (BMI) and lipid levels. But again RCTs did not show any change in liver fat in patients randomized on CPAP even when liver fat was quantified by magnetic resonance imaging and magnetic resonance spectroscopy [21].

Evidence of a potential beneficial role of CPAP in patients with NAFLD is even less convincing when authors tried to investigate the effect on the developement of liver fibrosis.

The Grenoble group randomized 103 patients to either receive CPAP treatment or sham-CPAP treatment for 6, 8, or 12 weeks. Liver fibrosis was assessed with the FibroMax score, a non-invasive method to assess liver injury [22].

At follow up, CPAP did not demonstrate any impact on reducing liver fibrosis, neither in the intention-to-treat nor in the per-protocol analysis, even when data were adjusted for gender, liver injury, BMI, CPAP compliance, and baseline apnea/hypopnea index.

Despite the relatively low number of studies, taken together these findings suggest that treatment of OSA by means of CPAP has only a modest effect in improving liver function and reduce the progression of NAFLD in liver fibrosis. Although this effect can be masked by the several confounders, it could be speculated that a greater beneficial effect of OSA treatment can be seen in early stages of NAFLD compared to the later stage, when liver fibrosis is already present.

In fact, a recent retrospective study on 17,374 patients followed up for 10 years showed that CPAP treatment significantly decreased cumulative incidence rate of developing liver disease, after adjusting for age, gender, urbanization level, and comorbidities [23].

Furthermore, it is important to note that the treatment duration in the RCTs was shorter than in prospective studies suggesting that perhaps a short duration of CPAP treatment does not lead to a significant observable effect whilst longer treatment period may eventually show a more consistent improvement.

References

[1] Lugaresi E, Cirignotta F, Coccagna G, et al. Some epidemiological data on snoring and cardiocirculatory disturbances. *Sleep* 1980;3:221-4.

[2] Bisogni V, Pengo MF, Maiolino G, Rossi GP. The sympathetic nervous system and catecholamines metabolism in obstructive sleep apnoea. *J. Thorac. Dis.* 2016;8(2):243-54.

[3] Fava C, Dorigoni S, Dalle Vedove F, et al. Effect of CPAP on blood pressure in patients with OSA/hypopnea a systematic review and meta-analysis. *Chest.* 2014;145(4):762-771.

[4] Schwarz EI, Schlatzer C, Rossi VA, Stradling JR, Kohler M. Effect of CPAP withdrawal on BP in OSA: data from three randomized controlled trials. *Chest.* 2016;150(6):1202-10.

[5] McEvoy RD, Antic NA, Heeley E, et al. CPAP for Prevention of Cardiovascular Events in Obstructive Sleep Apnea. *N. Engl. J. Med.* 2016;375(10):919-931.

[6] Kaneko Y, Floras JS, Usui K, Plante J, Tkacova R, Kubo T, Ando S, Bradley TD. Cardiovascular effects of continuous positive airway pressure in patients with heart failure and obstructive sleep apnea. *N. Engl. J. Med.* 2003; 348:1233-124.

[7] Bradley TD, Logan AG, Kimoff RJ, Sériès F, Morrison D, Ferguson K, Belenkie I, Pfiefer M, Fleetham J, Hanly P, Smilovitch M, Tomlinson G, Floras JS; CANPAP Investigators. Continuous positive airway pressure for central sleep apnea and heart failure. *N. Engl. J. Med.* 2005; 353:2025-2033.

[8] Momomura S, Seino Y, Kihara Y, Adachi H, Yasumura Y, Yokoyama H, Wada H, Ise T, Tanaka K; SAVIOR-C Investigators. Adaptive servo-ventilation therapy for patients with chronic heart failure in a confirmatory, multicenter, randomized, controlled study. *Circ. J.* 2015; 79:981-990.

[9] Cowie MR, Woehrle H, Wegscheider K, Angermann C, d'Ortho MP, Erdmann E, Levy P, Simonds AK, Somers VK, Zannad F, Teschler H. Adaptive servo-ventilation for central sleep apnea in systolic heart failure. *N. Engl. J. Med.* 2015; 373:1095-1105.

[10] Mattaliano P, Lombardi C, Sangalli D, et al. Impact of obstructive sleep apnea on cardiac organ damage in patients with acute ischemic stroke. *J. Hypertens.* 2018;36(6):1351-1359.

[11] Mehra R, Benjamin EJ, Shahar E, et al. Association of nocturnal arrhythmias with sleep-disordered breathing: The Sleep Heart Health Study. *Am. J. Respir. Crit. Care Med.* 2006;173(8):910-916.

[12] Holmqvist F, Guan N, Zhu Z, Kowey PR, Allen LA, Fonarow GC, Hylek EM, Mahaffey KW, Freeman JV, Chang P, Holmes DN, Peterson ED, Piccini JP, Gersh BJ; ORBIT-AF Investigators. Impact of obstructive sleep apnea and continuous positive airway pressure therapy on outcomes in patients with atrial fibrillation - results from the Outcomes Registry for Better Informed Treatment of Atrial Fibrillation (ORBIT-AF). *Am. Heart J.* 2015; 169:647-654.e642.

[13] da Silva Paulitsch F, Zhang L. Continuous positive airway pressure for adults with obstructive sleep apnea and cardiovascular disease: a meta-analysis of randomized trials. *Sleep Med.* 2019;54:28-34.

[14] Barbé F, Durán-Cantolla J, Sánchez-de-la-Torre M, Martínez-Alonso M, Carmona C, Barceló A, Chiner E, Masa JF, Gonzalez M, Marín JM, Garcia-Rio F, Diaz de Atauri J, Terán J, Mayos M, de la Peña M, Monasterio C, del Camp F, Montserrat JM; Spanish Sleep and Breathing Network. Effect of continuous positive airway pressure on the incidence of hypertension and cardiovascular events in nonsleepy patients with obstructive sleep apnea: a randomized controlled trial. *JAMA.* 2012; 307:2161-2168.

[15] Lyons, Inami, Perger. The effect of fluid overload on sleep apnoea severity in haemodialysis patients. *Eur. Respir. J.* 2017; 49: 4.

[16] Kinebuchi S, Kazama JJ, Satoh M, et al. Short-term use of continuous positive airway pressure ameliorates glomerular hyperfiltration in patients with obstructive sleep apnoea syndrome. *Clin. Sci.* (Lond) 2004;107:317-22.

[17] Koga S, Ikeda S, Yasunaga T, Nakata T, Maemura K. Effects of nasal continuous positive airway pressure on the glomerular filtration rate in patients with obstructive sleep apnea syndrome. *Intern. Med.* 2013;52:345-9.

[18] Marrone, Cibella, Fixed but not autoadjusting positive airways paressure attenuates the time-dependent decline in glomerular filtration rate in patients with OSA. *Chest* 2018.

[19] Loffler KA, Heeley E, Freed R, et al. Effect of Obstructive Sleep Apnea Treatment on Renal Function in Patients with Cardiovascular Disease. *Am. J. Respir. Crit. Care Med.* 2017; 196:1456-1462.

[20] Kohler M, Pepperell JC, Davies RJ, Stradling JR. Continuous positive airway pressure and liver enzymes in obstructive sleep apnoea: data from a randomized controlled trial. *Respiration*. 2009;78(2):141-146.

[21] Sivam S, Phillips CL, Trenell MI, et al. Effects of 8 weeks of continuous positive airway pressure on abdominal adiposity in obstructive sleep apnoea. *Eur. Respir. J.* 2012;40(4):913-918.

[22] Jullian-Desayes I, Tamisier R, Zarski JP, et al. Impact of effective versus sham continuous positive airway pressure on liver injury in obstructive sleep apnoea: Data from randomized trials. *Respirology*. 2016;21(2):378-385.

[23] Hang LW, Chen CF, Wang CB, Wu TN, Liang WM, Chou TC. The association between continuous positive airway pressure therapy and liver disease development in obstructive sleep apnea/hypopnea syndrome patients: a nationwide population-based cohort study in Taiwan. *Sleep Breath*. 2017;21(2):461-467.

In: Sleep Medicine in Critical Care
Editors: Antonio M. Esquinas et al.
ISBN: 978-1-53617-768-8

Chapter 11

NASAL HIGH FLOW THERAPY

Tristan Bonnevie[1], Antoine Cuvelier[2], MD, PhD
and Maxime Patout[2,*], MD

[1]Normandie Univ, Institute for Research and Innovation in Biomedicine (IRIB) and ADIR Association, Bois-Guillaume, France

[2]Normandie Univ, UNIRouen, Institute for Research and Innovation in Biomedicine (IRIB) and Rouen University Hospital, Service de Pneumologie, Oncologie thoracique et Soins Intensifs Respiratoires, Rouen, France

ABSTRACT

High flow therapy is a novel treatment that delivers warm, humidified air at a high flow. High flow therapy has numerous beneficial physiological effects and is now validated for the management of severe acute respiratory failure. Its use in the home setting is feasible. However, to date, the use of high flow therapy during sleep has only been shown to be effective for the management of obstructive sleep apnea in children.

Keywords: high flow therapy, hypoventilation, sleep apnea, sleep disordered breathing, COPD

---

* Corresponding Author's E-mail: France maxime.patout@chu-rouen.fr.

INTRODUCTION

High flow therapy is a novel treatment modality. High flow therapy is delivered through an electrically powered device that can generate a flow of air up to 60L/min. To avoid side effects of such level of flow, the delivered air is heated and humidified. Today, high flow therapy is mainly used with the adjunction of oxygen. As the generated flow is greater than patient's peak inspiratory flow, high flow therapy devices can provide an inspired fraction of oxygen up to 1.

In this chapter, we will first review the physiological benefits of high flow therapy. Then, we will review its current use and finally we will see how it could be used in the management of sleep disordered breathing.

PHYSIOLOGICAL BENEFITS OF HIGH FLOW THERAPY

In addition to the level of oxygen delivered, most high flow therapy devices allow adjustment of three parameters: the level of flow delivered, the temperature of the air delivered, and the humidity of the air delivered. These three parameters have different physiological effects.

Effects Related to High Flow Air Delivery

The flow generated by high flow therapy devices creates a positive pressure. The level of positive airway pressure is low and linearly correlated to the flow with a 1.16cmH2O per 10L/min of flow (Parke, Bloch, and McGuinness 2015). The level of positive airway pressure depends on month opening (Groves and Tobin 2007). It also varies according to upper airway dimension as it was shown that the level of positive airway pressure was higher in women when compared to men (Groves and Tobin 2007) and as a great intra-individual variability is observed (Parke, Bloch, and McGuinness 2015). The positive airway pressure produced by high flow therapy devices have in impact in lung volumes as it increase the end-expiratory lung volume (Parke, Bloch, and McGuinness 2015).

The flow generated also performs a wash-out of the upper airway as demonstrated by Moller et al., in an experimental model (Möller et al., 2015). Upper airway washout contributes to the decrease in capillary carbon dioxide seen in COPD patients (Bräunlich, Mauersberger, and Wirtz 2018).

Effects Related to Warmth and Humidified Air Delivery

In an animal tracheal explant model, it has been shown that humidity and temperature were key factors for tracheal ciliary beat frequency and mucus transport velocity. The best outcome was seen when temperature was set at 37°C and humidity at 100% (Kilgour et al., 2004).

These experimental results were confirmed:

- In patients admitted for acute respiratory failure. It was shown that standard oxygen therapy, delivered at 9L/min, was less comfortable than high flow therapy, delivered at 12L/min but at 37° C. Similarly, nose dryness was worst in the standard oxygen group (Cuquemelle et al., 2012).
- In newly tracheostomized patients for whom the administration of heated humidified air improved ciliary beat frequency and improved airway clearance (Birk et al., 2017).

Because of the humidification delivered and the warmth delivered, high flow therapy improves airway humidification and airway clearance.

Effects of High Flow Therapy on ventilation

The consequences of high flow therapy in the respiratory mechanics have been assessed in both acute and chronic patients.

The use of high flow oxygen therapy reduces the work of breathing in stable severe COPD patients (Pisani et al., 2017) and in patients with acute respiratory failure (Mauri et al., 2017; Delorme et al., 2017). This improvement in associated to an improvement in breathlessness (Pisani et al., 2017).

Despite reducing minute ventilation, high flow therapy reduces arterial carbon dioxide. This effect is explained by a reduction in dead space ventilation (Biselli et al., 2018).

Current Use of High Flow Therapy

In the Hospital Setting

High flow therapy is now well implemented in intensive care units for the management acute hypoxemic respiratory failure.

In a first large scale randomized clinical trial, it was shown that the use of high flow therapy improved mortality in the overall population and decreased intubation rate patients with P_aO_2 / F_iO_2 < 200mmHg (Frat et al., 2015). Similar benefit failed to be shown in immunocompromised patients (Azoulay et al., 2018). A meta-analysis that included 2093 patients from randomized controlled trials showed that high flow therapy decreased the need for tracheal intubation when compared to standard oxygen therapy (Rochwerg et al., 2019).

As high flow therapy reduces work of breathing, its use has been evaluated as an alternative to NIV. No benefit was shown prior to intubation when compared to non-invasive ventilation (Frat et al., 2019). Following extubation, there is conflicting results regarding the use of high flow therapy alone instead of non-invasive ventilation (Thille et al., 2019; Hernández et al., 2016). To date, there is no data suggesting a benefit in the use of high flow therapy in hypercapnic respiratory failure even if some non-randomized controlled trials suggest some efficacy (Bräunlich and Wirtz 2018; Lee et al., 2018).

In the Home Setting

In patients with chronic respiratory failure, the level of evidence supporting the use of high flow therapy is lower.

Rea et al., showed that the use of high flow therapy lengthened time to first exacerbation. This result was achieved in a heterogenous population of patients with COPD or bronchiectatic diseases. The use of high flow was low in this trial with a mean use of 1.6hours/day (Rea et al., 2010). Storgaard et al., showed a reduction of the number of acute exacerbations in a population of stable COPD patients. However, in that study, acute exacerbations were self-reported by the patient who was not blinded to of the treatment. In this study, compliance to treatment was 6hours/day over the study period. Finally, this study evaluated stable COPD which may have led to select a population with a low risk of acute exacerbation (Storgaard et al., 2018). If the impact of high flow therapy on exacerbation remains to be confirmed, both studies showed an improvement in quality of life and daytime carbon dioxide (Bonnevie et al., 2019).

We have shown that high flow therapy could be used in the home setting as part of patients care (Dolidon et al., 2019). Therefore, high flow therapy may be a treatment option in the home setting in order to treat sleep disordered breathing.

THE USE OF HIGH FLOW THERAPY DURING SLEEP

High flow therapy has not been validated for overnight use to date. However, this treatment modality is well tolerated and its home use associated with few to none side effects (Nagata et al., 2018).

High Flow Therapy in Patients with Sleep Apnea

In children, because of their smaller upper airway dimension, high flow therapy can provide sufficient pressure in order to provide an effective treatment to premature neonates (Sreenan et al., 2001). In children with obstructive sleep apnea, the use of high flow therapy at 20L/min has been shown to achieve similar control as continuous positive airway pressure (McGinley et al., 2009). Although, no randomized controlled has been conducted, several cohort studies have shown efficacy for the control of apneic events (Hawkins et al., 2017; Joseph et al., 2015).

In adults, very few data report the use of high flow therapy to treat obstructive sleep apnea. This can be explained by the fact that the level of pressure achieved to maintain upper airway patency is too low to control apneic events. However, in addition to the level of positive pressure, high flow therapy increases lung volume and therefore lower the risk of upper airway obstruction (Biselli et al., 2015). Small series have reported its use during the postoperative period in patients that were intolerant to continuous positive airway pressure (Gobindram, Singh, and Quek 2019) or in tracheostomized patients for which high flow therapy was delivered through the tracheostomy (Schneider et al., 2012).

High Flow Therapy in Patients with Nocturnal Hypoxemia

Nocturnal hypoxemia is mainly seen in patients with COPD. Treatment of nocturnal hypoxemia has not been shown to improve patient's outcome in COPD patients (Chaouat et al., 1999). In other conditions, such as lone obesity hypoventilation syndrome, nocturnal oxygen therapy has never been assessed.

During sleep, in COPD patients, nasal high flow therapy decrease the work of breathing during sleep (Biselli et al., 2017). It has also been shown that nasal high flow therapy reduced sympathetic activity during sleep in COPD patients (Fricke et al., 2018). Such effect was not seen in the same population with standard oxygen therapy and is therefore related to high-flow therapy itself. The clinical consequences of such findings remain to be evaluated.

Conclusion

High flow therapy has several physiological effects that may be beneficial during sleep. However, to date, the level of evidence supporting its use outside of intensive care units remains limited.

References

Azoulay, Elie, Virginie Lemiale, Djamel Mokart, Saad Nseir, Laurent Argaud, Frédéric Pène, Loay Kontar, et al., 2018. "Effect of High-Flow Nasal Oxygen vs Standard Oxygen on 28-Day Mortality in Immunocompromised Patients with Acute Respiratory Failure: the HIGH Randomized Clinical Trial." *JAMA: the Journal of the American Medical Association* 320 (20): 2099–2107. doi:10.1001/ jama.2018.14282.

Birk, Richard, Alexander Händel, Angela Wenzel, Benedikt Kramer, Christoph Aderhold, Karl Hörmann, Boris A Stuck, and J Ulrich Sommer. 2017. "Heated Air Humidification Versus Cold Air Nebulization in Newly Tracheostomized Patients." *Head & Neck* 39 (12): 2481–87. doi:10.1002/hed.24917.

Biselli, Paolo J C, Jason P Kirkness, Ludger Grote, Kathrin Fricke, Alan R Schwartz, Philip Smith, and Hartmut Schneider. 2017. "Nasal High-Flow Therapy Reduces Work of Breathing Compared with Oxygen During Sleep in COPD and Smoking Controls: a Prospective Observational Study." *J. Appl. Physiol.* 122 (1): 82–88. doi:10.1152/japplphysiol.00279.2016.

Biselli, Paolo, Kathrin Fricke, Ludger Grote, Andrew T Braun, Jason Kirkness, Philip Smith, Alan Schwartz, and Hartmut Schneider. 2018. "Reductions in Dead Space Ventilation with Nasal High Flow Depend on Physiological Dead Space Volume: Metabolic Hood Measurements During Sleep in Patients with COPD and Controls." *European Respiratory Journal* 51 (5): 1702251.

Biselli, Paolo, Peter R Grossman, Jason P Kirkness, Susheel P Patil, Philip L Smith, Alan R Schwartz, and Hartmut Schneider. 2015. "The Effect of Increased Lung Volume in Chronic Obstructive Pulmonary Disease on Upper Airway Obstruction During Sleep." *Journal of Applied Physiology* 119 (3): 266–71. doi:10.1152/ japplphysiol.00455.2014.

Bonnevie, Tristan, Mark Elkins, Clément Paumier, Clément Medrinal, Yann Combret, Maxime Patout, Jean Francois Muir, Antoine Cuvelier, Francis-Edouard Gravier, and Guillaume Prieur. 2019. "Nasal High Flow for Stable Patients with Chronic Obstructive Pulmonary Disease: a Systematic Review and Meta-Analysis." *Copd*, October, 1–10. doi:10.1080/15412555.2019.1672637.

Bräunlich, Jens, and Hubert Wirtz. 2018. "Nasal High-Flow in Acute Hypercapnic Exacerbation of COPD." *International Journal of Chronic Obstructive Pulmonary Disease* 13: 3895–97. doi:10.2147/ COPD.S185001.

Bräunlich, Jens, Friederike Mauersberger, and Hubert Wirtz. 2018. "Effectiveness of Nasal Highflow in Hypercapnic COPD Patients Is Flow and Leakage Dependent." *BMC Pulmonary Medicine* 18 (1): 14. doi:10.1186/s12890-018-0576-x.

Chaouat, A, E Weitzenblum, R Kessler, C Charpentier, M Ehrhart, R Schott, P Levi-Valensi, et al., 1999. "A Randomized Trial of Nocturnal Oxygen Therapy in Chronic Obstructive Pulmonary Disease Patients." *European Respiratory Journal* 14 (5): 1002–8. doi:10.1183/ 09031936.99.14510029.

Cuquemelle, Elise, Tai Pham, Jean-François Papon, Bruno Louis, Pierre-Eric Danin, and Laurent Brochard. 2012. "Heated and Humidified High-Flow Oxygen Therapy Reduces Discomfort During Hypoxemic Respiratory Failure." *Respiratory Care* 57 (10): 1571–77. doi:10.4187/ respcare.01681.

Delorme, Mathieu, Pierre-Alexandre Bouchard, Mathieu Simon, Serge Simard, and François Lellouche. 2017. "Effects of High-Flow Nasal Cannula on the Work of Breathing in Patients Recovering From Acute Respiratory Failure." *Critical Care Medicine* 45 (12): 1981–88. doi:10.1097/CCM.0000000000002693.

Dolidon, Samuel, Johann Dupuis, Luis-Carlos Molano Valencia, Mathieu Salaün, Luc Thiberville, Jean Francois Muir, Antoine Cuvelier, and Maxime Patout. 2019. "Characteristics and Outcome of Patients Set Up on High-Flow Oxygen Therapy at Home." *Therapeutic Advances in Respiratory Disease* 13 (January). SAGE Publications Sage UK: London, England: 1753466619879794. doi:10.1177/ 175346661 9879794.

Frat, Jean-Pierre, Arnaud W Thille, Alain Mercat, Christophe Girault, Stéphanie Ragot, Sébastien Perbet, Gwénael Prat, et al., 2015. "High-Flow Oxygen Through Nasal Cannula in Acute Hypoxemic Respiratory Failure." *The New England Journal of Medicine* 372 (23): 2185–96. doi:10.1056/NEJMoa1503326.

Frat, Jean-Pierre, Jean-Damien Ricard, Jean-Pierre Quenot, Nicolas Pichon, Alexandre Demoule, Jean-Marie Forel, Jean-Paul Mira, et al., 2019. "Non-Invasive Ventilation Versus High-Flow Nasal Cannula Oxygen Therapy with Apnoeic Oxygenation for Preoxygenation Before Intubation of Patients with Acute Hypoxaemic Respiratory Failure: a Randomised, Multicentre, Open-Label Trial." *The Lancet. Respiratory Medicine* 7 (4): 303–12. doi:10.1016/S2213-2600(19) 30048-7.

Fricke, K, H Schneider, P Biselli, N N Hansel, Z G Zhang, M O Sowho, and L Grote. 2018. "Nasal High Flow, but Not Supplemental O_2, Reduces Peripheral Vascular Sympathetic Activity During Sleep in COPD Patients." *International Journal of Chronic Obstructive Pulmonary Disease* 13: 3635–43.

Gobindram, Avinash, Prit Anand Singh, and Kelvin Howyow Quek. 2019. "Postoperative Use of High Flow Nasal Insufflation for Obstructive Sleep Apnea." *Korean Journal of Anesthesiology* 72 (6): 610–13. doi:10.4097/kja.d.18.00368.

Groves, Nicole, and Antony Tobin. 2007. "High Flow Nasal Oxygen Generates Positive Airway Pressure in Adult Volunteers." *Australian Critical Care* 20 (4): 126–31. doi:10.1016/j.aucc.2007.08.001.

Hawkins, Stephen, Stephanie Huston, Kristen Campbell, and Ann Halbower. 2017. "High-Flow, Heated, Humidified Air via Nasal Cannula Treats CPAP-Intolerant Children with Obstructive Sleep Apnea." *Journal of Clinical Sleep Medicine: JCSM: Official Publication of the American Academy of Sleep Medicine* 13 (8): 981–89.

Hernández, Gonzalo, Concepción Vaquero, Paloma González, Carles Subira, Fernando Frutos-Vivar, Gemma Rialp, Cesar Laborda, Laura Colinas, Rafael Cuena, and Rafael Fernandez. 2016. "Effect of Postextubation High-Flow Nasal Cannula vs Conventional Oxygen Therapy on Reintubation in Low-Risk Patients: a Randomized Clinical Trial. - PubMed - NCBI." *JAMA: the Journal of the American Medical Association* 315 (13): 1354.

Joseph, Leon, Shmuel Goldberg, Michal Shitrit, and Elie Picard. 2015. "High-Flow Nasal Cannula Therapy for Obstructive Sleep Apnea in Children." *Journal of Clinical Sleep Medicine: JCSM: Official Publication of the American Academy of Sleep Medicine* 11 (9): 1007–10. doi:10.5664/jcsm.5014.

Kilgour, Emma, Nigel Rankin, Stuart Ryan, and Rodger Pack. 2004. "Mucociliary Function Deteriorates in the Clinical Range of Inspired Air Temperature and Humidity." *Intensive Care Medicine* 30 (7): 1491–94. doi:10.1007/s00134-004-2235-3.

Lee, Myoung Kyu, Jaehwa Choi, Bonil Park, Bumjoon Kim, Seok Jeong Lee, Sang-Ha Kim, Suk Joong Yong, Eun Hee Choi, and Won-Yeon Lee. 2018. "High Flow Nasal Cannulae Oxygen Therapy in Acute-Moderate Hypercapnic Respiratory Failure." *The Clinical Respiratory Journal* 12 (6): 2046–56. doi:10.1111/crj.12772.

Mauri, Tommaso, Cecilia Turrini, Nilde Eronia, Giacomo Grasselli, Carlo Alberto Volta, Giacomo Bellani, and Antonio Pesenti. 2017. "Physiologic Effects of High-Flow Nasal Cannula in Acute Hypoxemic Respiratory Failure." *American Journal of Respiratory and Critical Care Medicine* 195 (9): 1207–15. doi:10.1164/ rccm. 201605-0916OC.

McGinley, B, A Halbower, A R Schwartz, P L Smith, S P Patil, and H Schneider. 2009. "Effect of a High-Flow Open Nasal Cannula System on Obstructive Sleep Apnea in Children." *Pediatrics* 124 (1): 179–88. doi:10.1542/peds.2008-2824.

Möller, Winfried, Gülnaz Celik, Sheng Feng, Peter Bartenstein, Gabriele Meyer, Eickelberg Oliver, Otmar Schmid, and Stanislav Tatkov. 2015. "Nasal High Flow Clears Anatomical Dead Space in Upper Airway Models." *J. Appl. Physiol.* 118 (12): 1525–32. doi:10.1152/ japplphysiol.00934.2014.

Nagata, Kazuma, Takashi Kikuchi, Takeo Horie, Akira Shiraki, Takamasa Kitajima, Toru Kadowaki, Fumiaki Tokioka, et al., 2018. "Domiciliary High-Flow Nasal Cannula Oxygen Therapy for Patients with Stable Hypercapnic Chronic Obstructive Pulmonary Disease. a Multicenter Randomized Crossover Trial." *Annals of the American Thoracic Society* 15 (4): 432–39. doi:10.1513/AnnalsATS.201706-425OC.

Parke, Rachael L, Andreas Bloch, and Shay P McGuinness. 2015. "Effect of Very-High-Flow Nasal Therapy on Airway Pressure and End-Expiratory Lung Impedance in Healthy Volunteers." *Respiratory Care* 60 (10): 1397–1403. doi:10.4187/ respcare.04028.

Pisani, Lara, Luca Fasano, Nadia Corcione, Vittoria Comellini, Muriel Assunta Musti, Maria Brandao, Damiano Bottone, Edoardo Calderini, Paolo Navalesi, and Stefano Nava. 2017. "Change in Pulmonary Mechanics and the Effect on Breathing Pattern of High Flow Oxygen Therapy in Stable Hypercapnic COPD." *Thorax* 72 (4): 373–75. doi:10.1136/thoraxjnl-2016-209673.

Rea, Harold, Sue McAuley, Lata Jayaram, Jeffrey Garrett, Hans Hockey, Louanne Storey, Glenis O'Donnell, Lynne Haru, Matthew Payton, and Kevin O'Donnell. 2010. "The Clinical Utility of Long-Term Humidification Therapy in Chronic Airway Disease." *Respiratory Medicine* 104 (4): 525–33. doi:10.1016/ j.rmed.2009.12.016.

Rochwerg, B, D Granton, D X Wang, Y Helviz, S Einav, J P Frat, A Mekontso-Dessap, et al., 2019. "High Flow Nasal Cannula Compared with Conventional Oxygen Therapy for Acute Hypoxemic Respiratory Failure: a Systematic Review and Meta-Analysis." *Intensive Care Medicine* 45 (5): 563–72. doi:10.1007/s00134-019-05590-5.

Schneider, Hartmut, Daniel J O'Hearn, karen Leblanc, Philip L Smith, Christopher P O'Donnel, David W Eisele, J H Peter, and Alan R Schwartz. 2012. "High-Flow Transtracheal Insufflation Treats Obstructive Sleep Apnea." *American Journal of Respiratory and Critical Care Medicine* 161 (6). American Thoracic Society New York, NY: 1869–76. doi:10.1164/ajrccm.161.6.9902061.

Sreenan, C, R P Lemke, A Hudson-Mason, and H Osiovich. 2001. "High-Flow Nasal Cannulae in the Management of Apnea of Prematurity: a Comparison with Conventional Nasal Continuous Positive Airway Pressure." *Pediatrics* 107 (5): 1081–83.

Storgaard, Line Hust, Hans-Ulrich Hockey, Birgitte Schantz Laursen, and Ulla Møller Weinreich. 2018. "Long-Term Effects of Oxygen-Enriched High-Flow Nasal Cannula Treatment in COPD Patients with Chronic Hypoxemic Respiratory Failure." *Copd* 13: 1195–1205.

Thille, Arnaud W, Grégoire Muller, Arnaud Gacouin, Rémi Coudroy, Maxens Decavèle, Romain Sonneville, François Beloncle, et al., 2019. "Effect of Postextubation High-Flow Nasal Oxygen with Noninvasive Ventilation vs High-Flow Nasal Oxygen Alone on Reintubation Among Patients at High Risk of Extubation Failure." *JAMA: the Journal of the American Medical Association* 322 (15): 1465. doi:10.1001/jama.2019.14901.

In: Sleep Medicine in Critical Care
Editors: Antonio M. Esquinas et al.
ISBN: 978-1-53617-768-8

Chapter 12

Options of Mechanical Ventilation in Sleep Related Breathing Disorders: Non-Invasive Mechanical Ventilation

Rebecca F. D'Cruz[1,*], MD
and Georgios Kaltsakas[2,†], MD
[1]Centre for Human and Applied Physiological Science,
School of Basic and Biomedical Science, King's College, London, UK
National Institute for Health Research Biomedical Research Centre, Guy's and St Thomas' NHS Foundation Trust and King's College, London, UK
[2]Lane Fox Clinical Respiratory Physiology Research Centre,
Centre for Human and Applied Physiological Science,
School of Basic and Biomedical Science,
King's College, London, UK

Abstract

Non-invasive ventilation delivers differential positive airways pressures during inspiration and expiration. It may be applied in the management of obesity hypoventilation syndrome, with or without severe obstructive sleep apnoea, and sleep-disordered breathing that occurs in association with chronic obstructive pulmonary disease and neuromuscular disease, including motor neurone disease, muscular dystrophies and chest wall deformities. Nocturnal application of NIV in these settings

* Corresponding Author's E-mail: Rebecca.DCruz@gstt.nhs.uk.
† Corresponding Author's E-mail: Georgios.Kaltsakas@gstt.nhs.uk.

may effectively abolish nocturnal hypoventilation and can improve patient-reported outcomes, including sleepiness and health status, and reduce healthcare utilisation. NIV should be delivered by trained specialists. Patients should be collaboratively involved in decisions relating to interfaces and ventilator settings and provided with access to technical support. All patients should undergo regular clinical follow-up at a specialist ventilation unit. This may be conducted in the outpatient department or, where resources permit, outreach services can deliver home-based care to patients unable to attend hospital appointments.

INTRODUCTION

Non-invasive ventilation (NIV) delivers differential pressures during inspiration and expiration which are termed inspiratory positive airway pressure (IPAP) and expiratory positive airway pressure (EPAP) respectively. Pressure support, which actively unloads respiratory muscles, is the difference between these two pressures. NIV has a wide range of applications in both the critical care and domiciliary settings. It may be applied as part of the management of sleep-related breathing disorders, including Obstructive Sleep Apnoea, Obesity Hypoventilation Syndrome and Central Sleep Apnoea. It may also confer benefits for patients with sleep-related breathing disorders that occur in association with other medical conditions, including neuromuscular diseases and Chronic Obstructive Pulmonary Disease. NIV should be implemented by experienced specialists who can identify patients who may benefit from it, and who are trained in its application.

Delivery of Non-Invasive Ventilation

Setup and delivery of non-invasive ventilation (NIV) should be undertaken by healthcare professionals trained in its application and management of troubleshooting. When establishing patients on NIV, consideration should be given to the type of interface and circuit used, the ventilator modes and its settings, whether humidification or supplementary oxygen should be concurrently administered, and what monitoring is required during setup and long-term delivery.

Interface

There are a range of interfaces through which positive airways pressure (PAP) therapy can be delivered. Oronasal and nasal masks are most commonly used in the management of sleep-related breathing disorders. Alternative available interfaces include full face masks, nasal pillows, mouthpieces and helmets, amongst others (Figure 1).

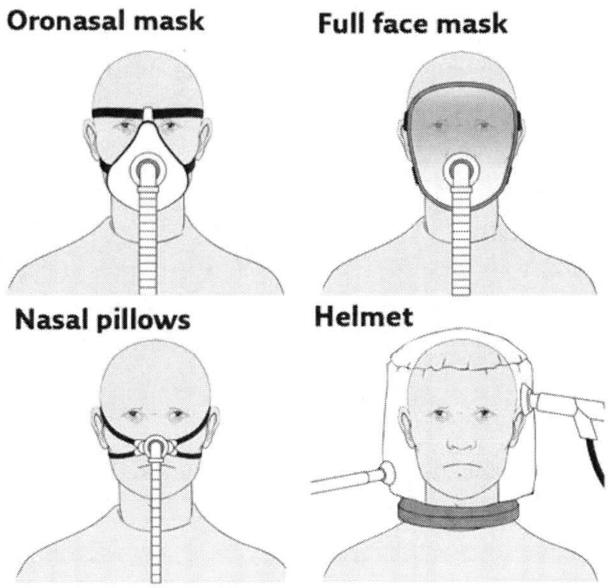

Figure 1. Interfaces for use with non-invasive ventilation.

Image of the Human Head by Patrick J. Lynch Reproduced from Wikimedia Commons under CC BY 2.5 Licence

Consideration must be given to maximize comfort and minimize leak to promote treatment efficacy and adherence. When selecting the interface, the clinician must consider patient-related factors, including the existence of an underlying respiratory disease, anticipated duration of treatment and patients' conscious level, face shape and breathing pattern (nose or mouth breather), and whether the patient experiences claustrophobia with certain interfaces. Local availability of equipment (ventilator models and interface types) and the ease with which patients' (or their caregivers) can apply the interface should be considered. Unlike in the acute setting, where rapid correction of ventilation is necessary, the clinical priority when delivering NIV in the management of sleep-related breathing disorders is treatment adherence. Therefore, although nasal masks and pillows do not achieve as effective short-term correction of $PaCO_2$ as oronasal or full face masks, they are better tolerated by patients [1] and permit oral intake, verbal communication and secretion clearance. They may therefore be considered for patients requiring long-term NIV, particularly those with both day and night ventilation requirements [2]. The choice of interface should involve collaboration with the patient, with the aims of therapy clearly identified. Face shape and patient preference may change during the course of therapy, and this should be addressed regularly and the interface changed if appropriate.

Circuit

Circuits used in the critical care setting are typically dual-limbed and require addition of a leak valve is used in a single limb. Home NIV devices typically use a single limb circuit with integrated leak to prevent carbon dioxide rebreathing. Not all leak systems offer the same properties, which is particularly relevant at low delivered pressures and therefore low flows [3]. Leak from the mask interface is superior in terms of dead space washout and therefore preferable [4].

Ventilator Modes and Settings

There are two principal modes of NIV delivery, pressure-targeted (in which inspiratory pressures are preset) and volume-targeted (in which tidal volume is preset). Volume-preset ventilation is less comfortable due to the pressure swings required to deliver a set tidal volume, and is less commonly employed than pressure-targeted ventilation [5, 6].

IPAP is the higher pressure delivered during inspiration which unloads inspiratory muscles and increases tidal volume and thus ventilation. EPAP is the lower pressure delivered during expiration which promotes upper airway patency and alveolar recruitment. EPAP (also referred to as positive end expiratory pressure, PEEP) may increase expiratory flow and promotes dead space CO_2 removal and, in the presence of intrinsic PEEP, can reduce work of breathing by overcoming this threshold load.

The modes that pressure-targeted ventilation may be delivered in are listed in Table 1:

Table 1. Common ventilator modes

Mode	Mechanisms of action
S (Spontaneous)	Positive pressures are preset and are only delivered in response to patient effort, which is detected by a change in airflow or fall in upper airways pressure.
ST (Spontaneous/Timed)	positive pressures, backup rate (BUR) and inspiratory time (Ti) are preset. Assisted breaths are delivered in response to patient effort and backup breaths if patients' respiratory rate falls below the preset level. The ventilator cycles from the inspiratory into the expiratory pressure after a preset time.
PCV (Pressure Control Ventilation)	positive pressures, BUR and Ti and I:E ratio are preset. The ventilator delivers inspiratory pressure for a preset time, therefore peak airway pressure remains constant.
Volume targeted pressure support modes (e.g., Average Volume Assured Pressure Support (AVAPS), and intelligent volume assured pressure support (iVAPS))	Target tidal volume and maximum inspiratory and expiratory pressures are preset. BUR may be preset or automatically determined by the ventilator. Positive airways pressures are automatically adjusted within a set range to deliver the preset tidal volume [7, 8]

Pressure support ventilation is associated with increased incidence of periodic breathing and central apneas amongst both healthy subjects during sleep and patients with sleep disordered breathing [9, 10]. A backup rate should therefore routinely be set when delivering PSV.

Trigger

There is significant variation in performance of ventilators in time from patient effort to pressure delivery and unloading of the respiratory muscles [17]. Some ventilators permit alterations in trigger sensitivity. With high trigger sensitivity, lower patient effort (change in flow or pressure) is needed for an assisted breath to be delivered.

Humidification

Airway dryness can occur as a result of positive airways pressure and is compounded in patients with a high respiratory rate and high inspiratory flow. Whilst humidification may affect trigger sensitivity and adds to dead space in the ventilator circuit, it has been shown to improve mucociliary function, secretion clearance and comfort [18, 19].

Supplementary Oxygen

Supplementary oxygen may be indicated despite adequate alveolar ventilation with positive airways pressures. Oxygen may be entrained into the circuit using air-oxygen blenders, which is typical of hospital ventilators, or may require connection between the ventilator and oxygen source, as with domiciliary devices. Direct connection of the oxygen source to the mask produces higher arterial oxygen saturation [20].

Location of NIV Setup

Setup of NIV in the management of sleep-related breathing disorders is conventionally undertaken in specialist ventilation centres. Overnight hospital admission with polysomnography is advocated, however limited respiratory polygraphy produces similar results and may be a more pragmatic alternative [21]. During NIV setup, patients are given the opportunity to acclimatize to the interface and settings and receive training on home use and troubleshooting. There is increasing evidence to support out-patient setup to reduce healthcare costs and improve patient access, and has been validated in the neuromuscular and COPD cohorts [22, 23]. Data from trials with patients with OHS (NCT02342899) [24] are pending.

Monitoring during NIV Delivery

NIV devices store a wealth of individual patient data including usage time, tidal volume, respiratory rate, inspiratory and expiratory time, minute ventilation, leak, patient triggered breaths and average pressures delivered (in automatically adjusting modes). Modern ventilators may also have the facility to connect to fingertip pulse oximeters, transcutaneous capnography and thoraco-abdominal belts which provides comprehensive physiological monitoring to assess of sleep-related breathing disorders during NIV delivery that can be performed in patients' homes [25]. Most ventilators provide data on residual apnoea-hypopnoea index, although the estimates they provide may be insufficiently sensitive compared to conventional polygraphy [26].

The data provided by ventilators and associated bespoke software may be utilised in clinical practice. In practice, although inpatient NIV setup is performed during a short hospital admission, it may take patients several weeks or even months for patients to acclimatize and become more compliant with the intervention. Home monitoring of NIV, using either data downloads at outpatient clinic appointments or remote monitoring enabled by wireless internet, may provide useful data to support clinicians in optimizing ventilator settings and the interface, monitoring adherence and identifying remediable factors impeding this [27].

Troubleshooting

Patient Selection

Careful patient selection is required to reduce risk of NIV failure and promote beneficial long-term clinical outcomes. Clinical indications for NIV in the management of sleep-related breathing disorders may include Obesity Hypoventilation Syndrome with or without severe Obstructive Sleep Apnoea, Central Sleep Apnoea and sleep-related breathing disorders associated with concurrent medical conditions, including neuromuscular disease and COPD. Although more applicable in the acute setting, contraindications to NIV should also be reviewed (Table 2).

Table 2. Contraindications to NIV

Relative	Absolute
pH 7.15 (or <7.25 with adverse features)	Haemodynamically unstable or severe acute underlying
Agitation	pathology
Inability to protect airway	Recent upper airway or upper gastrointestinal surgery,
	fixed upper airway obstruction
Aspiration risk	Facial burns

Unintentional Leak

Unintentional air leak may occur between the interface and patient's face or through the mouth when nasal interfaces are used. Consequences may include dry eyes, conjunctivitis and sleep fragmentation caused by the associated noise. Unintentional leak also reduces the pressures delivered to the upper airway and alveoli and can affect trigger sensitivity and cycling, which may lead to patient-ventilator asynchrony. In ventilators using oxygen added into the circuit, unintentional leak also significantly impacts on oxygen delivery [28].

Table 3. Causes of and solutions to unintentional leak

Problem	Solution
Incorrect interface size	Manufacturer guides aid interface size selection.
Unusual facial anatomy	Bespoke masks may be designed in special circumstances.
Excessive tightening	This undermines the interface seal and increases risk of pressure damage. Head straps should be loose enough for two fingers to fit between the patient's face and interface.
Mouth-breathing	Use a full face or oro-nasal mask or, where nasal interfaces are preferred, use a chin strap.

Feeling for air around the interface seal or mouth can aid identification of the site of leak. Some hospital ventilators can estimate leak using internal algorithms. Common causes and possible solutions are provided in Table 3.

Patient-ventilator Asynchrony

Patient-ventilator asynchrony (PVA) is the opposition of patients' ventilatory demand and respiratory muscles to inspiratory flow from the ventilator [29] which cause auto-triggering, ineffective patient inspiratory effort and delayed or premature cycling of the ventilator [29, 30]. Severe PVA is defined as a global asynchrony index of >10 [31] and affects up to 79% of patients during setup of home mechanical ventilation [29]. Those requiring higher pressures or who have higher respiratory rates are at increased risk [32].

Rudimentary assessment for PVA may be done at the bedside using clinical and ventilator-provided parameters, however detailed assessment requires measurement of patient effort from diaphragm electrical activity, oesophageal pressure swings or respiratory inductance plethysmography and ventilator-provided pressure and so are generally limited to specialist centres and research.

Skin Breakdown

Pressure-related skin damage is common and may become a barrier to NIV delivery. It may result from poor interface fit or excessive tightening and patients with co-morbid skin conditions, oedmea or sensory impairment and those who require prolonged ventilation are at higher risk. Interface type, size and fit and patients' skin must be reviewed and inspected regularly. Cushioning systems may be placed between the skin and interface to relieve pressure [33].

Use of Analgesia or Sedation

There is no international consensus on the use of analgesia or sedation to improve NIV adherence and indeed their use in combination is associated with increased risk of NIV failure, prolonged ICU admission and increased 28-day mortality [34]. Clinical practice varies widely according to geographic location and expertise [35]. Opioids and benzodiazepines, which have a rapid onset of action, are most commonly used and may be administered as intermittent boluses or continuous infusion [34]. However, they accumulate and have unpredictable effects, and may cause or exacerbate upper airway collapsibility and obstruction. Remifentanil, propofol and dexmedotomidine are more predictable. They are typically administered as continuous infusions, have a rapid onset of action and cause dose-dependent respiratory depression, however cannot be implemented outside the critical care environment. Given the paucity of evidence, sedation should be restricted to use by experienced clinicians in appropriate environments only in select cases.

NIV in the Management of Sleep-Related Breathing Disorders

Obstructive Sleep Apnoea

This is the occurrence of cyclical upper airway obstruction during sleep which is a consequence of reduced pharyngeal tone during sleep which causes upper airway occlusion. This results in transient and repeated episodes of hypoventilation and respiratory acidosis, which increases neural respiratory drive to overcome the obstruction. When daytime somnolence is present, this is collectively referred to as Obstructive Sleep Apnoea Syndrome (OSAS). OSA is defined as the presence of five or more obstructive events (hypopnoeas or apnoeas) hourly. The apnoea-hyponoea index (AHI), which can be ascertained using polysomnography, is used to grade severity [36].

Continuous positive airways pressure (CPAP), which delivers a relatively fixed positive pressure throughout the respiratory cycle, has been shown in numerous randomised studies to improve a range of patient-reported and physiological outcomes in OSAS compared to sham CPAP, usual care alone or mandibular advancement devices. Benefits have been shown to include improved quality of life and reduced sleepiness, anxiety and depression, lower AHI and 24-hour ambulatory mean arterial blood pressure [37-40].

There are a proportion of patients with OSA who may benefit from treatment with NIV rather than CPAP. Patients with OSA who are obese or those with severe OSA may fail CPAP threrapy, which may be a consequence of uncomfortably high pressures required to abolish upper airway obstruction. In these pressures, it is reasonable to trial a period of NIV, which permits delivery of lower therapeutic pressures which may be more acceptable to the patient [41].

Obesity Hypoventilation Syndrome

The pathophysiological mechanisms causing hypoventilation in obesity are related to:

1. Abnormal mechanical loads on the respiratory muscle pump. This reduces expiratory reserve volume and functional residual capacity [42], impairs lung

compliance and causes early airway closure which leads to development of intrinsic positive end expiratory pressure and basal atelectasis [43]

2. Blunting of the central neural response to hypercapnia. This may be attributable to renal buffering of recurrent brief periods of hypercapnia with raised serum bicarbonate [44] and changes in leptin sensitivity
3. Apnoea and hypopnoeas which are more prolonged than in pure obstructive sleep apnoea (OSA) [45], and rostral fluid shift whilst sleeping supine [46]. These prolonged periods of recurrent hypoventilation in conjunction with a blunted ventilatory response lead to diurnal hypercapnia [47].

Approximately three quarters of patients with OHS have concomitant severe OSA [48]. In these patients, both continuous positive airways pressure (CPAP) and NIV have been shown to improve a range of clinical outcomes, including improved ventilation and reduced sleepiness and healthcare utilisation [49, 50]. A recent randomised trial comparing NIV and CPAP to lifestyle modification alone in OHS patients with severe OSA (AHI ≥30 events/hour) demonstrated that after 2 months of treatment allocation, adherence between the two methods of delivering positive airways pressure were the same (5.3 hours daily), and that both produced similar improvements in arterial partial pressures of carbon dioxide, oxygen and bicarbonate, patient reported outcomes (including OHS symptoms, sleepiness and health related quality of life). Exercise capacity increased in both intervention groups, however 6-minute walk test distance improved more in the group receiving NIV [48]. Both CPAP and NIV appear to confer long-term benefits in these patient, with similar healthcare utilisation, arterial blood gas parameters, blood pressure, cardiovascular outcomes, patient-reported outcomes and spirometry reported after 5 years of treatment [51]. Given the higher device costs of NIV compared to CPAP, depending on local resources and experience, it may be preferable to commence CPAP as first line therapy for OHS patients with severe OSA. In OHS patients without severe OSA, short-term data have shown that NIV may improve $PaCO_2$, sleepiness and AHI and nocturnal oxygenation compared to lifestyle interventions alone after 2 months of treatment [52].

Central Sleep Apnoea

Central sleep apnoea (CSA), where there is cessation of airflow with no associated respiratory effort, may develop in a proportion of OSA patients treated with CPAP [53]. CSA may be classified as "treatment-emergent" if it resolves with ongoing CPAP therapy or "treatment-persistent" if it remains despite ongoing CPAP adherence. Management of CSA with positive airways pressure is controversial. Recent evidence from a randomised study suggests an increased mortality amongst CSA patients with symptomatic heart failure and impaired left ventricular ejection fraction who received adaptive servo-ventilation compared to the control arm [54] (ASV is a form of PAP therapy design to ameliorate the Cheynes-Stokes variant of CSA). Given the current paucity of data, these patients should be referred to specialist ventilation units for management.

Neuromuscular Disease

Amyotrophic Lateral Sclerosis

Amyotrophic Lateral Sclerosis (ALS) is one of the most common adult neurodegenerative diseases and is estimated to affect 4.7 per 100,000 people [55]. Sleep-related breathing disorders are a common complication, affecting between 17-76% of ALS patients [56], and are a consequence of progressive loss of motor neurones causing to respiratory muscle weakness. Patient typically experience altered sleep architecture, nocturnal hypoventilation and, in cases of bulbar involvement, OSA.

The development of sleep-related breathing disorders in ALS indicates respiratory muscle involvement and typically heralds the onset of daytime respiratory symptoms and chronic respiratory failure. Initiation of NIV in clinically stable ALS patients with demonstrable respiratory muscle weakness and normal or moderate bulbar function has been shown to improve survival and quality of life compared to standard multidisciplinary care alone. Those with severe bulbar dysfunction may be poorly tolerant of NIV and, although NIV may improve quality of life, it did not appear to confer a survival benefit in this subgroup [57]. NIV may also improve sleep architecture, with an observational study of ALS patients without bulbar involvement demonstrating improvements in sleep efficiency, arousal-awakening index, ventilation and duration of N3 and REM sleep stages one month after NIV initiation [58]. Given the established benefits in this cohort, NIV should be commenced in ALS patients exhibiting symptoms or signs of chronic respiratory failure and/or objective evidence of respiratory muscle weakness. Initiating NIV at the onset of sleep-related breathing disorders is less well established, however should be considered in clinical practice given the likely imminent onset of chronic respiratory failure.

Other Neuromuscular Diseases and Chest Wall Disease

Respiratory failure is a common complication of many progressive neuromuscular diseases and was uniformly fatal before the development of mechanical ventilation. Patients who develop symptomatic nocturnal hypoventilation or daytime hypercapnia should be commenced on NIV and be managed by specialist centres with multidisciplinary support of secretion management and nutrition [59]. NIV has been shown to improve nocturnal hypoventilation, improve survival and quality of life and reduce risk of hospitalisation in a range of conditions including Duchenne Muscular Dystrophy, Myotonic Dystrophy, Charcot-Marie-Tooth disease and Spinal Muscular Atrophy [60-63].

COPD

OSA is the most common sleep-related breathing disorder amongst COPD patients. There are currently no dedicated guidelines on the application of positive airways pressure in the management of COPD/OSA. Using disease-specific guidelines, it is recommended that CPAP be commenced in the management of non-hypercapnic patients with moderate to severe OSA [64], however caution should be exercised in patients with severe COPD in whom pressures above 10cmH_2O may worsen hyperinflation and increase work of breathing [65]. NIV should be commenced in patients requiring these higher CPAP pressures [65] and in hypercapnic COPD patients, irrespective of the presence of sleep-related breathing disorders [66, 67]. Auto-titrating NIV that can vary inspiratory and expiratory pressures and backup rate in response to patients' upper airway patency, tidal volume and respiratory rate have been evaluated in hypercapnic patients with COPD/OSA overlap syndrome [68]. Auto-titrating NIV was found to achieve as effective control of nocturnal hypoventilation and sleep-related breathing disorders as conventional fixed pressure-support NIV with similar sleep quality achieved when using either device. It was noted that adherence and patient-reported sleep comfort were higher during sleep with auto-titrating NIV.

CONCLUSION

Non-invasive ventilation delivers differential positive airways pressures during inspiration and expiration and is an effective adjunct in the management of obesity hypoventilation syndrome with or without severe obstructive sleep apnoea. It also has an evidence base in the management of sleep-disordered breathing that occurs in association with neuromuscular disease, including motor neurone disease, muscular dystrophies and chest wall deformities, and chronic obstructive pulmonary disease. NIV applied in these contexts may effectively abolish nocturnal hypoventilation, improve patient-reported outcomes and reduce healthcare utilisation. It should be delivered by specialists trained in its application and patients should be collaboratively involved in decisions relating to interfaces and ventilator settings, should be provided with access to technical support as required, and undergo regular clinical follow-up. For those patients unable to attend regular hospital-based outpatient appointments, many specialist ventilation units have the resources to employ outreach services to provide home-based support.

References

[1] Navalesi, P., et al., Physiologic evaluation of noninvasive mechanical ventilation delivered with three types of masks in patients with chronic hypercapnic respiratory failure. *Crit Care Med*, 2000. 28(6): p. 1785-90.

[2] Bach, J. R., et al., Mouth intermittent positive pressure ventilation in the management of postpolio respiratory insufficiency. *Chest*, 1987. 91(6): p. 859-64.

[3] Mehta, S., F. D. McCool, and N. S. Hill, Leak compensation in positive pressure ventilators: a lung model study. *Eur Respir J*, 2001. 17(2): p. 259-67.

[4] Stell, I. M., et al., Noninvasive ventilator triggering in chronic obstructive pulmonary disease. A test lung comparison. *Am J Respir Crit Care Med,* 2001. 164(11): p. 2092-7.

[5] Girault, C., et al., Comparative physiologic effects of noninvasive assist-control and pressure support ventilation in acute hypercapnic respiratory failure. *Chest*, 1997. 111(6): p. 1639-48.

[6] Struik, F. M., et al., Volume-targeted versus pressure-targeted noninvasive ventilation in patients with chest-wall deformity: a pilot study. *Respir Care,* 2011. 56(10): p. 1522-5.

[7] Murphy, P. B., et al., Volume targeted versus pressure support non-invasive ventilation in patients with super obesity and chronic respiratory failure: a randomised controlled trial. *Thorax,* 2012. 67(8): p. 727-34.

[8] Ekkernkamp, E., et al., Impact of intelligent volume-assured pressure support on sleep quality in stable hypercapnic chronic obstructive pulmonary disease patients: a randomized, crossover study. *Respiration*, 2014. 88(4): p. 270-6.

[9] Johnson, K. G. and D. C. Johnson, Bilevel positive airway pressure worsens central apneas during sleep. *Chest,* 2005. 128(4): p. 2141-50.

[10] Parreira, V. F., et al., Effectiveness of controlled and spontaneous modes in nasal two-level positive pressure ventilation in awake and asleep normal subjects. *Chest,* 1997. 112(5): p. 1267-77.

[11] Younes, M., Proportional assist ventilation, a new approach to ventilatory support. Theory. *Am Rev Respir Dis,* 1992. 145(1): p. 114-20.

[12] Hawkins, P., et al., Proportional assist ventilation as an aid to exercise training in severe chronic obstructive pulmonary disease. *Thorax*, 2002. 57(10): p. 853-9.

[13] Hart, N., et al., Comparison of proportional assist ventilation and pressure support ventilation in chronic respiratory failure due to neuromuscular and chest wall deformity. *Thorax,* 2002. 57(11): p. 979-81.

[14] Bianchi, L., et al., Lack of additional effect of adjunct of assisted ventilation to pulmonary rehabilitation in mild COPD patients. *Respir Med,* 2002. 96(5): p. 359-67.

[15] Demoule, A., et al., Neurally adjusted ventilatory assist as an alternative to pressure support ventilation in adults: a French multicentre randomized trial. *Intensive Care Med,* 2016. 42(11): p. 1723-1732.

[16] Ferreira, J. C., et al., Neurally Adjusted Ventilatory Assist (NAVA) or Pressure Support Ventilation (PSV) during spontaneous breathing trials in critically ill patients: a crossover trial. *BMC Pulm Med*, 2017. 17(1): p. 139.

[17] Richard, J. C., et al., Bench testing of pressure support ventilation with three different generations of ventilators. *Intensive Care Med,* 2002. 28(8): p. 1049-57.

[18] Hasani, A., et al., Domiciliary humidification improves lung mucociliary clearance in patients with bronchiectasis. *Chron Respir* Dis, 2008. 5(2): p. 81-6.

[19] Bhowmik, A., et al., Improving mucociliary clearance in chronic obstructive pulmonary disease. *Respir Med,* 2009. 103(4): p. 496-502.

[20] Simonds, A. K., ERS *Practical Handbook of Noninvasive Ventilation.* 2015: European Respiratory Soci.

[21] Patout, M., et al., Polysomnography versus limited respiratory monitoring and nurse-led titration to optimise non-invasive ventilation set-up: a pilot randomised clinical trial. *Thorax*, 2019. 74(1): p. 83-86.

[22] Chatwin, M., et al., Randomised trial of inpatient versus outpatient initiation of home mechanical ventilation in patients with nocturnal hypoventilation. *Respir Med,* 2008. 102(11): p. 1528-35.

[23] Duiverman, M. L., et al., Home initiation of chronic non-invasive ventilation in COPD patients with chronic hypercapnic respiratory failure: a randomised controlled trial. *Thorax*, 2019.

[24] Mandal, S., et al., Medium-term cost-effectiveness of an automated non-invasive ventilation outpatient set-up versus a standard fixed level non-invasive ventilation inpatient set-up in obese patients with chronic respiratory failure: a protocol description. *BMJ Open,* 2015. 5(4): p. e007082.

[25] Borel, J. C., A. Palot, and M. Patout, Technological advances in home non-invasive ventilation monitoring: Reliability of data and effect on patient outcomes. *Respirology*, 2019.

[26] Fernandez Alvarez, R., et al., Monitoring Noninvasive Ventilation in Patients with Obesity Hypoventilation Syndrome: Comparison between Ventilator Built-in Software and Respiratory Polygraphy. *Respiration*, 2017. 93(3): p. 162-169.

[27] Mansell, S. K., et al., Using domiciliary non-invasive ventilator data downloads to inform clinical decision-making to optimise ventilation delivery and patient compliance. *BMJ Open Respir Res,* 2018. 5(1): p. e000238.

[28] Schwartz, A. R., R. M. Kacmarek, and D. R. Hess, Factors affecting oxygen delivery with bi-level positive airway pressure. *Respir Care,* 2004. 49(3): p. 270-5.

[29] Ramsay, M., et al., Parasternal electromyography to determine the relationship between patient-ventilator asynchrony and nocturnal gas exchange during home mechanical ventilation set-up. *Thorax,* 2015. 70(10): p. 946-52.

[30] Vignaux, L., et al., Patient-ventilator asynchrony during non-invasive ventilation for acute respiratory failure: a multicenter study. *Intensive Care Med,* 2009. 35(5): p. 840-6.

[31] Thille, A. W., et al., Patient-ventilator asynchrony during assisted mechanical ventilation. *Intensive Care Med,* 2006. 32(10): p. 1515-22.

[32] Fanfulla, F., et al., Effect of sleep on patient/ventilator asynchrony in patients undergoing chronic non-invasive mechanical ventilation. *Respir Med,* 2007. 101(8): p. 1702-7.

[33] Nava, S., P. Navalesi, and C. Gregoretti, Interfaces and humidification for noninvasive mechanical ventilation. *Respir Care,* 2009. 54(1): p. 71-84.

[34] Muriel, A., et al., Impact of sedation and analgesia during noninvasive positive pressure ventilation on outcome: a marginal structural model causal analysis. *Intensive Care Med,* 2015. 41(9): p. 1586-600.

[35] Devlin, J. W., et al., Survey of sedation practices during noninvasive positive-pressure ventilation to treat acute respiratory failure. *Crit Care Med,* 2007. 35(10): p. 2298-302.

[36] Berry, R. B., R. Brookes, and C. E. Gamaldo, *The AASM Manual for the Scoring of Sleep and Associated Events: Rules, Terminology and Technical Specifications.* 2017, Darien, IL: American Academy of Sleep Medicine.

[37] Buchner, N. J., et al., Continuous positive airway pressure treatment of mild to moderate obstructive sleep apnea reduces cardiovascular risk. *Am J Respir Crit Care Med*, 2007. 176(12): p. 1274-80.

[38] Giles, T. L., et al., Continuous positive airways pressure for obstructive sleep apnoea in adults. *Cochrane Database Syst Rev,* 2006(3): p. CD001106.

[39] McDaid, C., et al., A systematic review of continuous positive airway pressure for obstructive sleep apnoea-hypopnoea syndrome. *Sleep* Med Rev, 2009. 13(6): p. 427-36.

[40] Haentjens, P., et al., The impact of continuous positive airway pressure on blood pressure in patients with obstructive sleep apnea syndrome: evidence from a meta-analysis of placebo-controlled randomized trials. *Arch Intern Me*d, 2007. 167(8): p. 757-64.

[41] Schafer, H., et al., Failure of CPAP therapy in obstructive sleep apnoea syndrome: predictive factors and treatment with bilevel-positive airway pressure. *Respir Med,* 1998. 92(2): p. 208-15.

[42] Hodgson, L. E., P. B. Murphy, and N. Hart, Respiratory management of the obese patient undergoing surgery. *J Thorac Dis*, 2015. 7(5): p. 943-52.

[43] Masa, J. F., et al., Obesity hypoventilation syndrome. *Eur Respir Rev,* 2019. 28(151).

[44] Norman, R. G., et al., Transition from acute to chronic hypercapnia in patients with periodic breathing: predictions from a computer model. *J Appl Physiol* (1985), 2006. 100(5): p. 1733-41.

[45] Levy, P., et al., Obstructive sleep apnoea syndrome. *Nat Rev Dis Primers,* 2015. 1: p. 15015.

[46] White, L. H. and T. D. Bradley, Role of nocturnal rostral fluid shift in the pathogenesis of obstructive and central sleep apnoea. *J Physiol,* 2013. 591(5): p. 1179-93.

[47] Ayappa, I., et al., Hypercapnia and ventilatory periodicity in obstructive sleep apnea syndrome. *Am J Respir Crit Care Med,* 2002. 166(8): p. 1112-5.

[48] Masa, J. F., et al., Efficacy of Different Treatment Alternatives for Obesity Hypoventilation Syndrome. Pickwick Study. *Am J Respir Crit Care Med,* 2015. 192(1): p. 86-95.

[49] Salord, N., et al., Continuous positive airway pressure in clinically stable patients with mild-to-moderate obesity hypoventilation syndrome and obstructive sleep apnoea. *Respirology*, 2013. 18(7): p. 1135-42.

[50] Priou, P., et al., Long-term outcome of noninvasive positive pressure ventilation for obesity hypoventilation syndrome. *Chest,* 2010. 138(1): p. 84-90.

[51] Masa, J. F., et al., Long-term clinical effectiveness of continuous positive airway pressure therapy versus non-invasive ventilation therapy in patients with obesity hypoventilation syndrome: a multicentre, open-label, randomised controlled trial. *Lancet,* 2019. 393(10182): p. 1721-1732.

[52] Masa, J. F., et al., Non-invasive ventilation in obesity hypoventilation syndrome without severe obstructive sleep apnoea. *Thorax*, 2016. 71(10): p. 899-906.

[53] Randerath, W., et al., Definition, discrimination, diagnosis and treatment of central breathing disturbances during sleep. *Eur Respir* J, 2017. 49(1).

[54] Cowie, M. R., et al., Adaptive Servo-Ventilation for Central Sleep Apnea in Systolic Heart Failure. *N Engl J Med,* 2015. 373(12): p. 1095-105.

[55] Mehta, P., et al., Prevalence of Amytrophic Lateral Sclerosis - United States, 2012-2013. *MMWR Surveill Summ,* 2016. 65(8): p. 1-12.

[56] Gaig, C. and A. Iranzo, Sleep-disordered breathing in neurodegenerative diseases. *Curr Neurol Neurosci Rep,* 2012. 12(2): p. 205-17.

[57] Bourke, S. C., et al., Effects of non-invasive ventilation on survival and quality of life in patients with amyotrophic lateral sclerosis: a randomised controlled trial. *The Lancet Neurology*, 2006. 5(2): p. 140-147.

[58] Vrijsen, B., et al., Noninvasive ventilation improves sleep in amyotrophic lateral sclerosis: a prospective polysomnographic study. *J Clin Sleep Med*, 2015. 11(5): p. 559-66.

[59] Hull, J., et al., British Thoracic Society guideline for respiratory management of children with neuromuscular weakness. *Thorax,* 2012. 67 Suppl 1: p. i1-40.

[60] Bolton, C. E., et al., British Thoracic Society guideline on pulmonary rehabilitation in adults. *Thorax,* 2013. 68 Suppl 2: p. ii1-30.

[61] Ishikawa, Y., et al., Duchenne muscular dystrophy: survival by cardio-respiratory interventions. *Neuromuscul Disord,* 2011. 21(1): p. 47-51.

[62] Oskoui, M., et al., The changing natural history of spinal muscular atrophy type 1. *Neurology,* 2007. 69(20): p. 1931-6.

[63] Ward, S., et al., Randomised controlled trial of non-invasive ventilation (NIV) for nocturnal hypoventilation in neuromuscular and chest wall disease patients with daytime normocapnia. *Thorax*, 2005. 60: p. 1019-1024.

[64] Patil, S. P., et al., Treatment of Adult Obstructive Sleep Apnea with Positive Airway Pressure: An American Academy of Sleep Medicine Clinical Practice Guideline. *J Clin Sleep Med*, 2019. 15(2): p. 335-343.

[65] O'Donoghue, F. J., et al., Sleep hypoventilation in hypercapnic chronic obstructive pulmonary disease: prevalence and associated factors. *Eur Respir J*, 2003. 21(6): p. 977-84.

[66] Kohnlein, T., et al., Non-invasive positive pressure ventilation for the treatment of severe stable chronic obstructive pulmonary disease: a prospective, multicentre, randomised, controlled clinical trial. *Lancet Respir Med*, 2014. 2(9): p. 698-705.

[67] Murphy, P. B., et al., Effect of Home Noninvasive Ventilation with Oxygen Therapy vs Oxygen Therapy Alone on Hospital Readmission or Death After an Acute COPD Exacerbation: A Randomized Clinical Trial. *JAMA*, 2017. 317(21): p. 2177-2186.

[68] Murphy, P. B., et al., Safety and efficacy of auto-titrating noninvasive ventilation in COPD and obstructive sleep apnoea overlap syndrome. *Eur Respir J,* 2015. 46(2): p. 548-51.

In: Sleep Medicine in Critical Care
Editors: Antonio M. Esquinas et al.
ISBN: 978-1-53617-768-8

Chapter 13

PATTERNS OF RESPONSE TO NON-INVASIVE POSITIVE PRESSURE VENTILATION (NIPPV) IN SLEEP-RELATED BREATHING DISORDERS

Giuseppe Fiorentino[1,*], Anna Annunziata[1] and Antonio M. Esquinas[2]
[1]Respiratory Unit, AO Ospedali dei Colli Monaldi, Naples, Italy
[2]Intensive Care Unit, Hospital Morales Meseguer, Murcia, Spain

ABSTRACT

Sleep-related disorders are life-threatening conditions. The optimal level of treatment should be decided in a sleep laboratory.Side effects directly influencing the patient's adherence to treatment are known. Unintentional leaks are very common in NIV. Leakage may be absent or minimum when the patient is awake, but may worsen during sleep as a result of the loss of voluntary control and reduced muscle tone. Every effort should be made to minimise air leaks, maximise patient comfort and optimise patient-ventilator interaction. The interface is of predominant relevance for adherence to NIV therapy. A variety of masks are now accessible, and producers continue to improve mask design. During NIV, a variable resistance developed by the Upper Airway (UA) is included between the ventilator and the lungs. The UA may change its opposition to airflow, compromising the delivery of an adequate tidal volume to the lungs. Intermittent obstruction of the UA is prevalent during NIV and may be correlated or to obstructive events at the oropharyngeal level.

Keywords: arousal, artificial respiration, critical illness, mechanical ventilator, sleep

---

* Corresponding Author's E-mail: giuseppefiorentino1@gmail.com.

ABBREVIATIONS

AHI	apnea-hypopnea index
ASV	assisted synchronized ventilation
CPAP	continuous positive airway pressure
CSA	central sleep apnoea
EPAP	expired positive pressure
ICU	intensive care unit
IPAP	inspired positive pressure
OHS	obesity-hypoventilation syndromes
OSA	obstructive sleep apnoea/hypopnea syndrome
PAV	proportional assisted ventilation
RDI	respiratory disturbance index
SDB	Sleep-disordered breathing
UA	upper airway resistance

INTRODUCTION

The Sleep-disordered breathing (SDB) comprises several sleep-related breathing disorders: snoring, the obstructive sleep apnoea/hypopnea syndrome (OSA), central sleep apnoea(CSA), hypoventilation syndromes and other rarer forms of disturbed breathing.

OSA is a common disorder that is characterised by repeated episodes of partial or complete closure of the upper airway resultant in disordered breathing during sleep. It is related to decreased quality of life and comorbidities. Untreated OSA can lead to a host of cardiovascular diseases, comprising coronary artery disease, stroke, and atrial fibrillation. Overall, 10% of breathing disorders during sleep are derived from CSA. It is more common in the elderly population and males.

The motive for this remark may lie in the fact that women have a lower apnoeic threshold which stabilises respiration [1]. The term CSA incorporates several different disorders characterised by either hypoventilation or hyperventilation and sensitivity to CO2.These are principal CSA, Cheyne-Stokes respiration, CSA secondary to high-altitude (periodic breathing), CSA secondary to brain-stem lesions and also secondary to drugs (i.e., opioid). Snoring is not a characteristic of this situation unless upper airway obstruction is also present.

Clinical presentation of patients with CSA will also diverge concerning the underlying disease. The hypercapnic CSA patients are typical of people with brain stem lesions, congenital central hypoventilation, opioids, obesity hypoventilation, neuromuscular disorders and chest wall syndromes. Non-hypercapnic or eucapnic forms of CSA include Cheyne-Stokes respiration and idiopathic CSA [1, 2].

The hypoventilation syndromes are characterised by a PaCO2 >45 mmHg on arterial blood gas during sleep, which eventually shows as abnormally raised PaCO2 during wakefulness. Arterial oxygen desaturations less than 90% for longer than 5 minutes during the sleep period with a nadir of less than 85% also characterise hypoventilation.

Hypoventilation beginning is apparent in REM-sleep, and as it advances, will happen during all sleep stages.

A complex of obesity, hypersomnolence and awake hypercapnia in the absence of an alternative neuromuscular, mechanical or metabolic explanation for hypoventilation are the cornerstones of this diagnosis. OHS deserves special attention as it is increasingly prevalent with a large amount of patients showing to sleep clinics in industrialised nations varying from 10% to 20%.

Eighty to 90% of people with OHS also have upper airway obstruction [2].

The Complex Sleep Apnea (CSA) is to designate a condition initially identified as OSA. This syndrome is characterised (while CPAP is being used) by the numerous episodes of central apnea after reduction (<5 events for an hour) or elimination of obstructive events. Rather than starting additional proceedings, it is useful to evaluate whether CPAP pressure is too high and is a problem of CSA.

The COPD overlap syndrome is defined as a combination of COPD and obstructive apnea-hypopnea syndrome [3]. Nevertheless, the coincidence of these situations can lead to severe events of desaturation during sleep (particularly during REM-sleep), thus increasing the possibility of hypoxemia, daytime hypercapnia and pulmonary hypertension.

Overnight polysomnography is the popular universally used method for the diagnosis of sleep-related respiratory disorders.

Currently, it is recognised as the "gold standard" by which newer developments in the measurement of breathing during sleep have been evaluated.

The respiratory disturbance index (RDI) is used synonymously with the apnea-hypopnea index (AHI) unless stated otherwise. Mild, moderate and severe OSA is defined according to criteria used in the accompanying review paper: Mild, $5 \leq RDI \leq 15$; Moderate, $15 \leq RDI \leq 30$; Severe, $RDI > 30$ episodes per hour of sleep. Several studies have reported severe sleep disruption in patients with both COPD and neuromuscular/chest wall deformity, and this can be improved with NIV [3, 4].

POSITIVE AIRWAY PRESSURE

Positive pressure available therapies include continuous positive airway pressure (CPAP), bilevel positive airway pressure, and auto-titrating positive airway pressure.

CPAP

CPAP is the most generally used mode of non-invasive ventilation in the treatment of OSA and of disordered breathing associated with chronic heart failure. The action of CPAP prevents intermittent narrowing and collapse of the airways in patients with obstructive sleep apnea-hypopnea syndrome; it counteracts auto-positive end-expiratory pressure, which decreases respiratory muscles load, the work of breathing and daytime PaCO2 in patients with overlap syndrome; it improves lung function, particularly the functional residual capacity, daytime gas exchange and improves systolic function of the left ventricle in patients with heart failure coexisting with OSA. CPAP has not only been shown to strengthen quality-of-life and sleep indices in patients with OSA, but also to lower blood pressure and rates of arrhythmia and stroke, to improve left ventricular ejection fraction in patients with heart failure, and to improve the rates of fatal and nonfatal cardiovascular events [5].

Standard practice involves pressure adjustment during attended laboratory polysomnography to eliminate obstructive respiratory-related events (apneas, hypopneas, oxygen desaturations, snoring, respiratory effort-related arousals). The best pressure value of CPAP is the value which decreases each apnea, hypopnea, arterial desaturation, snoring, respiratory effort-related arousal (RERA) in each stage of sleep and body position. The final assessment of pressure is always a balance between the patient's adherence, the absolute value of pressure reached, and the clinical benefits derived.

Automatic Adjustment of the Level of Continuous Positive Airway Pressure

Automatic adjustment of the level of CPAP (auto-CPAP) is performed through a self-titrating CPAP device, which applies algorithms to recognise variations in the degree of obstruction and regulates the pressure level to reestablish normal breathing. Auto-CPAP compensates for factors that change the upper airway collapsibility, such as body position during sleep, stage of sleep, use of alcohol, and drugs that alter upper airway muscle tone. It is not recommended in the diagnosis of OSA and titrating continuous pressure during split-night. The auto-CPAP can be utilised during polysomnography or cardiorespiratory monitoring to titrate a individual pressure value to be applied later with fixed CPAP for the treatment of OSA in patients without comorbid conditions.

The application of auto-CPAP is reserved only for those patients with sleep apnea syndrome only present during REM or respiratory events related to the position, in whom constraining positional manoeuvres are poorly tolerated.

Bilevel

Bilevel positive airway pressure may be considered in patients who need high pressure, who hypoventilate during sleep, and who have difficulty exhaling against a fixed pressure. Bilevel positive airway pressure is also used for sleep-related disorders, but its main indication is in pathological conditions associated with hypoventilation. The BIPAP devices deliver a higher-pressure during inspiration (IPAP) and a lower pressure during expiration (EPAP). The gradient between IPAP and EPAP is crucial in maintaining adequate alveolar ventilation and reducing PaCO2. The IPAP also acts in reducing the work of breathing and EPAP has the function of keeping the patency of the upper airway, to control obstructive apnea and to improve the functional residual capacity. BIPAP is now recommended for the patients who require high expiratory pressures to manage obstructive sleep apnea-hypopnea, but who cannot tolerate expiring against a high-fixed CPAP pressure. Other indication of BIPAP are the treatment of coexisting central apnea or hypoventilation, the obesity-hypoventilation syndrome, the overlap syndrome and neuromuscular disorders.Although the patient should be capable to sustain spontaneous breathing, it is used to set a back-up rate possibility for those patients whose ventilation during sleep may be particularly reduced (neuromuscular disorders, complex sleep apnea, central apnea in chronic heart failure, obesity-hypoventilation syndrome). A deficiency of pressure ventilation is that it cannot ensure a tidal volume delivered to the patient.

Patients with CSA most often respond to positive airway pressure, but the obstruction cannot be dismissed without producing central apnea. A potential preventive action is the so-called permissive flow-limitation: the pressure is set at a level that allows a mild degree of airway obstruction, without disturbing ventilator control mechanisms. Also, oxygen administration may lead to a reduction in the hypoxic ventilatory response. Also, BiPAP in the spontaneous-timed (ST) mode or adaptive servo-ventilation (ASV) can be useful in the treatment of CSA [5, 6].

Average Volume-Assured Pressure Support Ventilation (AVAPS)

Average volume-assured pressure support ventilation (AVAPS) is applied in patients with chronic hypoventilation and in particular with obesity hypoventilation syndrome, neuromuscular diseases, and sometimes, in chronic obstructive pulmonary disease. In this mode, a target tidal volume is set; the device regulates the pressure support which to influence the selected tidal volume. It supports a delivered tidal. In this mode, a target tidal volume is established; the device regulates the pressure support to reach the set tidal volume. The benefit of this mode is that it guarantees a delivered tidal volume regulated notwithstanding variability in the patient effort, airway resistance, and lung or chest wall compliance.

A particular advantage of this mode is that it may be adjusted as the disease progresses (as it occurs in neuromuscular disorders). This modality links elements of pressure and volume ventilation. The ventilator calculates the delivered tidal volume and modifies its parameters to ensure a predetermined target tidal volume. Volume targeting is a feature recently made available on specific bi-level ventilators which aims to solve this limitation: the ventilator measures or estimates delivered tidal volume (VT) through a built-in pneumotachograph and adjusts pressure support within a preset range to provide a VT as close as possible to a target VT set by the clinician. Although indexes of sleep fragmentation were unaffected by VT targeting, awakenings >20 s were more frequent. Subjectively patients described BPPV with VT targeting as less comfortable, with a more frequent perception of receiving too much air, and an increased understanding of leaks. The concept of VT targeting is attractive, especially in patients with severe OHS, because of the low compliance of their respiratory system, and the difficulty in controlling nocturnal hypoventilation in these patients [7].

Volume-Targeted Ventilation (VTV)

In this modality, the ventilator performs a fixed volume during a given period and will produce whatever pressure is required to manage this, regardless of the patient contribution to ventilation.

Pressure in the airways (Paw) is not fixed and results from the interaction between ventilator settings, compliance and resistance of the respiratory system and spontaneous inspiratory efforts. It should be stressed that any additional inspiratory effort will not influence to changes in dispensed volumes or flows but only occur in a reduction in Paw.

As each breath is provided with the same planned flow-time profile and as the area under the flow-time curve denotes the volume, the benefit of this modality is the powerful performance, in the absence of leaks, of the present volume, whatever the values of compliance and resistance. A significant disadvantage of VTV is precisely that delivery of this fixed ventilatory assistance does not allow the account to be taken of patients' varying requirements.

Another difficulty is that, if there is a leak, there will be no improvement in flow rate to compensate for it and the produced pressure will be lower so that the effectively delivered volume will be reduced in proportion. Conventional ventilation provides fixed pressure or volumes rates. Some new modes use a more physiological delivery of assistance following the spontaneous inspiratory signal coming from the patient. Hence, they are supposed to improve patient-ventilator synchronism.

Pressure-Targeted Ventilation (PTV)

In this modality, the ventilator is set to generate airflow by making a predefined positive pressure in the airways for a given time. Airflow is therefore adjusted to establish and maintain a constant Paw. Continuous analysis of the flow rate and airway pressure commands the flow variations required to support a flat or 'square wave' pressure. Flow is active at the beginning of inspiration when the gradient between the circuit pressure and the pressure target is notable. As this gradient narrows the flow decelerates until driving pressure no longer exists, and flow ceases. Thus, for a given patient, the volume produced is not determined and will depend on the interaction between the preset pressure, patient inspiratory effort, the physical characteristics of the respiratory system and inspiratory time. An essential advantage of PTV is the ability to compensate for mild to moderate leaks. One of these modes, proportional assisted ventilation (PAV), relies on the inspiratory flow of the spontaneously breathing pattern and adds fixed proportional assistance. If the patient's flow increases, the aid increases proportionally. The degree of support is defined by the practitioner based on estimations of the patient's resistance and compliance. Even if PAV explains to work according to theoretical presuppositions, clinical studies using this mode both in invasive ventilation and NIV missed to show any clear advantages of this mode over others.

Adaptive Servo-Ventilation (ASV)

The adaptive servo-ventilation (ASV) has been produced for the therapy of Cheyne-Stokes respiration-central apnea syndrome in patients with chronic heart failure who have a breathing pattern characterised by periods of crescendo-decrescendo variation in tidal volume. This more complex device can utilise patient expiratory positive airway pressure (EPAP) level sufficient to control the obstructive apnea. The machine then automatically adjusts the inspiratory pressure support for each inspiration within a pre-specified range, to maintain moving-target ventilation set at 90% of the patient's recent average ventilation. The aim is the stabilisation of breathing patterns and the reduction of the respiratory alkalosis, which can trigger apnea reentry cycles.

Clinical Implications

Management of Non-Invasive Ventilation

When doctors set the ventilator during the daytime, they do not save it on whether a patient is asleep or awake. In clinical practice, the level of pressure support is set following the patient's respiratory rate, which produces plausible supervision as to a patient's inspiratory effort. The empirical setting of the ventilator during wakefulness is effective in improving gas exchange, but that it may cause patient-ventilator asynchrony during sleep, and this is associated with sleep disruption.The improvement of sleep quality during NIV setting was demonstrated by an increased amount of REM sleep and a reduced number of arousals. The minimum required is registering SpO2 on room air, assessing that the normalisation of SpO2 accompanies the normalisation or at least the improvement in PaCO2. A full polysomnography recording SpO2 and PtcCO2 or PetCO2, flow, tidal volume, airway pressure, rib cage and abdomen excursion and sleep-staging allow a complete assessment. When the sources are not possible, fewer parameters may be utilised [8].

Nocturnal monitoring of NIV is far more complicated, and unexpected problems occur for many reasons: (1) sleep can produce profound ventilatory variations, in particular in patients with respiratory insufficiency; (2) these ventilatory variations are also increased by the interactions with a preset devised the ventilator can produce sleep disturbances by itself; (3) physicians considering for these patients may vary significantly in their methods of evaluatingthe impacts of NIV from a single blood gas measurement to full polysomnography.

Patient-Ventilator Desynchrony

Patient-ventilator desynchrony or a particular ventilator mode might also lead to sleep disruption. Pressure support predisposes to an irregular breathing pattern, specifically central apneas with consequent hyperpnea. Meza and coworkers demonstrated that healthy subjects develop central apneas during pressure support when their carbon dioxide tension (Pco2) decreases by a few torrs below the apnea threshold. Whether pressure support effects apneas in critically ill patients and whether the apneas lead to disruption of sleep are unknown. Unlike pressure support, assist-control ventilation produces a fixed tidal volume on every breath, and it can be set to release breaths when a patient neglect to make an effort. The back-up rate will prevent the development of apneas, and perhaps reduce arousals.If pressure support produces central apneas by lowering arterial Pco2 under the apnea threshold, then attaching a dead space to the ventilator circuit might also reduce both the apneas and arousals [9].

A second object was to decide whether adding dead space during pressure support would reduce sleep fragmentation as a result of reducing the frequency of central apneas.

These apneas can worsen sleep fragmentation; adding dead space reduces the incidence of central apneas and sleep fragmentation during pressure support; and in critically ill patients, the patterns of breathing and gas exchange during sleep change from those during wakefulness, and these variations are more significant with pressure support as compared with assist-control ventilation. Variations in sleep depth are thought to be more significant than the poor frequency of disruptions in causing daytime sleepiness in patients with obstructive sleep apnea. Although daytime sleepiness may not be an interest in critically ill patients, sleep fragmentation can negatively influence the cardiorespiratory and autonomic nervous systems. A large number of apnea-related arousals and awakenings happened during pressure support. These events were reduced by adding dead space and completely abolished with assist-control ventilation. At first glance, it might seem that categorising arousals and awakenings as apnea or non-apnea related would lead to predictable results (because the back-up rate on assist-control ventilation should inhibit apnea-related arousals). The classification, however, highlights that all other (non-apnea-related) arousals and awakenings were evenly common during assist-control ventilation and pressure support [9, 10].

Nevertheless, a variance in the ventilator mode from assist-control ventilation to pressure support can further worsen sleep disruption. The existence of central apneas during pressure support is not uncommon to patients with heart failure. Central apneas can happen in healthy subjects receiving pressure support. Moreover, pressure support has inherent oscillatory behaviour that predisposes to substantial variations in tidal volume even when the patient effort is constant. This instability, linked with higher levels of pressure support influences to central apneas and following sleep fragmentation in patients without heart failure and may reveal the existence of apneas in patients who did not have heart failure. The lack of apneas may have happened from depressing of the chemical control system secondary to abnormal respiratory mechanics and elevated dead space; a low functional residual capacity and low levels of pressure support may have also contributed.

Influence of Type of Exhalation Device and Connecting Circuits

Whereas ICU ventilators classically utilise a double circuit with a combined expiratory valve, two different kinds of circuits can be utilised to give NIV. The first uses a similar construction to those used in ICU devices and incorporates either single or double tubing in which inspiration and expiration are parted, and a correct expiratory valve is present so that carbon dioxide (CO2) rebreathing is not a notable problem. A second type does not have a correct exhalation valve and often uses a single-limb circuit with a risk of rebreathing. For avoid the rebreathing, this system includes a calibrated leak (called an intentional leak) either at the mask level or in the circuit. Single circuit pressure-targeted ventilators equipped with a calibrated leak (called bilevel ventilators) are usually utilised for NIV nowadays. These machines cycle between a higher IPAP and a lower EPAP that can be individually regulated.

With these devices, a smallest mandatory EPAP level of 4 cm H2O is needed to ensure an adequate washout of CO2 [11].

Interestingly, the exhalation port position influences CO2 rebreathing with a more efficient CO2 washout when the leak is positioned within the mask. A low EPAP maybe just insufficient to counterbalance upper airway collapse possibly induced by positive airway pressure. First, increasing the EPAP seems to be the most promising option to prevent upper airway collapse, but higher IPAP settings may be necessary to maintain tidal volume and minute ventilation. Adjustment of the EPAP can be achieved by increasing a fixed EPAP or switching to a variable EPAP mode [12].

It is, therefore, essential to evaluate NIV efficacy. However, as NIV is generally employed for several hours during sleep, more specific and sophisticated monitoring is needed to determine overnight patient-machine 'agreement' and efficacy of ventilation. The most accessible and easy monitoring can be made from flow and pressure curves. Understanding the importance of non-invasive ventilator roles on the occurrence of abnormal respiratory events and a relevant knowledge of the possible instruments for monitoring NIV during sleep are necessities to a better perception of how patients and ventilators cooperate. Lately, a technique called "high-intensity NIV" has developed, utilising inspiratory pressure levels up to 28 cm H2O and high back-up respiratory rates to deliver pCO2 control in stable hypercapnic COPD patients. This procedure has been physiologically proven to reduce the inspiratory effort when compared to conventional ventilation strategies.

Furthermore, high-intensity NIV does not negatively impact sleep quality, and improves blood gases, lung function, hematocrit, and decrease COPD exacerbations rates. However, it remains questionable what influence the setting of the breathing frequency has on ventilation quality in COPD. If the results are not satisfying, modifications must be made to the settings. One may also modify the type of mask and ventilator. A back-up frequency set near to the spontaneous rate of the patient during sleep is a feasible step.

Effect of Dead Space

Hypocapnia can trigger central apneas in patients with heart failure, and the rise of hypocapnia can eliminate central apneas in patients with idiopathic central sleep apnea and central sleep apnea due to heart failure. Inspiratory assistance, pain, discomfort, and sepsis can produce chronic hyperventilation, which, in turn, may lower the Pco2 under the apnea threshold and produce central apneas. The level of pressure support and elastance of the respiratory system compared with the frequency of central apneas. Similarly, acute hyperventilation due to awakenings from sleep can also lower Pco2, and thereby cause central apneas [13].

As expected, the number of awakenings related with the number of central apneas. In line with the other conceptual structure, a smaller variation between the end-tidal CO2 and the apnea threshold point would happen in various central apneas. The increase of dead space allowed a mean improvement in end-tidal CO2 of 4.3 mm Hg, which happened in a reduction in the frequency of central apneas and sleep disruptions.

The Choice of the Mask

Every effort should be made to minimise air leaks, maximise patient comfort and optimise patient-ventilator interaction. The interface is of predominant relevance for adherence to NIV therapy. A variety of masks are now accessible, and producers continue to improve mask design. Nasal pillows or full-face masks are seldom utilised if nasal masks are a problem for the patient. The oronasal mask should be considered if the patient is a mouth breather to avoid leaks through the open mouth.

In patients with OSA receiving CPAP treatment, oronasal interfaces can increase the residual AHI compared to nasal masks. This finding was attributed to insufficient handling or fitting of the mask and increased leakage of air. Considering the kind of treatment designed and choosing masks which deliver positive pressure through both the nose and the mouth is of great importance [14].

In NMD patients initiated on NIV, oronasal masks may be preferred because of better oral leak control, especially if buccal weakness and mouth breathing are present. Potential disadvantages include claustrophobia, aspiration risk, increased dead space ventilation, and relevant compromise about eating and speaking. Therefore, substituting an oronasal by a nasal mask with a chin strap can be considered, especially when buccal weakness is present.

Influence of Unintentional Leaks

Unintentional leaks are very common in NIV. Leakage may be absent or minimum when the patient is awake, but may worsen during sleep as a result of the loss of voluntary control and reduced muscle tone. Leaks can be at the mouth or between the skin and the mask, and air could also be collected in the oropharyngeal reservoir and even flow into the digestive tract (internal leaks). Leaks can primarily affect ventilator triggering, pressurisation, volume delivered, rate of inspiratory pressuring and cycling function and induce sleep fragmentation. Leaks have been shown to disrupt sleep, though others have shown remarkably effective control of nocturnal ventilation, reasonable sleep quality and long-term acceptance in established users with considerable leak overnight. Nasal congestion will significantly accentuate the pressure drop with the leak. Hayes et al. showed that mouth leak caused a significant increase in nasal mucosal blood flow and a reduction in the lumen, largely preventable by humidification. Consequently, it might be speculated that in the absence of a heated humidifier, the effect of mouth leak on the effectiveness of ventilation might be more severe. The improvement is despite an increase in REM sleep, which of itself is a time of increasing PCO2 in subjects with hypercapnic respiratory failure [5, 6].

A variety of more or less adequate measures have been recommended to resolve the problem of leaks during NIV. These combine the restriction of neck flexion, the semi-recumbent positioning of the patient, the use of a chin rest or a cervical collar to restrict of the mouth opening, switching to controlled pressure mode, reducing the peak inspiratory pressure and enhancing the delivered volume, optimising the interface. The effectiveness of each of these actions must be verified during sleep recording. Humidification of delivered gas may increase these symptoms. Education of the patient is mandatory.

Leaks and upper airway resistance changes may, in turn, modify these patterns. The effect is complicated further because volume and pressure preset ventilators will respond differently in particular conditions and because the type of mask used will also have different effects on monitoring parameters [15].

Influence of the Upper Airway

During NIV, a variable resistance developed by the UA is included between the ventilator and the lungs. The UA may change its opposition to airflow, compromising the delivery of an adequate tidal volume to the lungs. Intermittent obstruction of the UA is prevalent during NIV and may be correlated or to obstructive events at the oropharyngeal level (UA collapse as a result of insufficient expiratory airway pressure) or to hyperventilation induced by NIV that may also provoke undesirable respiratory events by promoting active glottic closures and precipitate central apneas, affecting the efficacy of ventilation but also the quality of sleep.

As adding CO2 to the inspired air could widen the glottis, it was suggested that glottic narrowing could be caused by extreme hypocapnia, to attempt to reverse the hypocapnia induced by NIV. Glottic contraction as a result of NIV increased during sleep compared to wakefulness, and effective ventilation was also lower during sleep than during wakefulness. Besides, an extensive interindividual variability in glottis behavior and adequate ventilation is observed, especially during wakefulness. Although in lambs as well as in healthy subjects the glottis narrows with increasing inspiratory pressure during NIV, the results of the current study showed no closure of the glottis during NIV. Mechanical factors such as tidal volume and flow are known to trigger glottis closure, effected by receptors at laryngeal or upper airway level, to avoid hyperventilation in NIV.

CONCLUSION

Sleep-related disorders are life-threatening conditions. The optimal level of treatment should be decided in a sleep laboratory. Side effects directly influencing the patient's adherence to treatment are known. The most common are discomfort using the mask and leakages followed by nasopharyngeal symptoms, including improved congestion and rhinorrhea; these effects are correlated to decreased humidity of inspired gas. The clinical implications of sleep quality in the ICU are unclear. Some sleep alterations were associated with NIV failure. A lower activities-of-daily-living score, indicating more significant functional impairment, was found in the patients who subsequently failed NIV. Also, a higher respiratory frequency and more hours under NIV at polysomnography are data suggestive of more significant respiratory compromise. Absence of the typical EEG signs of sleep and wakefulness has been reported previously in ICU patients. In elderly patients who failed NIV, we found marked sleep disturbances with an abnormal EEG pattern, disruption of the circadian sleep cycle, and decreased REM sleep.

REFERENCES

[1] Nicolini, A., Banfi, P., Grecchi, B., Lax, A., Walterspacher, S., Barlascini, C. & Robert, D. (2014). Non-invasive ventilation in the treatment of sleep-related breathing disorders: A review and update. *Rev Port Pneumol.*, *20*, 324-35.

[2] Resta, O., Guido, P., FoschinoBarbaro, M. P., Picca, V.,Talamo, S.&Lamorgese, V. (2000). Sleep-related breathing disorders in acute respiratory failure assisted by non-invasive ventilatory treatment: utility of portable polysomnographic system. *Respiratory Medicine.*, *94*, 128-134.

[3] Eline Oppersma, Jonne Doorduin, Petra J. Gooskens, Lisanne H. Roesthuis, H.F.M., van der Heijden, Johannes G. van der Hoeven, Peter H. Veltink. & Leo, M.A. Heunks. (2019). Glottic patency during non-invasive ventilation in patients

with chronic obstructive pulmonary disease, *Respiratory Physiology & Neurobiology.*, *259*, 53–57.

[4] Owens, R. L. & Malhotra, A. (2010). Sleep-disordered breathing and COPD: the overlap syndrome. *Respir Care.*, *55*(10), 1333–1346.

[5] Gonzalez-Bermejo, J., Perrin, C., Janssens, J. P., Pepin, J. L., Mroue, G., Leger, P., Langevin, B., Rouault, S., Rabec, C., Rodenstein, D. & Somno, N. I. V. G. (2012). Proposal for a systematic analysis of polygraphy or polysomnography for identifying and scoring abnormal events occurring during non-invasive ventilation. *Thorax*, *67*, 546-552.

[6] Grossbach, I., Chlan, L. & Tracy, M. F. (2011). Overview of mechanical ventilatory support and management of patient- and ventilator-related responses.*Crit Care Nurse.*, Jun, *31*(3), 30-44.

[7] Ramar, K., Ramar, P. & Morgenthaler, T. I. (2012). Adaptive servo-ventilation in patients with central or complex sleep apnea related to chronic opioid use and congestive heart failure. *J Clin Sleep Med.*, *8*(5), 569–576.

[8] Berry, R. B., Chediak, A., Brown, L. K., et al. (2010). Best clinical practices for the sleep center adjustment of non-invasive positive pressure ventilation (NPPV) in stable chronic alveolar hypoventilation syndromes. *J Clin Sleep Med.*, *6*(5), 491–509.

[9] Fanfulla, F., Taurino, A. E., Lupo, N. D., Trentin, R., D'Ambrosio, C. & Nava, S. (2007). Effect of sleep on patient/ventilator asynchrony in patients undergoing chronic non-invasive mechanical ventilation. *Respir Med.*, *101*(8), 1702-7.

[10] Aarrestad, S., Qvarfort, M., Kleiven, A. L., Tollefsen, E., Skjønsberg, O. H. & Janssens, J. P. (2017). Sleep-related respiratory events during non-invasive ventilation of patients with chronic hypoventilation, *Respiratory Medicine*.

[11] Vignaux, L., Vargas, F., Roeseler, J., Tassaux, D., Thille, A. W., Kossowsky, M. P., Brochard, L. & Jolliet, P. (2009). Patient-ventilator asynchrony during non-invasive ventilation for acute respiratory failure: a multicenter study. *Intensive Care Med.*, *35*(5), 840–846.

[12] Younes, M., Brochard, L., Grasso, S., Kun, J., Mancebo, J., Ranieri, M., Richard, J. C. & Younes, H. (2007). A method for monitoring and improving patient: ventilator interaction. *Intensive Care Med.*, *33*, 1337–1346.

[13] Puyol, C. L., Larrosa, R., Luján, M. & Sayas, J. (2018). Trigger asynchronies induced by the introduction of external gas into the circuit in non-invasive ventilation: a bench study, *European Respiratory Journal.*, *52*, PA2402.

[14] Zhu, K., Rabec, C., Gonzalez-Bermejo, J., Hardy, S., Aouf, S., Escourrou, P. & Roisman, G. (2017). Combined effects of leaks, respiratory system properties and upper airway patency on the performance of home ventilators: a bench study, *BMC Pulmonary Medicine*, *17*, 145.

[15] Rabec, C., Rodenstein, D., Leger, P., Rouault, S., Perrin, C., Gonzalez-Bermejo, J. & Somno NIV group. (2011).Ventilator modes and settings during non-invasive ventilation: effects on respiratory events and implications for their identification *Thorax.*, *66*, 170-178.

In: Sleep Medicine in Critical Care
Editors: Antonio M. Esquinas et al.
ISBN: 978-1-53617-768-8

Chapter 14

NON-INVASIVE VENTILATION IN OBESITY HYPOVENTILATION SYNDROME

Irena Sarc[*]
Noninvasive Ventilation Department.
The University Clinic For Pulmonary And Allergic Diseases,
Golnik, Slovenia

ABSTRACT

Obesity hypoventilation syndrome (OHS) is defined by the presence of hypercapnia in an obese patient with sleep-disordered breathing. Obesity influences respiratory physiology by decreasing compliance of the respiratory system and reducing lung volumes. In addition, respiratory centres' responses are blunted. Patients with OHS most often present with acute hypercapnic failure with the need for noninvasive ventilation (NIV) or in sleep centres with typical symptoms of obstructive sleep apnea (OSA). An important feature of OHS is increased cardiometabolic morbidity and mortality. NIV is the initial treatment of acute hypercapnic respiratory failure (AHRF). When used in the correct patient by a skilled NIV team in a proper fashion NIV is successful in the majority of obese patients with AHRF. In a chronic setting, patients with OHS should be treated according to sleep study results. When severe OSA is present, continuous positive airway pressure (CPAP) is the first choice of treatment, if adequate physiological and clinical responses can be achieved. The rest of the patients should be treated with home NIV.

Keywords: obesity, noninvasive ventilation, acute hypercapnic respiratory failure

[*] Corresponding Author's E-mail: Irena.Sarc@klinika-golnik.si.

INTRODUCTION

In recent decades growing numbers of patients experience obesity-related respiratory complications as a consequence of obesity epidemic. Obstructive sleep apnea (OSA) and obesity hypoventilation syndrome (OHS) are the most common respiratory manifestations of obesity. OHS is commonly underdiagnosed, even when patients with severe obesity present with acute respiratory failure. Failure to recognize and manage OHS according to guidelines significantly influences the prognosis of OHS patients. In this review, key features of the syndrome are presented with the newest findings that inform the management of these patients, especially at and after an episode of acute hypercapnic respiratory failure.

Definition and Diagnosis of OHS

OHS is defined as the combination of obesity (body mass index (BMI) $\geq$ 30 kg/m^2) and daytime hypercapnia (awake resting arterial carbon dioxide tension (P_aCO_2) $\geq$ 45 mmHg) when other potential causes of hypercapnia are excluded (Masa et al., n.d.). Hypercapnia during the day is preceded by hypoventilation during sleep with intermittent nocturnal hypercapnia. The classic clinical presentation of OHS develops gradually. Recently, the European Respiratory Society (ERS) task force proposed a severity grading of OHS, highlighting that daytime hypoventilation indicates an already advanced phase of OHS (Randerath et al. 2017). In the early stages, without daytime hypercapnia, more extended periods of hypoventilation and/or sleep-disordered breathing overnight lead to increased daytime serum bicarbonate; a cutoff level > 27 $mmol \cdot l^{-1}$ indicates chronic nocturnal hypercapnia. However, serum bicarbonate < 27 $mmol \cdot l^{-1}$ excludes the diagnosis of OHS with a high degree of certainty (97% negative predictive value) (Masa et al., n.d.).

An important element of the diagnosis is concomitant sleep-disordered breathing, with a sleep study required to determine the exact pattern of disturbance. About 90% of patients with OHS have some degree of obstructive sleep apnea (OSA), with the majority of patients having severe OSA (Masa et al., n.d.). The remaining 10% of patients have non-apneic sleep hypoventilation. According to the American Academy of Sleep Medicine guidelines, sleep hypoventilation in adults in defined as arterial carbon dioxide tension (P_aCO_2) higher than 55 mmHg for > 10 min or an increase in P_aCO_2 more than 10 mmHg compared to an awake supine value to a value higher than 50 mmHg for > 10 min (Masa et al., n.d.). Instead of arterial P_aCO_2, a surrogate measure of transcutaneous carbon dioxide or end-tidal carbon dioxide can be used (Randerath et al. 2017).

Epidemiology

The obesity epidemic is a global phenomenon, impacting all ages. A recent cross-sectional analysis of the US population estimated that 39% of US adults are obese, and 7.6% are severely obese (BMI ≥ 40 kg/m²) (Hales et al. 2018). About half of severely obese adults have OSA. Severe obesity is a primary risk factor for the development of OHS. The prevalence of OHS linearly increases with BMI, with almost half of patients with BMI > 50 kg/m² having OHS (Nowbar et al. 2003). An estimate of the prevalence of OHS in the US population found that 0.4% of the US adult population has OHS (Hales et al. 2018).

In a population of patients referred to sleep centers, several studies reported a prevalence of OHS between 8 and 20% in obese patients.

A large Swedish registry of patients with OHS, with an approximately equal proportion of men and women, reported that the diagnosis of OHS is more delayed in women and that the disease is more advanced in women. When diagnosed, women were older, had a higher BMI and more hypercapnia, and were more frequently started on noninvasive ventilation (NIV) in an acute setting (Palm et al. 2016). Similar results were found in a recent study from Saudi Arabia, which examined a population referred to a sleep center and found that OHS women were significantly older, with almost a fourfold higher prevalence of OHS in women compared to men (Bahammam et al. 2016)

Pathophysiology of Obesity and OHS

The main features of respiratory physiology in obese patients are decreased compliance of the respiratory system and reduced lung volumes. Accumulation of fat has a direct mechanical effect on reduction of total respiratory system compliance with increased BMI (Masa et al., n.d.). This is partly due to decreased lung compliance, but primarily to reduced chest wall compliance linked to excessive fat around the ribs and diaphragm, and in the abdomen. Reduction of compliance is further exacerbated by supine position. Reduction of compliance in eucapnic obese patients compared to normal-weight individuals has been found to be around 20 and 60% reduction in OHS patients (Verbraecken and Mcnicholas 2015).

As a consequence of mass loading, obese patients have decreased lung volumes with a linear decrease in total lung capacity (TLC) relative to BMI and an exponential decrease in functional residual capacity (FRC) and expiratory reserve volume (ERV). Breathing at lower lung volumes, when ERV approaches the lung closing volume, leads to closure of small airways, causing air trapping with intrinsic positive end-expiratory pressure (PEEPi), especially in the supine position (Verbraecken and Mcnicholas 2015). The collapsibility of small airways at low lung volumes and positive pleural pressures due to accumulated fat cause decreased ventilation and atelectasis in the basal regions of the lungs, resulting in a ventilation/perfusion mismatch and decreased pO_2 (Masa et al., n.d.).

Reduced respiratory system compliance and increased lower airway resistance lead to increased work of breathing (WOB) and a shallow rapid breathing pattern (Masa et al., n.d.). Increased WOB is compensated with increased respiratory drive in order to maintain normocapnia in eucapnic obese patients (Verbraecken and Mcnicholas 2015).

Compared to eucapnic severely obese patients, OHS patients display more severe derangement of respiratory mechanics, including respiratory muscle weakness and blunted central responsiveness to hypercapnia and hypoxia (Verbraecken and Mcnicholas 2015). In an OHS patient, the increased respiratory drive is not maintained, leading to hypoventilation. In the early stage of development of OHS, hypoventilation initially develops during sleep, initially during rapid eye movement (REM) sleep. During REM sleep, the diaphragm is the primary inspiratory muscle due to loss of overall muscular activity. With decreased diaphragm function and reduced central sleep drive, hypoventilation ensues (Masa et al., n.d.). Interestingly, daytime sleepiness correlates with the severity of REM sleep hypoventilation (Randerath et al. 2017).

Hypoventilation during sleep causes secondary depression of respiratory centers through buffering of increased carbon dioxide (increased bicarbonate), leading to a further decrease of ventilation and eventually to daytime hypercapnia and OHS. It is hypothesized that one of the contributing mechanisms to the reduction in the central drive and central hypoventilation in obese patients could be leptin resistance. Leptin is an adipokine, secreted by adipocytes. Plasma leptin levels correlate closely with total body fat mass. Leptin acts on the central respiratory centers to stimulate ventilation. Increased levels of leptins in obese patients potentially protect the majority of them from hypoventilation. Serum leptin levels are higher in hypercapnic obese patients compared to normocapnic obese subjects, which suggests resistance to leptin effects. Interestingly, leptin levels fall after ventilation therapy initiation.

Up to 90% of patients with OHS have obstructive sleep apnea (OSA). In OSA accumulation of fat induces structural changes in the upper airway with the reduction of pharyngeal volume and increased collapsibility (Masa et al., n.d.). Furthermore, due to decreased lung volumes, loss of caudal traction on upper airway structures exacerbates upper airway collapsibility (Schwartz et al. 2010). During sleep, these changes lead to partial or complete closure of the upper airway: hypopneas and apneas. During apneas and hypopneas, which are relatively longer in OHS, loading of CO_2 occurs. Postevent ventilation in OHS is insufficient for unloading of CO_2 to occur due to reduced activity of the respiratory centers and reduced time between events (Berger et al. 2002). During these events, breathing at lower respiratory volumes also results in a rapid onset of hypoxemia and more pronounced dips in blood oxygen saturation. Hypoxemia could further aggravate sleep hypoventilation through complex mechanisms (Verbraecken and Mcnicholas 2015).

In the remaining 10% of OHS patients, the main sleep-disordered breathing feature is sleep hypoventilation without OSA.

CLINICAL PRESENTATION AND COMORBIDITIES IN PATIENTS WITH OHS

OHS is diagnosed in two clinical scenarios: 1) during an episode of acute-on-chronic hypercapnic respiratory failure, or 2) in a stable condition during a diagnostic workup in a sleep center. Several studies found that a sizable proportion of patients are diagnosed with OHS only when they present with acute respiratory failure (Borel et al. 2012). A study by Nowbar found that only 20% of OHS patients admitted to the hospital had a prior diagnosis of OHS; during a follow-up, 18-month mortality in largely positive airway pressure (PAP) untreated patients was 23% (Nowbar et al. 2003). Berg et al. found that OHS patients were frequently hospitalized in the 5 years prior to diagnosis and treatment of OHS; hospitalization days were substantially reduced after treatment with PAP was initiated (Berg et al. 2001). Surprisingly, OHS is misdiagnosed even in severely obese patients that present with acute hypercapnic respiratory failure (AHRF). In a series of OHS patients admitted to an intensive care unit (ICU), Malik et al. found that 75% of patients were erroneously diagnosed and treated for COPD in previous years (Marik and Desai 2014). These results highlight the fact that OHS is an underdiagnosed, misdiagnosed, and undertreated disease. The delay of diagnosis and treatment has serious prognostic implications for patients, negatively influencing healthcare utilization and potentially mortality.

Patients with OHS have the classic symptoms of OSA, including snoring, nocturnal gasping episodes, witnessed apneas, excessive daytime sleepiness, nocturia and morning headaches (Mokhlesi 2010) In addition and in contrast to OSA, patients with stable OHS frequently complain of dyspnea, with the prevalence of clinically significant dyspnea (MRC dyspnea scale ≥ 2) approximately 60% according to a recent study (Masa 2019). Many patients may have signs of cor pulmonale. Pulmonary hypertension in OHS is a common feature and is probably multifactorial. Increased pulmonary vascular resistance due to hypoxia-induced vasoconstriction and elevated left atrial pressure due to left heart dysfunction play an important role.

A recent ERS task force statement included cardiometabolic comorbidities as a feature of the most advanced stage of OHS (Stage IV), which is in line with observational data from many studies, all demonstrating a high prevalence of cardiovascular and metabolic diseases in OHS (Randerath et al. 2017). Comorbidities are commonly diagnosed before establishing a diagnosis of OHS. The prevalence of arterial hypertension in OHS is very high, ranging above 50% in most studies (Masa et al., n.d.). Metabolic syndrome, diabetes, and heart failure with preserved ejection fraction are all commonly associated with OHS (Masa et al. 2019).

ACUTE HYPERCAPNIC RESPIRATORY FAILURE IN OHS

Not surprisingly, in parallel with the obesity epidemic, obese patients with acute respiratory failure (ARF) are increasingly common in medical wards and critical care units all over the world, with some reports finding AHRF in OHS to be the second most frequent indication for acute NIV (Sequeira, Bahammam, and Esquinas 2016). NIV treatment is recommended in the setting of acute-on-chronic respiratory failure in OHS by British thoracic society 2016 guidelines; however, no prospective randomized controlled trials (RCT) are available demonstrating the efficacy of NIV in this clinical situation (Davidson et al. 2016). Nevertheless, using NIV in this clinical setting has become standard clinical practice. Observational studies report good results compared to exacerbations of COPD treated with NIV, with similar efficacy and better outcomes (Carrillo et al., n.d.).

Precipitating factors of AHRF in OHS such as infection or heart failure should be carefully investigated and aggressively treated (Masa et al., n.d.). About 50% of patients present with decompensated chronic respiratory failure without an apparent precipitating factor, sometimes termed decompensated OHS (Lemyze et al. 2014). Patients are frequently severely fluid overloaded at admission, with hypervolemia contributing to ventilatory failure and necessitating the application of diuretics concurrently with NIV (Davidson et al. 2016). However, excessive use of diuretics can aggravate metabolic alkalosis with aggravation of hypoventilation (Sequeira, Bahammam, and Esquinas 2016).

Importantly, severe obesity on its own is not a poor prognostic factor, as demonstrated by numerous studies, and it should not prevent patients from being escalated to invasive ventilation. Cardiometabolic comorbidities, rather than obesity drive the prognosis of patients with severe obesity treated in ICUs. Approximately 20% of those treated in ICUs are obese in the developed world. During treatment, obese patients are prone to more frequent complications, including hospital infections. Published meta-analyses do not indicate increased mortality of obese patients treated in ICUs compared to other patients treated in ICUs, but instead prolonged time on mechanical ventilation, difficult weaning, and longer treatment time for obese patients (Sequeira, Bahammam, and Esquinas 2016).

Patients with decompensated chronic respiratory failure with AHRF can be successfully treated with NIV. In a series of severely obese patients treated with NIV for

ARF, Lemynze et al. found that 17% of patients failed NIV. Multiple organ failure and pneumonia (28% of patients) were the strongest predictors of NIV failure and death in hypoxemic ARF in this study. In contrast, the strongest predictor of NIV success was AHRF due to decompensation of OHS (48% of patients), where NIV was universally successful, although sometimes delayed and requiring higher pressures (Lemyze et al. 2014). Carrillo et al. reported an NIV failure of 6% in a prospective study of patients with OHS having AHRF (Carrillo et al., n.d.). The differences in NIV failure rate could be attributed to different study populations' characteristics and different response to NIV in the contexts of hypoxemic versus hypercapnic ARF. The strongest predictors of NIV failure reported in patients established on home NIV was poor NIV adherence and high BMI (> 60 kg/m²) (Masa et al., n.d.). Taken together, these reports accentuate the need for careful initial assessment of patients and their risk for NIV failure through appropriate patient selection and level of care assignment.

NIV should be started early in AHRF if, despite optimal medical treatment and controlled oxygen therapy (maintenance of oxygen saturation between 88 and 92%), respiratory acidosis persists or worsens, usually as early as pH < 7.35 and pCO_2 > 6.5 kPa (Davidson et al. 2016). *Inappropriately* high administration of oxygen can worsen respiratory acidosis. The early use of NIV can prevent deterioration of the condition and the need for intubation and invasive ventilation. Access to NIV should be available within 1 hour of presentation and should be delivered by a trained and experienced NIV team (Masa et al., n.d.).

Oronasal masks are usually used in the treatment of AHRF because patients are commonly dyspnoic at presentation and breathing through the mouth. Oronasal mask is also linked to less leakage (Sequeira, Bahammam, and Esquinas 2016). Appropriate mask fitting is essential because a good fit and seal are key to effective NIV. Excessive leakage affects triggering, cycling, and patient synchronization with the ventilator and minute ventilation (Davidson et al. 2016).

The specific respiratory mechanics of obesity and OHS direct setting of NIV parameters. High expiratory positive airway pressure (EPAP) is applied to eliminate the upper airway obstruction by air splint and to increase FRC, prevent small airway closure, recruit collapsed lung, and improve oxygenation(Davidson et al. 2016) (Sequeira, Bahammam, and Esquinas 2016). The NIV team treating an OHS patient with AHRF should be sensitized to the occurrence of upper airway obstructive events when patients fall asleep, necessitating titration of EPAP by the bedside to ensure upper airway patency. The high impedance of the thorax can necessitate higher inspiratory pressures. Inspiratory positive airway pressure (IPAP) should be titrated to achieve adequate minute ventilation and unloading of the respiratory muscles (Davidson et al. 2016). Tidal volumes should be calculated according to ideal body weight. If the patient continues to have persistent hypoxemia despite the elimination of obstructive events and hypoventilation, oxygen should be administered to achieve oxygen saturation of 88 to 92%. A detailed protocol for NIV in AHRF in OHS is shown in Figure 1.

A review of published studies shows that the usual pressures required for adequate ventilation of these patients are IPAP of 18 + 3 cmH_2O and EPAP of 7 + 3 cmH_2O. Some extremely obese patients may require IPAP levels of up to and above 30 cmH_2O and EPAP levels higher than 10 cmH_2O for successful NIV (Sequeira, Bahammam, and Esquinas 2016). The need for high inspiratory pressures to achieve adequate minute ventilation and oxygenation can be reduced by appropriate patient positioning. A lateral recumbent position, or better still a reclining or sitting position, is recommended (Davidson et al. 2016).

During NIV, patients must be carefully monitored for comfort, level of consciousness, oxygen saturation, ventilatory parameters (pressures, respiratory volumes, leaks, and patient-ventilator synchrony), and vital signs (respiratory rate, pulse, and blood pressure). Arterial blood gas analysis is required within the first 2 hours of NIV to assess NIV effect (Davidson et al. 2016). Patients that are severely hypoxemic or experience severe drops in oxygen saturation after being temporarily disconnected from NIV are at higher risk and require intensive monitoring in the ICU and consideration of switching to invasive ventilation (Davidson et al. 2016).

Within the first 24 to 48 hours, NIV is used for as long as possible, including 20 hours and more per day. After clinical stabilization and resolution of acute acidosis, NIV is gradually reduced to only night use.

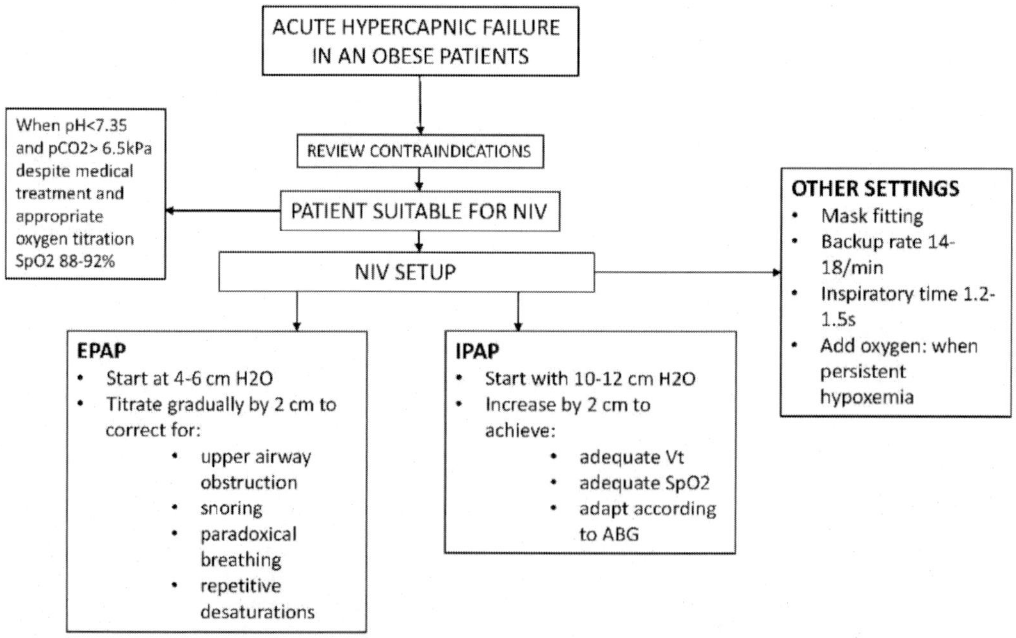

Figure 1. Algorithm for management of obese patients with AHRF with NIV.

Prognosis of OHS Patients Treated for AHRF

A study by Malik et al. described malignant OHS and reported very high in-hospital mortality for AHRF in OHS (18%) (Marik and Desai 2014), but Carrillo et al. found significantly lower in-hospital mortality rates (6%) (Carrillo et al., n.d.). These differences potentially reflect extreme parts of the severity spectrum of AHRF in OHS with patients differing in clinical characteristics and precipitating factor of AHRF.

Another critical issue is posthospitalization prognosis of these patients, especially in view of the prescription of PAP therapy at discharge. An ATS panel of experts recently analyzed data from 10 selected studies that included hospitalized patients with OHS. Altogether, the analysis included 1,162 patients with OHS that survived hospitalization for AHRF and were discharged. Of these, 119 (10%) were discharged without PAP and 1,043 (90%) on PAP. Patients without PAP were more often female, older, and more hypercapnic. Importantly, the vast majority of patients (92%) from the studies analyzed were discharged on NIV and not CPAP. At 3 months, 16.8% of patients that were discharged without PAP had died, as opposed to only 2.3% discharged with PAP (Mokhlesi et al. 2019). Although these are observational data, the posthospitalization prognosis of patients suspected to have OHS seems to depend strongly on whether NIV was prescribed for home use. On this basis, the ATS panel concluded that NIV should be considered the treatment of choice for patients with suspected OHS at discharge until further evaluation is performed, preferably within 3 months by a sleep specialist. When NIV is not available because of limited resources, the panel recommended discharging patients on CPAP.

Because several other studies reported low rates of patients being discharged with PAP therapy after AHRF (Sequeira, Bahammam, and Esquinas 2016), it is especially important to raise awareness among intensive care specialist to this growing group of patients.

Treatment of Stable OHS

Positive Airway Pressure (PAP) Treatment

PAP treatment (CPAP and NIV) is an established treatment modality for patients with stable OHS, although it is not based on definitive randomized trials comparing PAP versus no PAP therapy, but on a wealth of observational and nonrandomized data accumulated over the years demonstrating physiological and clinical effectiveness (Masa et al., n.d.). The central treatment objectives of PAP treatment in a patient with OHS are two: to reverse hypoventilation and hypercapnia and to address sleep-disordered breathing because most patients exhibit OSA.

Understandably, performing sleep studies (either polysomnography or polygraphy) is a crucial first step in the evaluation of these patients. There is no clear evidence of the superiority of polysomnography over respiratory polygraphy in this clinical situation (Windisch and Simon 2018). Sleep study results are broadly divided into three distinct phenotypes: 1) OHS with isolated severe OSA, 2) isolated OHS with sleep hypoventilation, and 3) a combination of OSA and OHS (Simonds et al. 2015), Figure 2.

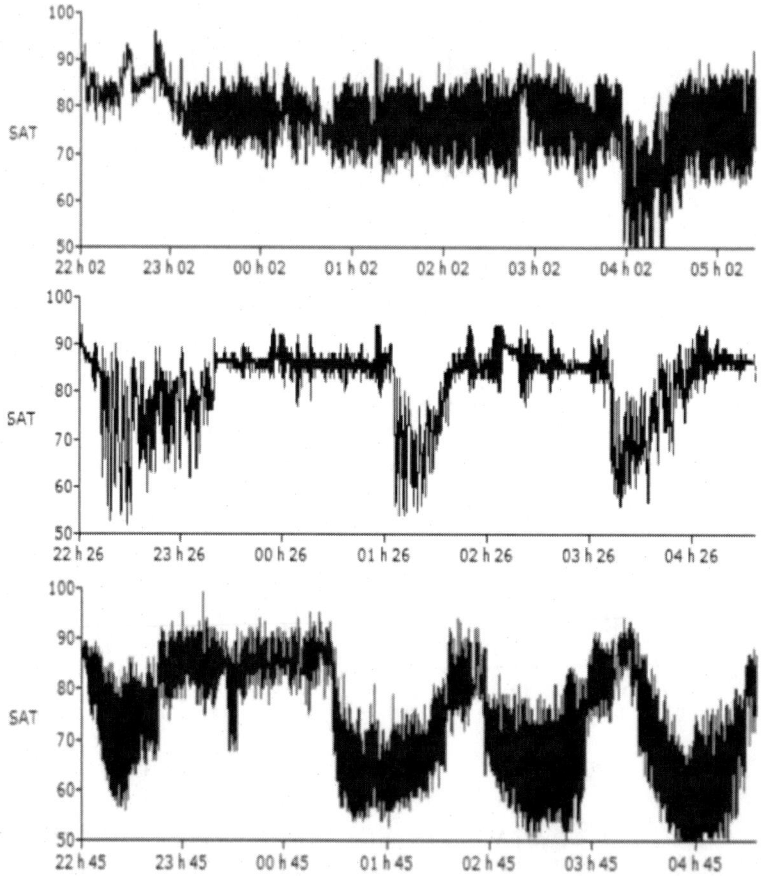

Figure 2. Phenotypes of OHS according to sleep study: 1) OHS with isolated severe OSA, 2) isolated OHS with sleep hypoventilation, and 3) a combination of OSA and OHS.

Generally, the first step in management is a CPAP titration trial, ideally under poly(somno)graphy or autotitration. The basic premise behind CPAP being effective in a patient with a severe OSA OHS phenotype is that, by eliminating obstructive upper airway events, CPAP prevents loading of CO_2 and improves the unloading of CO_2 that has accumulated during long obstructive events during sleep (Berger et al. 2002). In addition, CPAP improves lung volumes and offsets the closure of small airways, contributing to improved alveolar ventilation and reduced work and oxygen cost of breathing (Verbraecken and Mcnicholas 2015). In clinical practice, even one night of effective CPAP treatment can significantly improve gas exchange in a patient with a severe OSA phenotype. CPAP is not deemed effective, and switching to NIV is warranted in the case of one of the following under fully titrated CPAP: 1) a clinically relevant increase in nocturnal PCO_2, 2) persistent upper airway obstructive events, or 3) prolonged periods of desaturation ($\geq$ 10 min of SpO_2 < 80%) (Windisch and Simon 2018). Furthermore, if hypercapnia or symptoms persist (the patient is termed a CPAP nonresponder) at 3 months of CPAP treatment, a switch to NIV is warranted. A switch to NIV should also be considered if the patient experiences repeated episodes of AHRF under CPAP treatment (Masa et al., n.d.). Some national guidelines also suggest that severe hypercapnia and symptomatic comorbidities at initial presentation be considered, favoring the choice of NIV over CPAP (Windisch and Simon 2018). Patients with isolated OHS without OSA and a potentially mixed severe OSA OHS phenotype are more suitable candidates for NIV. Hypoventilation is better addressed with the use of positive inspiratory pressure, titrated to overcome hypoventilation (Mokhlesi et al. 2019).

In recent years, data from randomized trials have emerged that help guide decision-making on the exact treatment choices, mainly the decision between CPAP and NIV. Three trials have compared the effectiveness of CPAP and NIV. Piper et al. conducted the first trial to compare CPAP to NIV in a randomized fashion (Piper et al. 2008). The study recruited 36 stable OHS patients, excluding patients with severe desaturations ($\geq$ 10 min SpO_2 < 80%) or CO_2 retention under CPAP. In this trial, both CPAP and NIV appeared to be equally effective in improving daytime hypercapnia and sleepiness at 3 months. The NIV patient group reported improved subjective sleep quality and performed slightly better on a psychomotor vigilance task compared to CPAP. In a more recent trial by Howard et al., 60 participants with OHS were randomized to CPAP or NIV (Howard et al. 2017). Participants in this study were more hypercapnic. Again, both modalities were similarly effective in preventing the primary outcome of predefined treatment failure and in improving hypercapnia and quality-of-life measures, and achieving similar compliance. The largest study to date conducted by a multicentric Spanish group, Masa et al., recruited stable OHS patients with concomitant severe OSA (Masa et al. 2019). Again at 2 months, both CPAP and NIV produced similar results in improving daytime pCO_2, bicarbonate, and sleepiness. Both were significantly improved compared to lifestyle modification alone. Comparing the patient populations of the three randomized trials, the patients recruited differed in some characteristics. Howard et al. recruited patients with the highest degree of hypercapnia (c. +10 mmHg on average compared to the other two trials), and Masa et al. included patients with the lowest BMI (c. −10 kg/m^2 on average compared to the other two trials), demonstrating that the effectiveness of CPAP versus NIV does not necessarily depend on the level of baseline pCO_2 or BMI and can hence be potentially equally effective in a wider spectrum of stable OHS patients, at least in the short term. Nonetheless, Masa et al. found some differences between CPAP and NIV at 2 months. NIV was more effective than CPAP or lifestyle modification in improving pulmonary hypertension, left ventricular hypertrophy, and some functional outcomes, and importantly showed significant improvement in 6-minute walk distance. Pulmonary artery pressure decreased more in patients treated with NIV that had pulmonary hypertension at baseline (Masa, 2019). These results suggest a potential need to perform additional tests in stable OHS patients to better tailor treatment to individual risk profiles.

The patients in the Spanish study were followed for three additional years in the second phase of the study, where investigators only compared CPAP to NIV. The second phase of the study addressed the remaining question: whether similar short-term effectiveness of CPAP versus NIV would also be sustained long-term with similar effectiveness on more robust long-term outcomes, especially hospitalization rate and mortality. At 1 year the study found a stark reduction in clinically significant dyspnea (MRC scale ≥ 2) from the baseline rate of approximately 60% by about a half in both groups, an effect that developed over the 1st year of the study and was sustained over the study period of 3 years. Interestingly, the study demonstrated an improvement in lung function, specifically FVC and FEV1, which was independent of the treatment modality used. This effect is not completely explained, but it probably reflects the ability of PAP to reduce lung microatelectasis.

Both treatment modalities had a similar effect on health resource utilization, including ICU admissions during follow-up (Masa et al. 2019). No difference was detected in cardiovascular and all-cause mortality. Approximately half of the deaths in the mean follow-up of about 5 years were due to cardiovascular causes, further attesting to the fact that cardiovascular morbidity is driving prognosis in this patient group. Interestingly, a post hoc analysis demonstrated that the subgroup of patients with higher adherence had improved outcomes in healthcare utilization, including the risk of ICU admission and mortality, compared to the group with lower adherence. This suggests that, when adhered to, PAP therapy can reduce morbidity and mortality, although the healthy adherer effect has to be taken into account when interpreting these results. As expected, the CPAP group had a lower cost of treatment compared to the NIV group.

In view of the current evidence on newly diagnosed OHS, the option of de-escalation of treatment from NIV to CPAP in patients already established on NIV in the absence of weight reduction has to be considered. The question has been addressed by a recent study by Arrellano-Maric et al. (Arellano-maric et al. 2019). They found that out of 42 OHS patients that were switched from NIV to CPAP, 71% maintained normocapnia after 4 to 6 weeks. The switch to CPAP therapy was successful and safe even in patients that previously failed CPAP or were put on NIV after an episode of AHRF. Interestingly, 65% of patients preferred CPAP over NIV. Furthermore, switching patients from NIV to CPAP is an attractive option, especially given restricted healthcare budgets and the need for ever-increasing numbers of new OHS patients to be treated. Switching patients from NIV to CPAP is also warranted after successful weight reduction because the gas exchange will improve, and hypoventilation and AHI will decrease in parallel with weight reduction.

In summary, the available evidence supports the use of PAP therapy in patients with OHS. A sleep study in stable OHS is the initial step when deciding on a long-term therapy mode, depending on the sleep study phenotype of OHS. CPAP therapy should be fully titrated under poly(somno)graphy in OHS patients with a severe OSA phenotype. Responders to CPAP therapy will achieve appropriate and sustained physiological and clinical effects. In CPAP, responders' risk of hospital admissions and episodes of AHRF will be small and comparable to NIV. With a sleep hypoventilation phenotype without severe OSA, NIV should be considered first-line therapy.

Furthermore, patients that fail CPAP in the follow-up period should also be switched to NIV. In the case of substantial weight reduction, a switch from NIV to CPAP should be undertaken. Potentially, patients diagnosed with severe OSA and set up with NIV at initial presentation could be given a CPAP trial to undertake de-escalation from NIV to CPAP, but the long-term results of such de-escalation are not currently available.

Oxygen Therapy

In OHS patients not treated with PAP therapy, oxygen application alone aggravates hypoventilation, as has been demonstrated by several randomized studies. Furthermore, oxygen can precipitate acute respiratory failure (Randerath et al. 2017). Oxygen as monotherapy in OHS patients should be avoided whenever possible, and it should only be applied with NIV when required. A proportion of OHS patients will require oxygen supplementation after fully titrated PAP therapy, the rate probably depending on the level of inspiratory pressures applied. In a randomized trial comparing fixed pressure support to the hybrid volume targeted mode of ventilation, Murphy et al. found that only 12% of patients required supplemental oxygen when high NIV pressures were applied by a strict protocolized setup (mean EPAP 10 cmH_2O and IPAP 25 ± 3 cmH_2O)(Murphy et al., n.d.). In contrast, in the Spanish study in both the CPAP (mean CPAP 10.7 ± 2.6 cmH_2O) and NIV (mean IPAP 19.7 ± 4.3 cmH_2O and EPAP 8.2 ± 2.2 cmH_2O) arms of the trial, the proportion of patients requiring oxygen at initial setup was high (27 vs. 22%, respectively)(Masa et al. 2019).

Interestingly, patients in the study by Murphy had a higher BMI (52 ± 8 vs. 50 ± 8 kg/m^2) compared to the patients in the Spanish study (42.7 vs. 42.9 kg/m^2). This might explain why the pressures levels were different, but it can also point to the fact that the need for supplemental oxygen depends more on the level of aggressive pressure titration than on the level of obesity. How pressure range and supplemental oxygen influence the prognosis of patients is unclear.

Weight Reduction Strategies

Many studies have demonstrated that without substantial weight reduction key prognostically important features of OHS will not be sufficiently addressed, primarily metabolic and cardiovascular morbidity (Masa et al., n.d.). Interestingly, PAP therapy seems to have a divergent effect on weight when applied in eucapnic OSA, where it is associated with weight gain, or in OHS, where it is associated with weight loss (Masa et al., n.d.). The Spanish study demonstrated a small but statistically significant decrease of weight in NIV but not in the CPAP arm. The divergent effect is potentially linked to a different response to PAP therapy in terms of change in physical activity, with a couple of studies demonstrating increased daily activity of OHS patients after PAP initiation.

Nonetheless, even in OHS reduction of weight is small, and it is not likely to influence outcomes by itself. A study by Mandal recently explored the potential of a comprehensive rehabilitation program in addition to NIV to influence weight reduction, exercise capacity, and quality of life (Mandal et al. 2018). Intervention consisting of exercise and nutritional and motivational advice resulted in a significant reduction in weight and improvement in exercise capacity at 3 months, but the effect was not sustained at 12 months. Lifestyle modifications are generally not very successful in achieving significant and sustained weight reduction in this patient group. It appears that bariatric surgery is the only measure with a sustained effect on weight reduction.

In addition, bariatric surgery seems to have an acceptable risk profile in OHS patients with established PAP therapies. Recent clinical trials have demonstrated improvement in metabolic and cardiovascular indices, with a reduction in cardiovascular and all-cause mortality in obese patients undergoing bariatric surgery (Masa et al., n.d.). Recent guidelines suggest weight-loss interventions that will result in a sustained weight loss of 25 to 30% of body weight to achieve resolution of OHS, which is more likely to be achieved with bariatric surgery (Mokhlesi et al. 2019).

Key Points

1. Acute hypercapnic respiratory failure is a common presentation of OHS, requiring noninvasive ventilation in most cases and invasive ventilation in some patients

2. After an episode of acute hypercapnic respiratory failure has resolved, patients with OHS should be discharged with noninvasive ventilation until they undergo sleep studies in their stable state within 3 months
3. In stable OHS patients with severe OSA, CPAP is recommended as initial treatment; all other OHS patients should be started on home noninvasive ventilation
4. Weight reduction interventions are a crucial part of the management of these patients, with bariatric surgery providing substantial and sustained weight-loss

REFERENCES

Arellano-Maric, M., Aria, P., Hristine Hamm, C., Arieke L Duiverman, M., Arah Schwarz, S., Callegari, J. E. N. S., Storre, J. A. N. H., Laudia Schmoor, C. & Spielmanns, M. A. R. C. (2019). *Obesity Hypoventilation Syndrome Treated with Non-Invasive Ventilation : Is a Switch to CPAP Therapy Feasible ?*, 2019 (September). https:// doi.org/10.1111/resp.13704.

Articles, Ajrccm. (2019). *Authors*, 1–105. https://doi.org/10.1164/ rccm.201906-1122OC.

BaHammam, A. S., Pandi-Perumal, S. R., Piper, A., Bahammam, S. A., Almeneessier, A. S., Olaish, A. H. & Javaheri, S. (2016). *Gender differences in patients with obesity hypoventilation syndrome*, 445-53.

Berg, Greg, Kenneth Delaive, Jure Manfreda & Randy Walld. (2001). *The Use of Health-Care Resources in Obesity-Hypoventilation Syndrome*, 377–83. https://doi.org/10.1378/chest.120.2.377.

Berger, Kenneth I, Indu Ayappa, I Barry Sorkin, Robert G Norman, David M Rapoport, Roberta M Goldring, I Kenneth, et al. (2002). *Postevent Ventilation as a Function of CO 2 Load during Respiratory Events in Obstructive Sleep Apnea*, 917–24.

Borel, J. E. A. N. Hristian., Aure Borel, A. N. N. E., Enis Monneret, D., Enaud Tamisier, R., Atrick Levy, P. & Ouis Pepin, J. E. A. N. (2012). *Invited Review Series : Obesity And Respiratory Disorders Obesity Hypoventilation Syndrome : From Sleep-Disordered Breathing to Systemic Comorbidities and the Need to Offer*, no. October 2011, 601–10. https://doi.org/10.1111/j.1440-1843.2011.02106.x.

Carrillo, Andres, Miquel Ferrer, Gumersindo Gonzalez-diaz, Antonia Lopez-martinez, Noemi Llamas, Maravillas Alcazar, Lucia Capilla, & Antoni Torres. n.d. *Noninvasive Ventilation in Acute Hypercapnic Respiratory Failure Caused by Obesity Hypoventilation Syndrome and Chronic Obstructive Pulmonary Disease.* https://doi.org/10.1164/ rccm.201206-1101OC.

Davidson, A Craig, Stephen Banham, Mark Elliott, Daniel Kennedy, Colin Gelder, Alastair Glossop, Alistair Colin Church, et al. (2016). *BTS/ ICS Guideline for the*

Ventilatory Management of Acute Hypercapnic Respiratory Failure in Adults. https://doi.org/10.1136/thoraxjnl-2015-208209.

Hales, Craig M, Cheryl D Fryar, Margaret D Carroll, David S Freedman, Yutaka Aoki, & Cynthia L Ogden. (2018). *Differences in Obesity Prevalence by Demographic Characteristics and Urbanization Level Among Adults in the United States, 2013-2016*, 20782 (23), 2419–29. https://doi.org/10.1001/jama.2018.7270.

Howard, Mark E, Amanda J Piper, Bronwyn Stevens, Anne E Holland, Brendon J Yee, Eli Dabscheck, Duncan Mortimer, et al. (2017). *A Randomised Controlled Trial of CPAP versus Non-Invasive Ventilation for Initial Treatment of Obesity Hypoventilation Syndrome*, 437–44. https://doi.org/10.1136/thoraxjnl-2016-208559.

Lemyze, Malcolm, Pauline Taufour, Alain Duhamel, Johanna Temime, Olivier Nigeon, Nicolas Vangrunderbeeck, Stéphanie Barrailler, et al. (2014). "Determinants of Noninvasive Ventilation Success or Failure in Morbidly Obese Patients in Acute Respiratory Failure." *PLoS ONE, 9* (5), 5–11. https://doi.org/10.1371/journal.pone.0097563.

Mandal, Swapna, Eui-sik Suh, Rachel Harding, Anna Vaughan-france, Michelle Ramsay, Bronwen Connolly, Danielle E Bear, et al. (2018). *Nutrition and Exercise Rehabilitation in Obesity Hypoventilation Syndrome (NERO): A Pilot Randomised Controlled Trial*, 62–69. https://doi.org/10.1136/thoraxjnl-2016-209826.

Marik, Paul E. & Himanshu Desai. (2014). *Care Medicine.* https://doi.org/10.1177/0885066612444261.

Masa, Juan F, Babak Mokhlesi, Iván Benítez, Francisco Javier, Gomez De Terreros, Maria Ángeles Sánchez-quiroga, & Auxiliadora Romero. (2019). "Articles Long-Term Clinical Effectiveness of Continuous Positive Airway Pressure Therapy versus Non-Invasive Ventilation Therapy in Patients with Obesity Hypoventilation Syndrome : A Multicentre, Open-Label," *Randomised Controlled Trial, 6736* (18), 1–12. https://doi.org/10.1016/S0140-6736(18)32978-7.

Masa, Juan F, Jean-louis Pépin, Jean-christian Borel, Babak Mokhlesi & Patrick B Murphy. n.d. *Obesity Hypoventilation Syndrome*, 1–14. https://doi.org/10.1183/16000617.0097-2018.

Mokhlesi, Babak, Juan Fernando Masa, Jan L Brozek, Indira Gurubhagavatula, Patrick B Murphy, Amanda J Piper, Aiman Tulaimat, et al. (2019). *American Thoracic Society Evaluation and Management of Obesity Hypoventilation Syndrome An Of Fi Cial American Thoracic Society Clinical Practice Guideline*, 200 (3). https://doi.org/10.1164/rccm.201905-1071ST.

Murphy, Patrick Brian, Craig Davidson, Matthew David Hind, Anita Simonds, Adrian J Williams, Nicholas S Hopkinson, John Moxham, Michael Polkey & Nicholas Hart. n.d. *Volume Targeted versus Pressure Support Non-Invasive Ventilation in Patients with Super Obesity and Chronic Respiratory Failure : A Randomised Controlled Trial.* https://doi.org/10.1136/thoraxjnl-2011-201081.

Nowbar, Sogol, Kristin M Burkart, Ralph Gonzales, Andrew Fedorowicz, Wendolyn S Gozansky, Jon C Gaudio, Matthew R G Taylor & Clifford W Zwillich. (2003). *Hospitalized Patients : Prevalence, Effects, and Outcome*, 1–7. https://doi.org/10.1016/j.amjmed.2003.08.022.

Palm, Andreas, Bengt Midgren, Christer Janson & Eva Lindberg. (2016). "Gender Differences in Patients Starting Long-Term Home Mechanical Ventilation Due to Obesity Hypoventilation Syndrome." *Respiratory Medicine, 110*, 73–78. https://doi.org/10.1016/ j.rmed.2015.11.010.

Piper, A. J., Wang, D., Yee, B. J., Barnes, D. J., Grunstein, R. R. & Royal Prince Alfred. (2008). *Randomised Trial of CPAP vs Bilevel Support in the Treatment of Obesity Hypoventilation Syndrome without Severe Nocturnal Desaturation*, no. 2: 395–402. https://doi.org/10.1136/ thx.2007.081315.

Mokhlesi Babak. (2010). *Obesity Hypoventilation Syndrome. A State-of-the-Art Review*, 1347–65.

Randerath, Winfried, Johan Verbraecken, Stefan Andreas, Michael Arzt, Konrad E. Bloch, Thomas Brack, Bertien Buyse, et al. (2017). "Definition, Discrimination, Diagnosis and Treatment of Central Breathing Disturbances during Sleep." *European Respiratory Journal*, *49* (1). https://doi.org/10.1183/13993003.00959-2016.

Simonds Anita. (2015). *Handbook Noninvasive ventilation*. London: European respiratory society.

Schwartz, Alan R, Susheel P Patil, Samuel Squier, Hartmut Schneider, Jason P Kirkness & Philip L Smith. (2010). *Obesity and Upper Airway Control during Sleep*, 430–35. https://doi.org/10.1152/ japplphysiol.00919.2009.

Sequeira, Telma C. A., Ahmed, S Bahammam. & Antonio, M Esquinas. (2016). *Noninvasive Ventilation in the Critically Ill Patient With Obesity Hypoventilation Syndrome: A Review*. https://doi.org/ 10.1177/0885066616663179.

Verbraecken, Johan & Walter T Mcnicholas. (2015). *Respiratory Mechanics and Ventilatory Control in Overlap Syndrome and Obesity Hypoventilation*, 1–17.

Windisch, Wolfram & Karsten Simon. (2018). *German National Guideline for Treating Chronic Respiratory Failure with Invasive and Non-Invasive Ventilation – Revised Edition*, 2017, Part 2, 171–203. https://doi.org/10.1159/000488667.

In: Sleep Medicine in Critical Care
Editors: Antonio M. Esquinas et al.
ISBN: 978-1-53617-768-8

Chapter 15

SLEEP-RELATED BREATHING DISORDERS IN CHRONIC NEUROMUSCULAR DISEASES

Jacek Nasiłowski**, MD, PhD
Department of Internal Medicine, Pulmonary Diseases and Allergy, Medical University of Warsaw, Warsaw, Poland

ABSTRACT

Sleep-related breathing disorders are a frequent phenomenon in patients with neuromuscular diseases. There are many mechanisms which predispose the occurrence of respiratory events during sleep. The principal pathomechanisms are weakness of respiratory muscles (mainly diaphragm), impaired breathing control and restriction of the chest. There are three main types of sleep-related breathing disorders: hypoventilation, central events and obstructive events. The gold standard for the diagnosis is full polysomnography, with concomitant measurement of transcutaneous partial pressure of O2 and CO2. Non-invasive ventilation is a treatment of choice and should be started in a hospital setting in order to adequately titrate the settings. Inadequate treatment is a risk factor of a worse prognosis. Tolerability of long-term non-invasive ventilation may be an issue in neuromuscular patients.

Keywords: sleep-related breathing disorders, neuromuscular diseases, obstructive sleep apnea, polysomnography, hypoventilation

* Corresponding Author's E-mail: jnasilowski@wum.edu.pl.

ABBREVIATIONS

AHI	apnoea/hypopnea index
ALS	amyotrophic lateral sclerosis
EPAP	expiratory positive airway pressure
FRC	functional residual capacity
IPAP	inspiratory positive airway pressure
NIV	non-invasive ventilation
NMD	neuromuscular diseases
PSG	polysomnography
RDI	respiratory disturbance index
SCI	spinal cord injury
SMA	spinal muscle atrophy
SRBD	sleep-related breathing disorders
VC	vital capacity

INTRODUCTION

The common context of respiratory problems in patients with neuromuscular diseases (NMD) is awake hypoventilation due to weakness of inspiratory muscles and cough inefficacy due to impairment of expiratory muscles and/or bulbar involvement, which may lead to chronic respiratory failure and recurrent respiratory infections. The majority of the diagnostic and treatment effort is focused on these issues. While the presence of sleep-related breathing disorders (SRBD) in this population is usually ignored as having less impact on quality of life and mortality. While SRBD in NMD patients are very frequent and may play a significant role on the course of the disease.

The prevalence of SRBD in NMD patients is not well established. There is a paucity of surveys which aim to assess their prevalence and type. Moreover, the progressive character of NMD makes it even more difficult. The number and types of events may coincide with the continuing decline in vital capacity (VC) and muscle strength. In the 90's Labanowski et al. investigated SRBD in a cohort of 50 adults and 10 children with various disorders, mainly: myopathy, amyotrophic lateral sclerosis (ALS) and muscular dystrophy. They found that as much as 83% had a respiratory disturbance index (RDI) of 5 or more, 63% of 10 or more, and 42% of 15 or more, which proved a very high prevalence of SRBD in this group of patients. More interestingly, they found that most of them (90%) had scored as hypopneas and only 1,5% as apneas of which 68% were non-obstructive. The reason for the predominance of non-obstructive events may be a weakness of the diaphragm in order to generate enough negative pressure to collapse the airway. Interestingly, a majority of SRBD occurred in a non-supine position, which is contrary to SRBD in the general non-NMD population.

However, SRBD are not the only phenomenon characterized for hereditary NMD. The prevalence of SRBD in patients with spinal cord injuries (SCI) is very high and reaches more than 90% of the subjects in cervical SCI. The central type of event is predominant in cervical SCI, while in the thoracic SCI obstructive events are more frequent.

The presence of SRBD should be screened in all NMD patients. Taking into account the progressive type of NMD, a schedule of a regular follow-ups should be set up for every patient. The heterogeneity of SRBD requires evaluation by a medical staff with experience in sleep medicine.

PATHOPHYSIOLOGY

There are three main types of SRBD: hypoventilation, central events and obstructive events. Hypoventilation is often manifested in so-called diaphragmatic or pseudo-central events, which are unique for NMD. The type of SRBD usually depends on the distribution of muscle involvement. The predominant impairment of the diaphragm predisposes individuals to hypoventilation and central events, while in the case of involvement of intercostal and upper airway muscles, obstructive events predominate.

Hypoventilation

Nocturnal hypoventilation may be induced by several underlying conditions, which can be grouped into two: restriction of the chest and sleep-related factors.

Restriction of the chest is caused by the following mechanism:

1. Respiratory muscle weakness, mainly the diaphragm, is the most important mechanism responsible for hypoventilation. In order to optimize the work of breathing and avoid muscle fatigue a patient changes the pattern of breathing and takes breaths of a small volume not to generate high transdiaphragmatic pressure. At the same time the respiratory rate has to be increased in order to preserve minute volume. This particular pattern of breathing, called "rapid shallow breathing", increases the ratio death space volume to tidal volume, which decreases alveolar ventilation.
2. Chest wall deformities. The weakness of other muscles than respiratory ones: dorsal, chest and abdominal can be a reason for chest wall deformities (e.g., scoliosis), which coexists often in the course of NMD and further aggravates

respiratory system dysfunction. The magnitude of hypoventilation is augmented by the increase in respiratory load as a consequence of the decrease in compliance of the thorax and contractibility of the muscles.

3. Increased stiffness of the rib cage joint cartilages due to permanent reduction in its expansion range reduces compliance of the chest wall even if the deformity has not developed yet.

Sleep related factors refer to:

1. horizontal position during sleep, which has deleterious impact on ventilation due to reduction in VC and functional residual capacity (FRC), particularly in the case of diaphragmatic weakness or paralysis.
2. reduction in tidal volume during the stage 2 sleep period
3. reduction in muscle tone of additional inspiratory and expiratory muscles during REM sleep
4. reduction in chemosensitivity of respiratory control centres particularly during REM sleep
5. increase in upper airway resistance, which negatively impacts on minute ventilation

Diaphragmatic or Pseudo-Central Events

These unusual events are characteristic features of patients with severe impairment of the diaphragm. During REM sleep there is a significant relaxation of the tone of all muscles except the diaphragm. However, when the function of the diaphragm is impaired then the amplitude of the movement of the thorax and the abdomen may be so small that this is not registered by polysomnography signals. As a result, the pattern of central apnea or hypopnea occurs in polysomnography (PSG). To avoid misdiagnosis diaphragm electromyography should be used as a method of choice. However, monitoring of esophageal pressure or pulse transit time maybe useful as well.

Central Events

Central events are common findings in NMD patients particularly with diaphragmatic involvement and cardiomyopathy. They can be in the form of separate apneic or hyponeic events, or have a regular pattern of periodic breathing, or Cheyne-Stokes respiration. The main mechanisms of susceptibility to central events is impaired control of breathing during sleep, which refers to enhanced ventilatory responses to CO2, a lower awake and sleep CO2 level, and circulatory delay.

Obstructive Events

Obstructive events are characteristic features of disorders with preserved diaphragmatic functions and impaired muscles of upper airways and the rib cage. Typically, they are present in the early phase of muscular dystrophy. The main underlying mechanisms predisposing patients to obstructive events refers to:

1. Bulbar dysfunction, common in various NMD (ALS, spinal muscle atrophy (SMA), myasthenia gravis), which may impair the patency of upper airways.
2. Reduction in activity of pharyngeal dilators due to the decrease in genioglossal and tensor palatine muscles caused probably by suppression of pharyngeal and laryngeal nerves during sleep
3. Pharyngeal neuropathy may be an element of certain NMDs, like Charcot-Marie-Tooth disease.
4. Anatomic predisposition, like macroglossia, may play an important role in the occurrence of obstructive events. This phenomenon is frequent in muscular dystrophy or Pompe disease especially during childhood, when the diameter of pharynx is relatively smaller.

DIAGNOSIS

The diagnosis of SRBD is based on the same rules as in the general population. Most typical symptoms include diurnal (excessive daytime sleepiness, morning headache, and restless sleep) and nocturnal (snoring, awaking with choking, nightmares and enuresis) complaints.

Interestingly, some authors do not found the correlation between quantity of nocturnal events and variables indicating progression of the disease (vital capacity or strength of inspiratory and expiratory muscles). However, patient with impaired muscle strength and reduced VC below 1-1.5 litre are more likely to desaturate during sleep.

Typical screening tools like Epworth Sleepiness Scale or STOP-BANG questionnaire could be used in NMD, however they have never been validated in this group of patients and its specificity and sensitivity should be questionable. The British group invented and validated the self-administered 5-item questionnaire - SiNQ-5, particularly for NMD patients with diaphragm paralysis. Each item is scored between 0 and 2 and a score of 5 or more points indicates increased likelihood of associated SRBD.

The gold standard for the diagnosis of SRBD is a full PSG with transcutaneous monitoring of CO_2 to reveal hypoventilation. As mentioned above, sometimes this equipment should be enhanced with diaphragm electromyography or esophageal pressure catheters. Access to such sophisticated investigations are limited only to specialized centres. That is why the diagnosis may be established on the basis of more simple tools like unattended polygraphy with four channels. In case of a negative result or a result not corresponding with severity of symptoms, a full PSG should be obtained.

TREATMENT

The principal method of treatment of SRBD in NMD patients is non-invasive ventilation (NIV) because of the high prevalence of hypoventilation and central events. CPAP therapy may be used in the early stages of such diseases, like muscular dystrophy or Pompe disease with a picture of the obstructive syndrome alone.

The initiation of NIV should be managed in a hospital setting with careful adjustment of the interface and ventilator settings, and if necessary oxygen flow and the use of a humidifier. The time to accept NIV treatment differs between patients from a few days to a few months and is much worse with bulbar involvement. In extreme cases, a patient may not accept NIV treatments at all and the only option is then ventilation via tracheostomy if the patient will accept such an invasive approach. Usually a few days in the hospital should be enough to adapt the best interface and to titrate initial settings. Titration of the settings should be made on the basis of the analysis of the built-in device software with the combination of overnight transcutaneous monitoring of pO2 and pCO2 levels. Optionally, in the most complex cases, a full PSG during NIV treatment may be used to reveal potential pitfalls, and to assess efficacy for the restoration of normal sleep architecture.

The diversity of interfaces provided by the equipment company allows for broad possibility in interface choice. Some patients, usually more active, prefer smaller interfaces, like nasal pillows, which does not disrupt communication and eating. Others prefer oronasal interfaces which allow for breathing through the nose and mouth. However, attention has to be paid to make sure the oronasal mask will not provoke obstructive events.

The initial settings should be set at a low level, e.g., EPAP 2 - 4 cmH_2O, IPAP 8 - 10cmH_2O, in order to let the patient familiarize themselves with breathing with positive pressures. The rise time should not be very short. Subsequently, the inspiration time and the back-up rate should be titrated to maintain inspiration to expiration time ratio between 1:1 to 1:2. Further increase in respiratory pressures should be made on the basis of their effectiveness. Usually, low pressure support is needed to obtain adequate tidal volume, unless the severe deformity of the chest exists and decreases chest compliance. In cases of severe obstructive syndrome, high EPAP is necessary; however, its application may be difficult, because of the lack of tolerability. To improve tolerability the mode with automatic EPAP may be used. However, in some patients adequately effective pressure cannot be set up and the compromise between efficacy and tolerability has to be discussed with the patient.

Ventilation modes with a back-up rate is more effective than spontaneous modes in improvement in gas exchange, correction of SRBD and the quantity of patient-ventilator asynchrony.

Efficacy of the treatment of SRBD have an impact on the clinical outcome. Georges et al. proved that ALS patient with suboptimal control of respiratory events during NIV have a worse prognosis than patients with adequate treatment. Moreover, Gonzales-Bermajo et al. found that inadequate ventilation in the first month of treatment is the main (?) independent risk factor of mortality in ALS patients.

KEY POINTS

1. SRBD are frequent in patients with NMD. The types of SRBD include nocturnal hypoventilation, central events and obstructive events.
2. The best method of diagnosis is full polysomnography with simultaneous transcutaneous monitoring of pO2 and pCO2.
3. NIV is the treatment of choice, which improves quality of life, sleep quality and survival.
4. NIV should be started in a hospital setting with adequate setting titration, optimally under the control of PSG and transcutaneous monitoring of pO2 and pCO2.
5. Inadequate quality of NIV is the risk factor of worse prognosis.

REFERENCES

[1] Gonzalez-Bermejo, J., Morelot-Panzini, C., Arnol, N., Meininger, V., Kraoua, S., Salachas, F., Similowski, T. Prognostic value of efficiently correcting nocturnal desaturations after one month of non-invasive ventilation in amyotrophic lateral sclerosis: a retrospective monocentre observational cohort study. *Amyotroph. Lateral Scler. Frontotemporal Degener.,* 2013 Sep.; 14(5 - 6):373 - 9.

[2] Georges, M., Attali, V., Golmard, J. L., Morélot-Panzini, C., Crevier-Buchman, L., Collet, J.-M. et al. Reduced survival in patients with ALS with upper airway

obstructive events on non-invasive ventilation. *J. Neurol. Neurosurg. Psychiatry,* 2016; 87:1045 - 50.

[3] Janssens, J. P., Borel, J. C., Pépin, J. L. Nocturnal monitoring of home non-invasive ventilation: the contribution of simple tools such as pulse oximetry, capnography, built-in ventilator software and autonomic markers of sleep fragmentation. *Thorax,* 2011; 66:438 - 45.

[4] Vrijsen, B., Buyse, B., Belge, C., Vanpee, G., Van Damme, P., Testelmans, D. Randomized cross-over trial of ventilator modes during non-invasive ventilation titration in amyotrophic lateral sclerosis. *Respirology,* 2017 Aug.; 22(6):1212 - 1218.

[5] Labanowski, M., Schmidt-Nowara, W., Guilleminault, C. Sleep and neuromuscular disease: frequency of sleep-disordered breathing in a neuromuscular disease clinic population. *Neurology,* 1996; 47(5): 1173 - 1180.

[6] Loutfi, S. Aboussouan, Eduardo Mireles-Cabodevila. Sleep-Disordered Breathing in Neuromuscular Disease. Diagnostic and Therapeutic Challenges. *Chest,* 2017; 152(4):880 - 892.

[7] Mohamad Ammar Albdewi, Liistro, Giuseppe, El Tahry, Riëm. Sleep-disordered breathing in patients with neuromuscular disease. *Sleep Breath,* (2018) 22:277 - 286.

[8] Steier, J., Jolley, C. J., Seymour, J., Teschler, H., Luo, Y. M., Polkey, M. I. and Moxham, J. Screening for sleep-disordered breathing in neuromuscular disease using a questionnaire for symptoms associated with diaphragm paralysis. *Eur. Respir. J.,* 2011; 37: 400 - 405.

[9] Sankari, Abdulghani, Bascom, Amy T., Susmita Chowdhuri and M. Safwan Badr. Tetraplegia is a risk factor for central sleep apnea. *J. Appl. Physiol.,* 116: 345 - 353, 2014.

[10] Bart Vrijsen, Bertien Buyse, Catharina Belge, Dries Testelmans. Upper Airway Obstruction during Noninvasive Ventilation Induced by the Use of an Oronasal Mask. *J. Clin. Sleep Med.,* 2014; 10(9):1033 - 1035.

In: Sleep Medicine in Critical Care
Editors: Antonio M. Esquinas et al.
ISBN: 978-1-53617-768-8

Chapter 16

SLEEP-RELATED BREATHING DISORDERS: INVASIVE MECHANICAL VENTILATION (NON-PERIOPERATIVE)

Ebru Ortac Ersoy*[1,*]*, MD Mehmet Yildirim*[1]*, MD
Medical Intensive Care Unit, Hacettepe University, Ankara, Turkey

ABSTRACT

Sleep abnormalities are common problems in patients who are mechanically ventilated in the intensive care unit (ICU). Causes of sleep disturbances in ICU patients are multifactorial. Mechanical ventilation typically disturbs and disrupts sleep. The severity of the disease, the endotracheal tube, mask, nasogastric tube, aspiration, physical restraints, and mouth patches in patients undergoing mechanical ventilation cause sleep deprivation. Ventilator modes applied in mechanical ventilation also affect sleep quality and cause sleep related breathing disorders. Ventilator settings and modes affect sleep quality and can cause sleep related breathing disorders, especially if patient ventilator asynchrony exists.

Keywords: Sleep, mechanical ventilation, ventilator modes

1. INTRODUCTION

Invasive mechanical ventilation is frequently used in intensive care units for improving blood gas parameters, protection of airway and reduction of work of breath.

---

[*] Corresponding Author's E-mail: ebru.ortac@hacettepe.edu.tr.

Mechanically ventilated patients have changes in sleep architecture and they have severe sleep fragmentation [1]. Although sleep disorders can be easily missed for these critical ill patients, sleep disruption, low sleep quality have been more reported in mechanicaly ventilated patients than other critical ill patients [2, 3]. However almost 60% of the mechanically ventilated intensive care survivors suffer from sleep disturbances after hospital discharge at 2 months [4]. Disrupted sleep is associated with increased morbidity and mortality. Several studies have shown sleep disorders in patients receiving mechanical ventilation. Patient-ventilator asynchrony, inappropriate ventilator modes, environmental noise and light, sedation and critical illness itself are major causes of sleep disorders for invasive mechanical ventilated patients [2, 5, 6].

2. Sleep Related Breathing Disorders and Ventilator Modes

2.1. Invasive Mechanical ventilation

Invasive Mechanical ventilation is used quite often in intensive care and life saving treatment method. The severity of the disease, the endotracheal tube, mask, nasogastric tube, aspiration, physical restraints, and mouth patches in patients undergoing mechanical ventilation cause sleep deprivation. Mechanical ventilation is also cause sleep disturbances because of applying positive pressure or volume. Sedation during mechanical ventilation can cause sleep deprivation.

Cooper et al. were first to measure sleep in critically ill patients receiving mechanical ventilation objectively. They studied on 20 mechanically ventilated patients and none of them demonstrated normal sleep on 24-h polysomnography [3]. Cortical breath alert disappears during sleep and chemoreceptors are only stimulant factors to continue ventilation. PCO2 is the most important stimulant for chemoreceptors. Therefore mechanism of central apnea is decreasing PCO2 levels below the threshold [7]. Central apnea development can occur due to mechanical ventilation. and leads poor cardiovascular outcomes especially in critically ill patients.

2.2.Ventilator Modes and Sleep

Ventilator modes applied in mechanical ventilation also affect sleep quality and can cause sleep related disorders alone.

2.2.1. Pressure Support Ventilation, Assist Control Ventilation:

Central apnea leads to sleep disruptions and apneas oftenly occur during ventilation with pressure support mode (PSV) [8, 9]. Because higher levels of pressure support result in hyperventilation, high minute ventilation and hypocapnia. Finally hypocapnic stimulation of chemoreceptors responds with apnea. Parthasarathy and Tobin studied on 11 mechanically ventilated patients and observed that 6 of the patients had central apneas during PSV. Among the 6 patients who developed apneas, adding dead space decreased the frequency: 4±2 versus 53±8 apneas/hour. Sleep fragmantations, arousals, awakenings were more frequent during PSV than asist control ventilation (ACV). During PSV, addition of dead space decreased the frequency of arousals and awakenings and reduced central apneas (4 ± 2 versus 53 ± 8 apneas/hour) [10]. On the other hand during sleep, high support levels of PSV can lead hypocapnia, central apneas and sleep fragmantations, thus back up mode of ventilation (ACV) can be activated. ACV may maintain periodic breathing during sleep, although putting the respiratory muscles excessively at rest might be the downside [11]. Therefore, minimum support level which maintains optimum gas exchange, patient comfort and sleep quality should be set on PSV and apneic effect of high support levels should not be ignored.

2.2.2. Proportional Assist Ventilation

Proportional assist ventilation (PAV), was designed to improve patient-ventilator synchrony for patients with spontaneous respiratory efforts. In this mode patient's inspiratory effort determines the support given. The ventilator amplifies the patient's inspiratory effort without any preselected target volume or pressure. PAV adjusts flow and volume based on respiratory resistance, elastance, and inspiratory effort. There are limited studies about the relationship between PAV and sleep quality. Bosma et al. randomized thirteen patient to receive pressure support ventilation or proportional assist ventilation on the first night and then crossed over to the alternative mode for the second night. During PSV arousals per hour were 16 and 9 during PAV. Sleep quality was significantly improved with PAV. PAV was associated with increased REM. During the night increasing of PCO2 was greater on PAV, therefore minute ventilation were lower [12]. In chronic obstructive lung disease when compared to PSV, PAV with load adjustable gain factor (PAV+) was associated with better patient-ventilator synchrony. However in these patients, there were no significant difference between PAV+ and PSV in sleep quality [13]. Further studies are needed to understand the effectiveness of PAV on sleep quality.

2.2.3. Neurally Adjusted Ventilatory Assist

Neurally adjusted ventilatory assist (NAVA), provides to maintain patient ventilator synchrony using transdiaphragmatic pressure to deliver ventilatory assist. Electrical activity of diaphragm is recorded through an esophageal probe. Similar to PAV, patient determines pressure support for every breath [14]. Delisle et al. studied on 14 patients to determine sleep quality during NAVA in mechanically ventilated patients. They compared PSV and NAVA. NAVA showed a normal percentage of REM and important decrease in fragmentation and better patient-ventilator synchrony compared to PSV [15].

On the other hand, in an observational study, total sleep time of patients who received mechanically ventilation was higher and median arousal indices were fewer than the patients who did not [16]. Roche-Campo et al. evaluated the direct impact of the mechanical ventilator on sleep quality in diffucult to wean intensive care patients. They found longer sleeping hours during mechanical ventilation and no significant impact of mechanical ventilator mode on sleep quality. This study may demonstrate that mechanical ventilation could improve sleep quality by decreasing work of breathing, anxiety and dyspnea during spontaneous ventilation [17].

Conclusion

We have not yet clearly understood the effects of mechanical ventilation on sleep. There are not any randomized controlled trial with large patient groups. To improve sleep quality and also reduce the central apneas in the patients who receive invasive mechanical ventilation using low support levels seems reasonable. As PAV and NAVA are more similar to normal physiology, they may give the opportunity of more physiological sleep. There are not enough studies on this subject in the literature. The future widescale studies should enlighten this subject.

Invasive mechanical ventilation can cause sleep related breathing disorders. Ventilator modes are important for preventing sleep disorders. Modes such as ACV, PAV and NAVA appear to be associated with better sleep.

References

[1] Ortac Ersoy, E., Ocal, S., Kara, A., Ardıç, S., Topeli, (2016); A. Sleep in Mechanically Ventilated Patients in the Intensive Care Unit. *J. Turk. Sleep Med.,* 3:10 - 13.

[2] Freedman, N. S., Kotzer, N., Schwab, R. J. (1999);Patient perception of sleep quality and etiology of sleep disruption in the intensive care unit. *Am. J. Respir. Crit. Care Med.,* 159(4): 1155 - 1162.

[3] Cooper, A. B., Thornley, K. S., Young, G. B., Slutsky, A. S., Stewart, T. E., Hanly, P. J. (2000); Sleep in critically ill patients requiring mechanical ventilation. *Chest,* 117(3): 809 - 818.

[4] Choi, J., Hoffman, L. A., Schulz, R., Tate, J. A., Donahoe, M. P., Ren, D., Given, B. A., Sherwood, P. R. Self-reported physical symptoms in intensive care unit (ICU) survivors: pilot exploration over four months post-ICU discharge. *J. Pain Symptom Manage,* 2014; 47:257 - 270.

[5] Bourne, R. S., Mills, G. H. (2004); Sleep disruption in critically ill patients-pharmacological considerations. *Anaesthesia,* 59(4): 374 - 384.

[6] Thille, A. W., Rodriguez, P., Cabello, B. Lellouche, F. And Brochard, L. (2006); Patient-ventilator asynchrony during assisted mechanical ventilation. *Intensive Care Med.,* 32: 1515 - 1522.

[7] Ortaç Ersoy, E., Demir, A. U., Topeli, A. (2016); Sleep in Intensive Care: Is there or not? *Journal of Medical and Surgical Intensive Care Medicine,* 7:28 - 33.

[8] Skatrud, J. B. and Dempsey, J. A. (1983); Interaction of sleep state and chemical stimuli in sustaining rhythmic ventilation. *J. Appl. Physiol.,* 55: 813 - 822.

[9] Ohayon, M. M., Carskadon, M. A., Guilleminault, C., Vitiello, M. V. (2004);Meta-analysis of quantitative sleep parameters from childhood to old age in healthy individuals: Developing normative sleep values across the human lifespan. *Sleep,* 27: 1255 - 1273.

[10] Parthasarathy, S., Tobin, M. J. (2002);Effect of ventilator mode on sleep quality in critically ill patients. *Am. J. Respir. Crit. Care Med.,*; 166: 1423 - 1429.

[11] Rittayamai, N., Wilcox, E., Drouot, X., Mehta, S., Goffi, A., Brochard, L. (2016); Positive and negative effects of mechanical ventilation on sleep in the ICU: a review with clinical recommendations. *Intensive Care Med.,* 42:531 - 541.

[12] Bosma, K., Ferreyra, G., Ambrogio, C., Pasero, D., Mirabella, L., Braghiroli, A., Appendini, L., Mascia, L., Ranieri, V. (2007); Patient-ventilator interaction and sleep in mechanically ventilated patients: pressure support versus proportional assist ventilation. *Crit. Care Med.,* 35(4): 1048 - 1054.

[13] Alexopoulou, C., Kondili, E., Vakouti, E., Klimathianaki, M., Prinianakis, G., Georgopoulos, D. (2007); Sleep during proportional-assist ventilation with load-adjustable gain factors in critically ill patients. *Intensive Care Med.,* 33(7):1139 - 1147.

[14] Younes, M., Puddy, A., Roberts, D., Light, R. B., Quesada, A., Taylor, K., Oppenheimer, L., Cramp, H. (1992); Proportional assist ventilation. Results of an initial clinical trial. *Am. Rev. Respir. Dis.,* 145: 121 - 129.

[15] Delisle, S., Ouellet, P., Bellemare, P., Tétraul, J. P., Arsenault, P. (2011); Sleep quality in mechanically ventilated patients: comparison between NAVA and PSV modes. *Ann. Intensive Care,*; 1: 42.

[16] Elliott, R., McKinley, S., Cistulli, P., Fien, M. (2013); Characterisation of sleep in intensive care using 24-hourpolysomnography: an observational study. *Crit. Care,* 17: R46.

[17] Roche-Campo, F., Thille, A. W., Drouot, X., Galia, F., Margarit, L., Córdoba-Izquierdo, A., Mancebo, J., d'Ortho, M., Brochard, L. (2013); Comparison of Sleep Quality with Mechanical Versus Spontaneous Ventilation during Weaning of Critically Ill Tracheostomized Patients. *Crit. Care Med.,* 41:1637 - 1644.

In: Sleep Medicine in Critical Care
Editors: Antonio M. Esquinas et al.
ISBN: 978-1-53617-768-8

Chapter 17

Airway Management in Sleep-Related Breathing Disorders: Key Practical Approach

Eda Macit Aydın**, *MD
Department of Anesthesiology and Reanimation, Division of Critical Care Medicine,
Gazi University Faculty of Medicine Ankara, Turkey

Abstract

Sleep related breathing disorders" are respiratory failure during sleep and associated with narrowing or closing of the upper airway in many cases. The degree of respiratory disorders ranges from a partial obstruction of the airway to apnea asssociated with recurrent hypoxemia. Sleep-related breathing disorders include: obstructive sleep apnea (OSAs) disorders, central sleep apnea (CSA) syndromes, sleep-releated hypoventilation disorders and sleep-releated hypoxemia disorder. The decrease of chest wall compliance, lung capacity(functional residual volume) in patients with sleep-related respiratory disorders may cause difficulties in airway control. This condition, these patients may require intense perioperative management because of prolonged respiratory depression potential due to residual anesthetic agents and increases concerns about the application of general anesthesia. It is important to plan a perioperative anesthesia management for potential adverse events such as airway management, difficult mask ventilation and difficult intubation. In the postoperative period, close hemodynamic monitoring, blood oxygen level and continuous positive airway pressure (CPAP) should be provided and respiratory support should be provided.

---

* Corresponding Author's E-mail: edamct@hotmail.com.

Keywords: difficult airway, positive airway pressure, sleep related breathing disorder

INTRODUCTION

Sleep-related breathing disorders, due to changes in respiratory pattern (e.q., apnea, hypopnea, or respiratory effort related arousal) or abnormal reduction of gas exchange (e.q., hypoventilation) during sleep, are a common group of diseases with harmful consequences for health. Sleep-related breathing disorders are classified in four major categories: OSA disorders, CSA syndromes, sleep-related hypoventilation disorders and sleep-related hypoxemia disorders [1]. The most common sleep-related breathing disorder is OSA, which is characterized by a significant reduction in airflow in the presence of respiratory effort due to partial or complete collapse of upper respiratory tract that often leads to oxygen value in the blood during sleep. The predisposition to collapsibility is due to anatomical factors such as excessive adipose tissue surrounding the airway, weak bony skeletal structure, inadequate function of the upper respiratory muscles, and edema of oropharyngeal (uvula, tongue, softpalate) structures. Collapsibility is associated with an increased incidence of pulmonary complications including respiratory failure and oxygen desaturation. These complications are associated with a significantly increased risk of planless transfer to a post-anesthtesic care unit or an ICU [2, 3]. All these factors are also associated with severe complications such as stroke, hypertension in patients with OSA. A less common form, namely CSA, is distinguished from other types with recurrent apneic episodes in the absence of upper airway obstruction during sleep. Sleep-related hypoventilation disorders (e.q., obesity hypoventilation syndrome, idiopathic central alveolar hypoventilation, congenital central alveolar hypoventilation syndrome, late-onset central hypoventilation with hypotalamic dysfunction, disorders primarily affecting the respiratory pump including neuromuscular and skeletal disorders) are characterized with insufficient ventilation that can cause an elevation of $PaCO_2$ during sleep. Hypercapnia and hypoxemia due to alveolar hypoventilation exacerbate the clinical manifestations of hypoventilation syndromes [3].

The most common comorbidities in these patients are metabolic and cardiovascular diseases including heart failure, coronary disease and pulmonary hypertension. Sleep has a negative effect on respiration by affecting the pharyngeal wall compliance, upper airway resistance and ventilation response to hypoxia and hypercapnia. This situation, which has an adverse effect on lung mechanics such as functional residual capacity and ventilation perfusion disorders, becomes more apparent due to the effect of anesthetic agents and patient position [4].

There is a need for special intraoperative and postoperative anesthesia management in patients with known or suspected sleep-related respiratory disorders to avoid adverse events such as difficult airway, which is one of the most important causes of perioperative morbidity and mortality. The major international guidelines support OSA screening as part of pre-anesthesia assesment in order to eveluate the gas exchange abnormalities such as pulmonary hypertension, hypoventilation syndromes, and resting hypoxaemia. Because of concers for general anesthesia in these patients; intensive perioperative management due to potential for prolonged respiratory depression caused by residual anesthetic agents is needed [5-7].

PREOPERATIVE ASSESSMENT

In patients with OSA; collapse of the upper airway causes some clinical symptoms and generally is accompanied by hypoxemia and hypercapnia. Therefore, it should be managed according to the "Practice Guidelines for Management of the Difficult Airway: An Updated Report.

People with OSA have clinical features such as obesity (particularly central, body mass index > 30 $kg.m^{-2}$), pharyngeal critical closure pressure, small mandible, small maxilla, retrognathia (back-set jaw), dental malocclusion and overbite, large neck circumference (17"/43.2 cm in men, 16"/38.1 cm in women), reduced nasal patency, high and narrow hard palate, elongated and low-lying uvula, enlarged tonsils and adenoids, makroglassia (large tongue), reduced thyroid-mental distance, limited head extension and craniofacial abnormalities. Therefore, detailed physical examination before operation should include evaluation of all these features, including Mallampati score, in the presence of difficult airway probability [8].

Preoperative preparation includes; implementation of continuous positive airway pressure (CPAP) theraphy during the preoperative and postoperative period [5, 6].

Many anesthetic drugs (intravenous induction agents, inhalation anesthesia, sedatives, opioids, neuromuscular blocking agents) used in the preoperative period inhibit respiratory muscle tone and disturb wakefulness response. As patients are sensitive to the depressant effects of these anesthetic drugs; respiration should be continuously monitored with oximetry and capnography during interventions under general anesthesia. In these patients, who receive oxygen supplementation and have two types of ventilation responses such as central apnea and obstructive apnea, monitoring only oxygenation does not mean that enough ventilation is also monitorized [2].

Intraoperative Assessment

Before anesthesia induction; airway management should be planned against potential difficulties such as difficult mask ventilation and difficult intubation. Routine and emergency airway equipments (tracheal tube guides, fiberoptic intubation equipment, retrograde intubation, transtracheal jet ventilation, emergency cricothyroidotomy, surgical or percutaneous tracheostomy) should be available and advanced intubation techniques (e.g., video laryngoscopy) should be used when necessary. Laryngeal masks and supraglottic airway devices (SGA) are life-saving alternative airway management tools that can be used in patients with difficult mask ventilation and difficult intubation. In awake intubation, which is another method, it should be remembered that topical anesthetic agents applied to the oropharyngeal and upper airways will disrupt airway protective reflexes and increase the risk of airway obstruction after extubation [8, 9].

Desaturation during apnea can be delayed by preoxygenating the patient with 100% oxygen in the presence of properly placed face-masks and nasopharyngeal airway equipment. In addition, patients should be in a semi-upright or lateral position during this oxygenation period in order to minimize compression of the diaphragm. This position is also important in improving the laringoscopic imaging by aligning the horizontal axis of the pharyngeal, laryngeal and respiratory tract in patients with difficult ventilation and difficult intubation [2, 4]. A second person may be needed to ensure adequate ventilation in patients with difficult mask ventilation. The first person ensures that the mask is seated in the correct position and the second person provides ventilation for the patient [4].

Short-acting anesthetic agents such as propofol, remifentanil should be preferred since respiratory depression and respiratory muscle inhibition will continue in the post-operative period.

Since residual neuromuscular blockade in the postoperative period may cause an increase in pulmonary complications such as airway obstruction, hypoxemia due to apnea-hypoapnea; It is important to verify that the effect of the neuromuscular block is reversed using train of four and, if necessary, reversal agents, and then safely extubated after evaluating that the patient is fully alert, providing airway patency [8, 9].

Upper Airway Edema and Fluid Management

During extubation and postoperative period, patients should be kept in the semi-upright position. Because the apnea-hypoapnea index (AHI) is higher in the supine position when compared with lateral position in these patients [2].

Continuous positive airway pressure treatment should be continued considering intra-operative anesthetic agents and upper respiratory edema that may develop after extubation. Supine position, perioperative excessive intravenous infusion of normal saline, and immobility, as well as fluid shift from the lower extremities to the neck can cause parapharyngeal edema which can lead to an increase in AHI. Ventilator drive in patients with a collapsible upper airway can low or high variations. These changes can occur by mechanisms such as reduction of pharyngeal muscle activation and production of negative inspiratory pressures [2, 5].

Key Points

- Prepare for difficult airway management and adequate pre-oxygenation
- Consider optimal positioning (Head Elevated Laryngoscopy Position) prior to anesthesia-induction in order to improve functional residual capacity
- Verify full reversal of neuromuscular blockade and extubate the patient when he/she is fully conscious and cooperative
- Non-supine posture for extubation and recovery

References

[1] Sateia MJ. International classification of sleep disorders-third edition: highlights and modifications. *Chest.* 2014 Nov;146(5):1387-1394. doi: 10.1378/chest.14-0970.

[2] Wood KL, Besecker BY. Perioperative issues and sleep-disordered breathing. *Crit. Care Clin.* 2015 Jul;31(3):497-510. doi: 10.1016/ j.ccc.2015.03.008.

[3] Masa JF, Pépin JL, Borel JC, et al. Obesity hypoventilation syndrome. *Eur. Respir. Rev.* 2019 Mar 14;28(151). doi: 10.1183/ 16000617.0097-2018.

[4] McNicholas WT, Hansson D, Schiza S, et al. Sleep in chronic respiratory disease: COPD and hypoventilation disorders. *Eur. Respir. Rev.* 2019 Sep 25;28(153).doi: 10.1183/16000617.0064-2019.

[5] Leong SM, Tiwari A, Chung F, et al. Obstructive sleep apnea as a risk factor associated with difficult airway management - A narrative review. *J. Clin. Anesth.* 2018 Mar;45:63-68. doi: 10.1016/j.jclinane. 2017.12.024.

[6] Chung F, Memtsoudis SG, Ramachandran SK, et al. Society of Anesthesia and Sleep Medicine Guidelines on Preoperative Screening and Assessment of Adult Patients with Obstructive Sleep Apnea. *Anesth. Analg.* 2016;123(2):452-73. doi: 10.1213/ANE.00 00000000001416.

[7] American Society of Anesthesiologists Task Force on Perioperative Management of Patients with Obstructive Sleep Apnea. Practice guidelines for the perioperative

management of patients with obstructive sleep apnea: an updated report by the American Society of Anesthesiologists Task Force on Perioperative Management of Patients with Obstructive Sleep Apnea. *Anesthesiology* 2014;120(2): 268-86. doi: 10.1097/ALN.0000000000000053.

[8] Practice guidelines for management of the difficult airway: An updated report by the American Society of Anesthesiologists Task Force on Management of the Difficult Airway. *Anesthesiology* 2013;118:251–70. doi: 10.1097/ ALN.0b013e31827773b2.

[9] Edwin Seet, Tee Lik Han, Frances Chung, Perioperative Clinical Pathways to Manage Sleep-Disordered Breathing, *Sleep Med. Clin.* 8 (2013) 105–120 http://dx.doi.org/10.1016/j.jsmc.2012.11.005.

In: Sleep Medicine in Critical Care
Editors: Antonio M. Esquinas et al.
ISBN: 978-1-53617-768-8

Chapter 18

ANALGESIA/SEDATION MECHANICAL VENTILATION: KEY PRACTICAL APPROACH

Lindsay A. Arrandale*, MD
Consultant Anaesthetist,
Guy's and St. Thomas' NHS Foundation Trust, London UK

ABSTRACT

Sedation and analgesia can result in increased mechanical ventilation requirements. Careful pre-procedure planning should include a multi-disciplinary assessment of benefit balanced against risks of proposed procedures.

Individualised assessment must include potential airway management issues, cardio-respiratory limitations, metabolic considerations, medication and functional issues affecting positioning for the procedure.

Checklists encourage a standardised approach for best and safest peri-procedural course.

Choice of sedation technique includes intermittent bolus or titrated continuous infusions selected for patient factors, ease of use and recovery profile.

Planning analgesia takes into account existing pain management requirements, a multi-modal approach with local, regional and central neuraxial techniques. Routes of parenteral analgesia depend on the patient's ability absorb medications. A stepwise approach with an escalating and de-escalating regime for acute pain is employed.

Careful monitoring and support of the patient, with available resuscitation equipment and expertly trained staff is mandatory.

* Corresponding Author's E-mail: Lindsay.Arrandale@gstt.nhs.uk.

Preparation for delivering safe anaesthesia and effective analgesia, in a population of patients with an often higher than average risk profile, should begin with a multi-disciplinary assessment. The benefit of the operative procedure proposed will be balanced against generic and specific risks to the individual patient. Risk profiles can be managed with careful planning and pre-optimisation, particularly by cardio-respiratory assessment and pharmacological rationalisation.

Techniques may be considered for long periods of mechanical ventilation in a critical care setting e.g., whilst recovering from critical illness, or for short interventions where sedation and analgesia are needed for a finite operative procedure e.g., invasive line insertion, where increased mechanical ventilation requirements can result.

Pre-Operative Assessment

Each patient will require an individualised anaesthetic assessment. This is best used as a broad review to decide if there are any patient factors which preclude the use of specific techniques or mandate the use of others particularly safety considerations for airway management such as awake fibre-optic intubation for a known difficult airway [1, 2]. It will include a systematic approach to identify, and plan for management of: airway issues; cardio-respiratory limitations; metabolic considerations such as renal or liver handling of metabolites; regular drugs which should be continued or paused, especially thromboprophylaxis [3]; and functional issues relating to obesity/extreme under-weight with concomitant risk of injury/fracture in positioning for procedure.

Checklists

Following a standardised approach within unit-based patient groups for common procedures can be beneficial for reducing missed steps and assuring the best and safest peri-procedural course is followed. A care plan can be written (see Appendix) which follows the preparation time course from a set time prior to procedures e.g., 1 week or 24 hours, and includes multiple steps undertaken by different members of the team. This type of task-based approach can be used as a prompt for incorporation of a WHO checklist [4] adapted for specific use. It can helpfully include recovery and post-procedural advice on specific management steps.

PRINCIPLES OF SEDATION

Options for administering sedation fall into two broad categories: intermittent bolus administration or titrated continuous infusions, each has benefits to the physician and patient in terms of ease of use and recovery profile.

Intermittent boluses e.g., midazolam etc. are easy to give but care should be taken to use small incremental dosing in order to avoid overdose to a drug-nieve patient.

Infused sedation e.g., Propofol etc. commonly given via a mechanical infusion pump which can include modifiable algorithms incorporating patient sex/wt./ht. to fine tune the mass of drug administered which ideally optimises recovery time.

PRINCIPLES OF ANALGESIA

Options for analgesia will be dictated by the procedure being undertaken and resultant pain experienced by the patient. Existing pain management requirements need to be taken into account and built upon in order to step up analgesia at the time of intervention. A multi-modal approach is best employed where possible.

Local anaesthesia, where a small area of the patient is rendered insensate, is used for discrete procedures e.g., Dental extractions. Where applicable, this technique removes the need for sedative analgesics which would inhibit respiration and may impact cardiac or metabolic function. The known, finite duration of action of each local anaesthetic will allow for a rescue analgesia plan to be formed to treat post-procedural pain.

Regional and central neuraxial techniques allow for more major procedures to be undertaken painlessly. These techniques often include a combination of agents e.g., Local anaesthetic with opioid agents for caesarean section (Figure 1. Non-invasive ventliation during cesarean section under epidural anaesthesia). The need for sedative use will be mitigated but associated adverse cardio-respiratory effects of positioning and adjacent neuromuscular weakness, invariably increase ventilatory difficulties which should be supported by carefully titrating non-invasive mechanical ventilatory pressures.

Local anaesthetic infusion catheter techniques allow for repeated doses of local anaesthetic to be infused over a prolonged course of peri-procedural pain e.g., Epidural catheter at the time of labour or laparotomy. Neuromuscular weakness is to be expected in the dermatomal distribution of analgesia and again will require close supervision of ventilatory support.

Parenteral analgesia can be administered via varying routes depending on the patient's ability to swallow or enterally/ parenterally absorb medications: oral/enteral route, subcutaneous, intramuscular, intravenous route by either bolus or infusion.

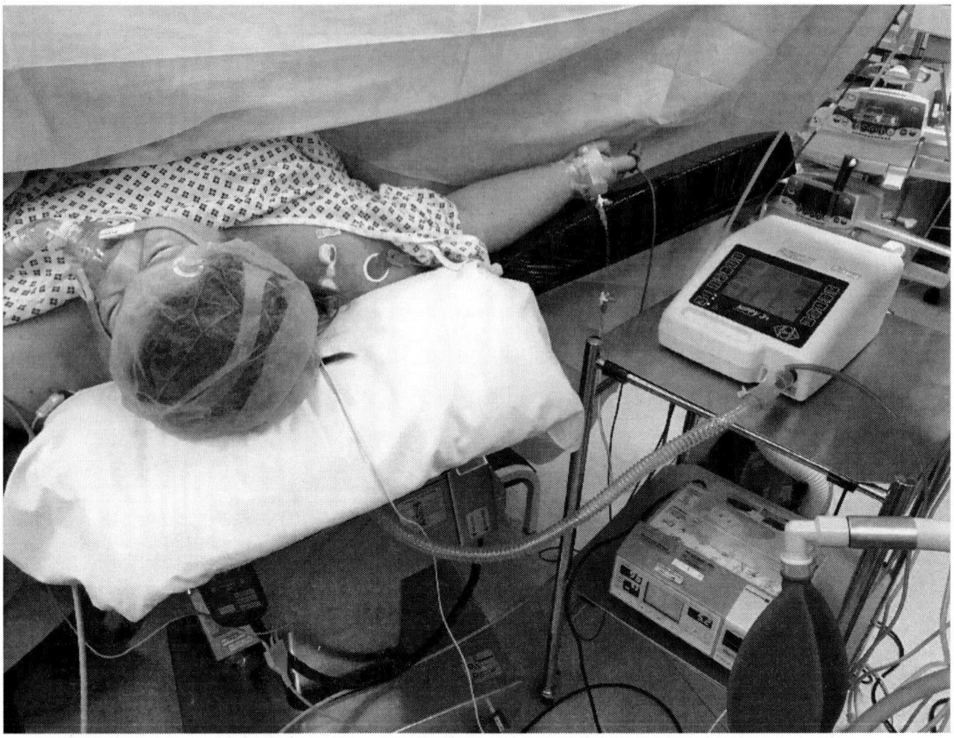

Figure 1. Non-invasive ventliation during cesarean section under epidural anaesthesia

A stepwise approach to analgesia should be followed according to locally adapted guidelines mostly based on WHO cancer pain analgesic ladder [5, 6], to maintain an escalating and de-escalating regime for acute pain ideally with time limited prescriptions requiring review and weaning.

Intravenous analgesia is principally divided into non-opioid and opioid agents. Various non-opiod drugs are used for their non-sedating effects e.g., Paracetamol or NSAIDs. Titrated strong opioid infusions are often used for critical care analgesia accepting the cardio-respiratory suppressant effects will require enhanced monitoring and ventilatory support.

Throughout the administration of all options for analgesia and sedation care must be taken to appropriately monitor and support the patient. Locally agreed minimum monitoring standards [7] should be followed in the knowledge that conscious level, respiratory and haemodynamic effects result from these techniques may result.

Resuscitation and airway management equipment plus expertly trained medical and nursing staff should be immediately accessible and available if required [8].

REFERENCES

[1] Major complications of airway management in the UK: results of the Fourth National Audit Project of the Royal College of Anaesthetists and the Difficult Airway Society. Part 1: Anaesthesia† T. M. Cook 1*, N. Woodall 2 and C. Frerk 3, on behalf of the Fourth National Audit Project *British Journal of Anaesthesia* 106 (5): 617-31 (2011).

[2] Major complications of airway management in the UK: results of the Fourth National Audit Project of the Royal College of Anaesthetists and the Difficult Airway Society. Part 2: intensive care and emergency departments† T. M. Cook 1*, N. Woodall 2, J. Harper 3 and J. Benger 4, on behalf of the Fourth National Audit Project. *British Journal of Anaesthesia* 106 (5): 632-42 (2011).

[3] Gogarten W., Vandermeulen E., Van Aken H., et al., Regional anaesthesia and antithrombotic agents: recommendations of the European Society of Anaesthesiology. *Eur J Anaesthesiol* 2010;27:999-1015.

[4] A Surgical Safety Checklist to Reduce Morbidity and Mortality in a Global Population, List of authors. Alex B. Haynes, MD., MPH, Thomas G. Weiser, M. D., MPH., William R. Berry, MD., MPH, Stuart R. Lipsitz, ScD., Abdel-Hadi S. Breizat, M. D., PhD., E. Patchen Dellinger, M. D., Teodoro Herbosa, M. D., Sudhir Joseph, M. S., Pascience L. Kibatala, M. D., Marie Carmela M. Lapitan, M. D., Alan F. Merry, M. B., Ch. B., FANZCA, FRCA, Krishna Moorthy, MD., FRCS, et al., for the Safe Surgery Saves Lives Study Group, *N Engl J Med* 2009; 360:491-49.

[5] World Health Organization. Traitement de la douleur cancéreuse. Geneva, Switz: *World Health Organization*; 1987.

[6] National Institute for Health and Care Excellence. *Clinical knowledge summaries: analgesia - mild-to-moderate pain.* 2015. Available at: https://cks.nice.org.uk/ analgesia-mild-to-moderate-pain#!scenarioRecommendation:1 (accessed December 2019).

[7] RCOA monitoring - Association of Anaesthetists of Great Britain and Ireland. Recommendations for standards of monitoring during anaesthesia and recovery 2015. *Anaesthesia* 2016; 71: 85-93. This guideline can be viewed online via the following http://onlinelibrary.wiley.com/doi/10.1111/anae.13316/full.

[8] *Guidelines for the Provision of Anaesthetic Services*. London: The Royal College of Anaesthetists, 2019. https://www.rcoa.ac.uk/safety-standards-quality/guidance-resources/guidelines-provision-anaesthetic-services.

APPENDIX

Patient Details: (Affix Label)
Name
Hospital No.______________
Date of Birth______________

Guy's and St Thomas' NHS
NHS Foundation Trust

Percutaneous Endoscopically Inserted Gastrostomy (PEG) Insertion Protocol for Lane-Fox Unit

<table>
<tr><th colspan="4">Checklist</th></tr>
<tr><th></th><th>Responsibility</th><th>Completed</th><th>Date</th></tr>
<tr><td colspan="4">Day before procedure (/ /)</td></tr>
<tr><td>• Full set of Bloods Results Available (including FBC, Renal profile, Liver profile, Bone profile, Magnesium, and Clotting)</td><td>Nurse</td><td>☐</td><td></td></tr>
<tr><td>• Chest x-ray</td><td>SpR/SHO</td><td>☐</td><td></td></tr>
<tr><td>• IV Cannula - inserted</td><td>Nurse/SHO/SpR</td><td>☐</td><td></td></tr>
<tr><td>• Airway and Respiratory Assessment (including overnight TcO2, SPO2 monitoring)</td><td>SpR/SHO</td><td>☐</td><td></td></tr>
<tr><td>• ECG</td><td>Nurse</td><td>☐</td><td></td></tr>
<tr><td>• Weight and Nutrition Screening Tool</td><td>Nurse</td><td>☐</td><td></td></tr>
<tr><td>• EPR referral form completed</td><td>SpR/SHO</td><td>☐</td><td></td></tr>
<tr><td>• Prophylactic anticoagulation stopped 24 hours pre procedure</td><td>SpR/SHO</td><td>☐</td><td></td></tr>
<tr><td>• Prescribe IV fluids to start at midnight</td><td>SpR/SHO</td><td>☐</td><td></td></tr>
<tr><td colspan="4">Day of procedure (/ /)</td></tr>
<tr><td>• Start IV fluids at midnight (40 – 80 ml/hour)</td><td>Nurse</td><td>☐</td><td></td></tr>
<tr><td>• NBM from midnight / Stop NG feeding at midnight</td><td>Nurse</td><td>☐</td><td></td></tr>
<tr><td>• Patient washed and ready for procedure</td><td>Nurse</td><td>☐</td><td></td></tr>
<tr><td>• Prophylactic antibiotics prescribed</td><td>SpR/SHO</td><td>☐</td><td></td></tr>
<tr><td>• Prophylactic antibiotics given immediately before procedure</td><td>Nurse</td><td>☐</td><td></td></tr>
<tr><td>• Appropriate consent form ready and available at bedside</td><td>Nurse/Ward Clerk</td><td>☐</td><td></td></tr>
<tr><td>• Ensure speaking valve removed from tracheostomy circuit</td><td>Nurse</td><td>☐</td><td></td></tr>
<tr><td>• Document bloods<table><tr><td>Hb</td><td></td></tr><tr><td>Platelets</td><td></td></tr><tr><td>INR</td><td></td></tr><tr><td>APTR</td><td></td></tr><tr><td>Creatinine</td><td></td></tr><tr><td>Potassium</td><td></td></tr></table></td><td>Nurse</td><td>☐</td><td></td></tr>
<tr><td>• Obtain consent from the gastroenterologist or Lane Fox SpR/Consultant if patient is incapable of giving consent</td><td>Gastroenterologist</td><td>☐</td><td></td></tr>
</table>

During procedure			
• Patient Monitoring ○ Attach to cardiac monitor (HR, BP, RR, ECG, SPO2) ○ TOSCA	Nurse	☐ ☐	
• Ventilation ○ Ventilator (NIPPY3+) ○ Settings (PC Mode) ○ Mask (Nasal Mask)	Nurse	☐ ☐ ☐	
• Supplemental oxygen including tubing and connector appropriate to patient's ventilator available	Nurse	☐	
• Emergency Equipment ○ Working bedside suction Unit ○ Emergency airway equipment ○ Bag Valve mask device/Mappleson Circuit	Nurse	☐ ☐ ☐	
• Prepare medications as per anaesthetist	Nurse	☐	
• Record Observations every 5 minutes	Nurse	☐	

PEG PROCEDURE SAFETY CHECKLIST

SIGN IN Gastroenterologist to lead

BEFORE INDUCTION

Has a team briefing taken place for this patient? YES ☐

Has the patient confirmed:

Identity ☐

Procedure ☐

Consent ☐

Is the ventilator and medication check complete? YES ☐

Does the patient have any allergies? YES ☐ NO ☐

If yes, what? ______

Does the patient have a safe airway plan in case of difficult airway?

YES ☐ N/A ☐

If yes, is any equipment needed?

______

Local anaesthetic checked? YES ☐ N/A ☐

Prophylactic antibiotic given? YES ☐ N/A ☐

Is the endoscope in date, sterile and the correct scope associated with the patient? YES ☐ NO ☐

Is the required equipment available and fully functioning without problems? YES ☐ NO ☐

Any patient concerns? YES ☐ NO ☐

Name of practitioner: ______

Signature: ______

Designation: ______

Date: ______ **Bleep:** ______

SIGN OUT Nursing staff to lead

AT THE END OF THE PROCEDURE

Has the planned procedure (s) been completed?

YES ☐

Has the name of the procedure(s) been recorded?

YES ☐ N/A ☐

Have the line extensions been flushed?

YES ☐ N/A ☐

Has the appropriate post-operative antibiotics been agreed and prescribed?

YES ☐ N/A ☐

Has the specimen been labelled?

YES ☐ N/A ☐

Were there any equipment problems?

YES ☐ N/A ☐

If yes, what?

______

Key concerns for recovery:

______

Any other issues for follow up:

______

Name: ______

Signature: ______

Designation: ______

Date: ______ **Bleep:** ______

AFFIX PATIENT LABEL or:

Patient name: ______

DOB: ______

Hospital number: ______

PEG Protocol

Patient Details: (Affix Label)
Name
Hospital No.______________
Date of Birth______________

Guy's and St Thomas' NHS
NHS Foundation Trust

Tube Information	
Date of Insertion:	**Time of insertion:**
Tube Type (Tick box below)	
• 15Fr Freka (*Fresenius Kabi)* bumper retained) ☐ • Other tube …………………………………………	
External Fixator Position (refer to endoscopy report if not documented): [cm] (Do not move external fixator plate and contact gastroenterologist/IR if any concerns)	

POST PEG INSERTION PROTOCOL

- IF THERE IS PAIN ON FEEDING
- PROLONGED OR SEVERE PAIN POST-PROCEDURE
- FRESH BLEEDING
- EXTERNAL LEAKAGE OF GASTRIC CONTENTS

STOP FEED/MEDICATION DELIVERY IMMEDIATELY. OBTAIN SENIOR ADVICE URGENTLY AND CONSIDER CT SCAN.

Monitoring Post PEG insertion			
15 minutes for 1 hour	30 minutes for the next 2-4 hours	Hourly for the next 4-6 hours	4th Hourly after 6 hours for the next 24 hours
Monitor patient 24 - 48 hours for signs of			
• Bowel perforation • Haemorrhage	• Aspiration pneumonia	• Wound leakage • Peritonitis	• Wound infection
• Provide pain relief if required (IV analgesics) o Add IV paracetamol (N.B. dose reduction in DMD patients)			

PEG Protocol

Feeding post insertion		
0 - 6 hours	..............to..............	Nil by mouth and PEG tube (consider IV fluids)
6 - 12 hours	..............to..............	Sterile water @ 30ml/hr via PEG Remain Nil by mouth
12 - 18 hours	..............to..............	Nutrison Standard (1.0 kcal/ml) @ 30ml/hr Recommence oral intake (if no contraindications)
18 - 24 hours	..............to..............	Nutrison Standard (1.0 kcal/ml) @ 50ml/hr
From 24 hours		Follow feeding regimen as per dietetic entry

Daily Aftercare (days 1-3 post procedure)

1. **Preparation**
   - Wash hands and wear gloves. Use aseptic technique (ANTT) and explain to patient
2. **Inspect**
   - Check for signs of inflammation and/or irritation (offensive discharge, pain, heat, redness, swelling)
   - If any signs of infection e.g. discharge, swab the site
   - Change dry dressing daily for first 24 hours. Remove the dressing around the PEG after 24 hours and leave exposed. Further dressing only required if exudate is excessive
3. **Cleaning**
   - Clean using sterile gauze and normal saline: around the stoma, underneath external fixation plate (lift the edges to access) and feeding tube and port. Dry stoma site using a dry sterile gauze
   - There should not be any tube movement and it must not 'pinch' the skin, risking necrosis

Day post insertion	Stoma site		Additional comment	Date dd/mm/yy	Sign
	Inspected [✓]	Cleaned [✓]			
1			Remove dressing after 24 hours		
2					
3					

In: Sleep Medicine in Critical Care
Editors: Antonio M. Esquinas et al.
ISBN: 978-1-53617-768-8

Chapter 19

POST-OPERATIVE MANAGEMENT AND CLINICAL RESULTS

***İlim Irmak**, MD**
Department of Chest Diseases,
Hacettepe University School of Medicine, Ankara, Turkey

ABSTRACT

Postoperative period is a critical process that requires careful approach for Sleep-Related Breathing Disorders (SRBDs) patients. In addition to sensitivity to post-surgical medication, complications such as cardiac, neurological and comorbidities, especially respiratory, may occure. Therefore, close follow-up and implementation of the necessary precautionary strategies in accordance with the recommendations may provide successful management of the postoperative process.

Keywords: sleep-related breathing disorders, postoperative conditions, management

INTRODUCTION

SRBDs range from upper airway obstruction and habitual snoring to sleep apnea disorders. Obstructive sleep apnea syndrome (OSA) is the most common disorder in SRBDs characterized by repetitive obstruction of the upper airway often resulting in oxygen desaturation and arousals from sleep and increased risk of diabetes mellitus, hypertension, and cardiovascular disorders [2]. Presence of OSA is not recognised in a

* Corresponding Author's E-mail: ilimirmak@hotmail.com.

significant ratio of surgical patients during surgery process. Therefore, apnea-induced hypoxemia and unexpected cardiac events may develop in postoperative period in patients with no diagnosis. Many of studies demonstrated that SRBD patients undergoing different types of surgery have an increased rate of postoperative complications including; oxygen desaturation, cardiac events, extended length of stay, intensive care unit transfers and hemodynamic instability [3, 1]. Furthermore, there are several conditions that people with OSA might have increased sensitivity to, such as respiratory depressant effects of anesthetic drugs, opioid analgesics, and sedative medications. For this reason, American Society of Anesthesiologists (ASA) and American Academy of Sleep Medicine (AASM) have developed protocols for perioperative management of these patients which recommend screening tests [4]. Hence, in postoperative period, approaches that take presence of SRBD into account and in line with the recommendations on medication, follow-up and possible complications are of extreme clinical importance.

RESPIRATORY CONDITIONS

Respiratory problems in surgical patients with SRBD can be counted among critical complications in postoperative period. Oxygen desaturation is the most common complication in OSA [1]. Patients are susceptible to hypoxemia due to high rate of obesity, tendency to apnea- hipoventilation, SRBD associated pulmonary hypertension and comorbid conditions. The presence of other forms of SRBD such as sleep hypoventilation syndrome increases postoperative respiratory failure risk [5]. Several studies have reported that both OSA patient groups with oxygen desaturation index ≥5 and apnea-hypopnea index ≥5 prior to surgery, demonstrated higher incidence of postoperative complications [6]. A meta-analysis by Kaw et al. has shown that patients with OSA were 2 to 4 times more likely to experience acute respiratory failure and oxygen desatuation was found to be 2 - 3 times higher in these patients at postoperative period [5].

Most SRBD patients require oxygen during postoperative care. Since the increase in partial oxygen pressure with excessive oxygen support will suppress peripheral chemoreceptor response, it may delay detection of apnea and hypoventilation in these patients. Accordingly, patients should be followed up with minimal oxygen supplementation along continuous saturation and apnea monitoring.

Continuous positive airway pressure (CPAP) is the most widely used treatment in patients with SRBD to improve lung volume, reduce apnea-hypopnea, and thus reduce hypoxemic and hypercarbic events. Because of their tendency to develop atelectasis and oropharyngeal collapse in the postoperative period, the need for positive pressure may increase in these patients. CPAP also reduces the upper airway edema and atelectasis after surgery, eventually providing lung volume stability and upper airway patency in surgical patients [7]. Similarly, a recent study investigating the impact of SRBD on postoperative outcomes reported that the need for positive pressure such as emergant endotracheal intubation, mechanical ventilation and non invasive mechanical ventilation (NIMV) use was significantly increased in these patients [3]. ASA guideline recommends postoperative CPAP usage for patients with OSA in both hospital and home settings [4]. Several studies have shown that patients used CPAP before and after surgery had fewer postoperative respiratory events than non users [7]. Although there is limited evidence for patients who have not used CPAP earlier, postoperative CPAP is recommended for patients with high risk and significant perioperative screening test results. This way, it is ensured that patients with undiagnosed OSA are not overlooked and have a chance to receive treatment and necessary precautions for post-operative complications are taken. In patients with apnea and oxygen desaturation under CPAP after surgery, the pressure should be titrated until the respiratory events are controlled, the duration of treatment should be prolonged and patients should be monitored as closely as possible.

Surgical patients are usually monitored in supine position at reanimation units. Due to increased tendency to pharyngeal collapse in supine position, this position causes respiratory events to worsen in OSA patients. If possible, the patient should be positioned lateral, semi-upright or non-supine during the postoperative follow-up [8].

Cardiovascular Conditions

SRBD has high prevalence of cardiovascular manifestations such as heart failure, arrhytmias, hypertension, stroke and coronary disorders. Postoperative cardiac event risk increases in OSA patients. Postoperative pain and surgical stress may increase sympathetic activation, as well as changes in blood pressure due to OSA-related hypoxemia and anesthetics [9]. In patients with SRBD, postoperative process is particularly important, as the risk of sudden cardiac events increases due to apnea-induced hypoxemic injury. Although postoperative cardiac outcomes vary between different studies, majority of studies have shown that patients with SRBD are at high risk for atrial fibrillation after any type of surgery. The most frequently reported cardiac complications are minor events such as blood pressure changes and arrhythmias [3].

Long-term CPAP therapy reduces cardiovascular mortality and morbidity in severe OSA patients. In the perioperative period, CPAP treatment can improve cardiac comorbidity in addition to reducing postoperative cardiac complications [7].

Postanesthesia Care

Because of high sensitivity to drugs such as narcotics, general anesthetics and sedatives, postoperative period is critical for patients with SRBD. As the upper airway and other respiratory muscles are very sensitive to neuromuscular drugs applied in surgery, these drugs may cause pharyngeal collapse and as a result of general anesthetics and narcotics use, respiratory response to upper airway obstruction may decrease [10]. This might lead to apnea and hypoxemia attacks in postoperative period. Accordingly, the surgery and anesthesia team should be aware of the presence of SRBD and stay in favor of general anesthesia alternatives such as regional blocs, short acting opioids and non-opioid analgesics. If possible, long acting or bolus medications should be avoided and multimodal approach should be employed for pain control (such as nonsteroidal anti-inflammatory drugs, gabapentin, pregabaline, acetaminophen, tramadol, ketamine, dexmedetomidine, clonidine, dexamethasone) in postoperative follow-up. Since benzodiazepine and barbiturate-derived drugs reduce respiratory muscle tone, antidote agents should be available when using such drugs [4].

Postoperative Follow – Up

ASA recommends extended monitoring all patients with diagnosed or suspected OSA who have received general anesthesia in the postanesthetic care unit, however there is no evidence based optimal post operative follow-up duration. All surgical patients are most susceptible to respiratory events at first days after surgery. Especially the Rapid Eye Movement (REM) is the most risky sleep period in which respiratory events may develop. Recent studies reported that oxygen desaturation index, sleep architecture and apnea hypopnea index were the most observed parametres at postoperative first night in surgical patients with OSA and non-OSA, however it is established that post operative third day is when the respiratory parameters are worse in OSA patients [1].

Ambulatory approach may be employed for OSA patients who undergo minor or skin-deep surgery under local or regional anesthesia. Patients scheduled to be discharged on the same day should be followed up in the recovery room for up to 3 hours and apnea or desaturation events should be recorded. If an outpatient develops respiratory events within this 3 hour follow-up period, they should be admitted for observation overnight. One night observation should also be considered for outpatients requiring oral opioid treatment after surgery [2].

Low-risk patient being those with no need for opioids, patients with mild OSA and patients that did not have any respiratory events in recovery, can be admitted to ward after routine follow-up. However, follow-up in post-anesthesia care unit should be continued for patients underwent major surgery and in need of opioids and patients with severe OSA or respiratory complications until it is ensured that no respiratory complications develop.

Other Conditions

OSA weakens cerebral functions and may increase the tendency for postoperative apnea and hypoxemia attacks and neurophsyiatric complications. The most common neuropsychiatric complications are delirium and confusion with agitation [1]. The effects of comorbidities accompanying OSA on postoperative complications vary according to the studies. Howewer in most of them, it is shown that OSA patients had a higher prevalence of pre-existing comorbidities, including obesity, hypertension, gastroesophageal reflux disease, diabetes, hypothyroidism, chronic pulmonary diseases, Liao et al. demonstrated that pre-existing stroke in patients with OSA is a risk factor for re-occurence postoperative complications [1]. Therefore, presence of additional disease should be paid attention to, it should be questioned whether comorbidity control was established or not, and patients should be comprehensively evaluated for complications secondary to additional diseases.

Key Points

1 Oxygen desaturation is the most common complication in post-surgical patients with SRBD due to increased the tendency to apne-hypopnea. Patients should be followed up with minimal oxygen supplementation along continuous saturation and apnea monitoring. CPAP should be used for patients with high risk in both hospital and home settings.

2 Due to increased tendency to pharyngeal collapse in supine position, patients should be positioned lateral, semi-upright or non-supine during the postoperative follow-up.

3 If possible, long acting or bolus medications should be avoided and multimodal approach should be employed for pain control in postoperative follow-up.

4 Ambulatory patients should be followed up in the recovery room for up to 3 hours and apnea or desaturation events should be recorded. If an outpatient develops respiratory events within this 3 hour follow-up period, they should be admitted for observation overnight. Follow-up in post-anesthesia care unit should be continued for patients underwent major surgery and in need of opioids and

patients with high risk until it is ensured that no respiratory complications develop.

REFERENCES

[1] Liao, P., Yegneswaran, B., Vairavanathan, S., Zilberman, P. and Chung, F. (2009). Postoperative complications in patients with obstructive sleep apnea: a retrospective matched cohort study. *Canadian Journal of Anesthesia/Journal canadien d'anesthésie,* 56(11), 819.

[2] Wolfe, R. M., Pomerantz, J., Miller, D. E., Weiss-Coleman, R. and Solomonides, T. (2016). Obstructive sleep apnea: preoperative screening and postoperative care. *J. Am. Board Fam. Med.,* 29(2), 263 - 275.

[3] Mokhlesi, B., Hovda, M. D., Vekhter, B., Arora, V. M., Chung, F. and Meltzer, D. O. (2013). Sleep-disordered breathing and postoperative outcomes after elective surgery: analysis of the nationwide inpatient sample. *Chest,* 144(3), 903 - 914.

[4] Gross, J. B., Bachenberg, K. L., Benumof, J. L., Caplan, R. A., Connis, R. T., Coté, C. J., ... and Ydens, L. (2006). Practice guidelines for the perioperative management of patients with obstructive sleep apnea: a report by the American Society of Anesthesiologists Task Force on Perioperative Management of patients with obstructive sleep apnea. *Anesthesiology,* 104(5), 1081.

[5] Kaw, R., Bhateja, P., y Mar, H. P., Hernandez, A. V., Ramaswamy, A., Deshpande, A. and Aboussouan, L. S. (2016). Postoperative complications in patients with unrecognized obesity hypoventilation syndrome undergoing elective noncardiac surgery. *Chest,* 149(1), 84 - 91.

[6] Chung, F., Yegneswaran, B., Liao, P., Chung, S. A., Vairavanathan, S., Islam, S., ... and Shapiro, C. M. (2008). Validation of the Berlin questionnaire and American Society of Anesthesiologists checklist as screening tools for obstructive sleep apnea in surgical patients. *Anesthesiology: The Journal of the American Society of Anesthesiologists*, 108(5), 822 - 830.

[7] Nagappa, M., Mokhlesi, B., Wong, J., Wong, D. T., Kaw, R. and Chung, F. (2015). The effects of continuous positive airway pressure on postoperative outcomes in obstructive sleep apnea patients undergoing surgery: a systematic review and meta-analysis. *Anesthesia and Analgesia,* 120(5), 1013 - 1023.

[8] Chung, F., Liao, P., Elsaid, H., Shapiro, C. M. and Kang, W. (2014). Factors associated with postoperative exacerbation of sleep-disordered breathing. *Anesthesiology: The Journal of the American Society of Anesthesiologists,* 120(2), 299 - 311.

[9] Kaw, R., Chung, F., Pasupuleti, V., Mehta, J., Gay, P. C. and Hernandez, A. V. (2012). Meta-analysis of the association between obstructive sleep apnoea and postoperative outcome. *British Journal of Anaesthesia,* 109(6), 897 - 906.

[10] Cullen, David J. *Obstructive sleep apnea and postoperative analgesia--a potentially dangerous combination.* (2001): 83 - 85

In: Sleep Medicine in Critical Care
Editors: Antonio M. Esquinas et al.

ISBN: 978-1-53617-768-8

Chapter 20

EXTUBATION AND REINTUBATION FAILURE: IMPACT OF SLEEP DISORDERED BREATHING

Milind P. Sovani*, MD
Department of Respiratory Medicine,
Nottingham University Hospitals NHS Trust, Nottingham, UK

ABSTRACT

OSA/OHS is common in patients who undergo mechanical ventilation. Undiagnosed and untreated OSA/OHS is associated with increased risk of difficult intubation or extubation failure. Morbid Obesity, neck circumference >42 cm, STOP-Bang score >3, as well as craniofacial anatomical features such as retrognathia, macroglossia are also risk factors for OSA/difficult intubation. Submental ultrasound, cuff- leak test and post-extubation spirometry could be used in addition to sleep studies to identify those at high risk of upper airway collapse.

Minimising opioid use, avoiding deeper level of anaesthesia, using semi-upright position post extubation and prophylactic use of PAP therapy/NIV - are likely to reduce the risk of extubation failure. In those with hypercapnic respiratory failure and/or overlap of OSA and COPD the author would recommend NIV rather than CPAP.

Tracheostomy decanulation should be preceded by assessment and treatment of any upper airway pathology including OSA.

* Corresponding Author's E-mail: Milind.sovani@nuh.nhs.uk, msovani5@gmail.com.

ABBREVIATIONS

AHI	Apnoea Hypopnea Index
AHRF	acute hypercapnic respiratory failure
BMI	Body-Mass Index
CPAP	ContinuousPositive Airway Pressure
EDAC	expiratory dynamic airway collapse
NIV	Non Invasive Ventilation
NMD	neuromuscular diseases
OSA	Obstructive Sleep Apnoea
OHS	Obesity Hypoventilation Syndrome
PAP	positive airway pressure (PAP)
RDI	Respiratory Disturbance Index
SDB	sleep disordered breathing
UA	Upper Airway

INTRODUCTION

Obstructive Sleep Apnoea (OSA) is related to recurrent upper airway collapse during sleep. In mammals OSA is seen only in humans (apart from brachycephalic dogs) and is a price that we pay for our ability for advanced speech [1]. Craniofacial anatomical features such as retrognathia, (syndromic) macroglossia, maxillary hypoplasia, are important factors contributing to the development of OSA [2]. Obesity is another important risk factor and with obesity epidemic around the world, prevalence of OSA is increasing. A systematic review by Senaratna et al. reported that at apnoea hypopnoea index (AHI) ≥ 15 events/hour, the prevalence in the general adult population ranged from 6% to 17% wit men more susceptible than women [3].

Upper airway features such as large tongue, crowded oropharyngeal structures, narrow upper airway and greater neck circumference are all likely to contribute to difficulty in intubation. There are mixed reports, however, regarding effects of obesity and concurrent OSA on difficulty in intubation. In a systematic review and meta-analysis Nagappa et al. identified a 3 (three) fold increased risk in difficult mask ventilation and intubation in patients with OSA [4]. Whereas in morbidly obese patients mean Body Mass Index (BMI) ~ 50 kg/m^2, 68% patients had OSA (mean AHI 31 events/hour). The authors reported 3.3% difficult intubation rate. Increasing neck circumference was associated with difficult laryngoscopy whereas Mallamapati grade III or more predicted difficult intubation [5].

In patients who are mechanically ventilated, prevalence of OSA can vary widely depending on the population being studied. In a large observational study Bolona et al. reported that nearly 8% patients admitted to Intensive Care Unit had a pre-admission physician diagnosed OSA [6]. A number of studies have reported higher prevalence of sleep disordered breathing (SDB) - with more than 50% patients suffering from OSA in patients admitted with acute cardio-respiratory failure [7, 8]. Morbid obesity (and concomitant OSA) has been associated with prolonged ICU stay. In addition, issues specific to obesity pose additional challenges to mechanical ventilation such as reduced functional residual capacity with rapid desaturation and increased aspiration risk [9].

In addition to obesity and/or craniofacial susceptibility, there are other factors linked particularly to Critical Care settings such as upper airway oedema, secretions and inflammation, as well as drugs used to facilitate care. Timm et al. reported incidence of OSA (AHI > 5) in 71% during the first night after extubation in patients admitted to intensive care unit. Moreover each 10 mg of opioids given 24 hours prior to extubation was also associated with 15% increased risk of upper airway collapse [10]. The authors reported that opioid use was associated with obstructive rather than central apnoeas and postulated that this could be due to reduced upper airway dilator tone.

Chishti et al. reported that in surgical ICU patients without previous diagnosis of OSA who were ventilated for more than 48 hours, 25% patients were noted to have moderate to severe SDB post extubation [11]. These data highlight high prevalence of undiagnosed OSA post extubation in patients treated in intensive care units.

In an observational cohort study Diaz-Abad et al. reviewed data for 19 patients admitted to a long term acute care hospital for weaning from prolonged mechanical ventilation via tracheostomy. These patients were obese (mean BMI 44 kg/m^2). 18 out of 19 patients (94%) had SDB with a median Respiratory Disturbance Index (RDI) of 24 events/hour. The authors report that they were able to decanulate 17 patients of which with 14 patients were treated with positive airway pressure (PAP) therapy [12].

There are a number of case reports and case series about perioperative respiratory complications and deaths associated with untreated OSA. Subramani et al. reported that although most patients were treated with continuous positive airway pressure (CPAP) prior to surgery, they did not use (or were not treated with) CPAP in the postoperative period. Use of relatively small doses of opioids, e.g., 10 mg of Morphine, was associated with serious complications and deaths often within 24 hours of surgery [13]. It is therefore not surprising that undiagnosed OSA is associated with extubation failure. In a small study involving 29 patients in medical ICU, STOP-Bang score was used as a marker of OSA. The authors reported that in patients with STOP-Bang score 3 or more were twice as likely to experience extubation failure compared to those with score of 2 or less. The finding was however not statistically significant due to small sample siz [14].

A report by Royal College of Anaesthetists, UK states that 30% complications related to airway management occurs around extubation and is associated with increased morbidity and mortality. Recognising difficult airway is an important step in mitigating this risk. Laryngeal oedema can cause measure problems on extubation. Direct laryngoscopy as well as a 'cuff-leak test' are helpful to assess presence of laryngeal oedema [14]. Obesity and undiagnosed OSA pose risk of upper airway collapse particularly in presence of opioids or reduced consciousness. Extubation whilst patient is in a deep plane of anaesthesia has been used to reduce the risk of laryngospasm. This approach however will increase the risk of upper airway collapse is therefore to be avoided in those with a diagnosis of or at risk of OSA [15].

In addition to upper airway collapse, in a few cases airways distal to larynx are prone to collapse during expiration. This condition is termed as expiratory dynamic airway collapse (EDAC) and can be diagnosed on Computerize Tomography (CT) or during bronchoscopy when posterior trachea-bronchial wall is seen to collapse by more than 50% during exhalation, again seen in context of obesity and can lead to prolonged ventilation [16].

Polysomnography (PSG) remains the gold standard for diagnosis of OSA but it is not the most effective way to diagnose OSA in intubated patients. STOP-Bang questionnaire can be used to risk stratify, however, it can lead to both false positive and negative results [17]. Sub-mental Ultrasound measurement of upper airway is a noninvasive technique. Shu et al. combined this with neck circumference measurement to predict presence of sever OSA. They reported that retropalatal airway measurement during Muller Manoeuvre combined with neck circumference has high sensitivity for diagnosis of severe OSA [18]. Bedside spirometry post extubation has also been evaluated as a tool to predict upper airway collapse. UA obstruction during wakefulness defined as the ratio of maximum expiratory and inspiratory flows at 50% of vital capacity (MEF50/MIF50) ≥ 1 was shown to correlate strongly with AHI and obstructive as well as central apnoeas [11]. Overnight Oximetry is a readable available tool if more detailed sleep studies are not easily accessible.

Although there are plenty of data to support poor outcome when underlying OSA or Obesity Hypoventilation Syndrome (OHS) is not treated, there are no data from randomised controlled studies that treating these patients with PAP therapy improves outcome. In a perioperative study following orthopaedic procedures, 177 patients with mean BMI of 33 were randomised to Auto PAP (APAP) treatment or standard care. APAP controlled SDB and reduced hypoxaemia, however, there was poor compliance with PAP therapy. Incidence of serious adverse events was very low with no difference between groups [19].

OHS with acute hypercapnic respiratory failure (AHRF) presents another challenge for Intensive Care Physicians and Pulmonologists with patients often misdiagnosed as suffering from heart failure and treated with diuretics with little attention paid to hypercapnic respiratory failure. Marik et al. reported that over an 8 months period 61 patients with morbid obesity (mean BMI 49 kg/m^2) were admitted with AHRF to their intensive care unit with a high proportion (>50%) being treated for COPD or Asthma or heart failure. 38% needed to be mechanically ventilated due to failure of Noninvasive ventilation (NIV) and the authors report 18% in-hospital mortality [20]. Our own data confirm these findings with delayed recognition and 13% mortality in OHS patients with AHRF in our institution [21].

Identification and appropriate treatment of OHS can lead to improved outcomes. In a cohort study 62 Morbidly obese patients (Mean BMI 46 kg/m^2, 23% had OSA and 21% had chronic lung diseases) who were weaned from mechanical ventilation using a protocol and then given a trial of NIV. When compared to matched historical controls, NIV reduced risk of respiratory failure by 16% as well as significantly reducing length of stay on intensive care unit. In patients with hypercapnia, use of NIV led to reduced mortality as well [22]. Prophylactic NIV has also been shown to reduce the risk of extubation failure in mechanically ventilated patients with COPD and hypercapnia [23].

Patients with prolonged ventilation via tracheostomy are another important group to consider as they can have high prevalence of SDB [12]. These patients in effect are being treated for any potential upper airway obstruction or OSA. To assess for underlying OSA, these patients can undergo a sleep study with their tracheostomy capped (this needs cuff to be deflated as a pre-requisite or a cuff less tracheostomy). If OSA/SDB is proven or likely difficult difficult airway, e.g., in patients with neck circumference of more than 42 cm (24) then these patients can be initiated on PAP therapy (CPAP or bi-level as appropriate) and only once they are established then tracheostomy can be safely removed. In Author's institute, direct visualization of larynx prior to decanulation to rule out glottis pathology, as well as neck imaging rule out external compression of trachea is a pre-requisite in patients with previously failed attempts at decanulation.

Summary and Recommendation

OSA/OHS is common in patients who undergo mechanical ventilation. Undiagnosed and untreated OSA/OHS is associated with increased risk of difficult intubation or extubation failure. Morbid Obesity, neck circumference >42 cm, STOP-Bang score >3, as well as craniofacial anatomical features such as retrognathia, macroglossia are also risk factors for OSA/difficult intubation. Submental ultrasound, cuff-leak test and post-extubation spirometry could be used in addition to sleep studies to identify those at high risk of upper airway collapse.

Minimising opioid use, avoiding deeper level of anaesthesia, using semi-upright position post extubation and prophylactic use of PAP therapy/NIV - are likely to reduce the risk of extubation failure. In those with hypercapnic respiratory failure and/or overlap of OSA and COPD the author would recommend NIV rather than CPAP.

Tracheostomy decanulation should be preceded by assessment and treatment of any upper airway pathology including OSA.

REFERENCES

[1] Davidson TM. The Great Leap Forward: the anatomic basis for the acquisition of speech and obstructive sleep apnea. *Sleep Med*. 2003;4:185-94.

[2] Agha B and Johal A. Facial phenotype in obstructive sleep apnea - hypopnea syndrome: a systematic review and meta-analysis. *J. Sleep Res*. (2017) 26, 122-131.

[3] Senaratna CV, Perret JL, Lodge CJ et al. Prevalence of obstructive sleep apnea in the general population: A systematic review. *Sleep Med. Rev.* 2017 Aug;34:70-81. doi: 10.1016/j.smrv.2016.07.002. Epub 2016 Jul 18.

[4] Nagappa M, Wong DT, Cozowicz C, et al. Is obstructive sleep apnea associated with difficult airway? Evidence from a systematic review and meta analysis of prospective and retrospective cohort studies. *PLOS ONE* https://doi.org/10.1371/journal.pone.0204904 October 4, 2018.

[5] Neligan PJ, Porter S, Max B, et al. Obstructive Sleep Apnea Is Not a Risk Factor for Difficult Intubation in Morbidly Obese Patients. *Anesth. Analg*. 2009;109:1182-6.

[6] Bolona E, Hahn PY, Afessa B. Intensive care unit and hospital mortality in patients with obstructive sleep apnea. *J. Crit. Care*. 2015 Feb;30(1):178-80.

[7] Goring K, Collop N. Sleep disordered breathing in hospitalized patients. *J. Clin. Sleep. Med*. 2008;4(2):105-110.

[8] Ankit Gupta, Stuart F. Quan, Olaf Oldenburg et al. Sleep-disordered breathing in hospitalized patients with congestive heart failure: a concise review and proposed algorithm. *Heart Fail. Rev*. 2018 Sep; 23(5): 701-709.

[9] Malhotra A, Hillman D. Obesity and the lung: 3 Obesity, respiration and intensive care. *Thorax* 2008;63:925-931.

[10] Timm FP, Zaremba S, Grabitz SD, et al. Effects of Opioids Given to Facilitate Mechanical Ventilation on Sleep Apnea After Extubation in the Intensive Care Unit. *Sleep*, Vol. 41, No. 1, 2018.

[11] Chishti A, Batchelor AM, Bullock RE, et al. Sleep-related breathing disorders following discharge from intensive care. *Intensive Care Med.* 2000; 26(4): 426-433.

[12] Diaz-Abad M, Verceles AC, Brown JE, and Scharf SM. Sleep-Disordered Breathing May Be Under-Recognized in Patients Who Wean From Prolonged Mechanical Ventilation. *Respiratory Care* 2012: 57; 229-37.

[13] Subramani Y, Nagappa M, Wong J, et al. Death or near-death in patients with obstructive sleep apnoea: a compendium of case reports of critical complications. *British Journal of Anaesthesia*, 119(5): 885-99 (2017).

[14] Thanthitaweewat V, Muntham D, Chirakalwasan N. Obstructive Sleep Apnea Prevalence And Extubation Outcome In Medical ICU. *Respirology* 2017: 22(Suppl. 3), 125-26.

[15] Hagberg CA, Artime CA. Extubation of the perioperative patient with a difficult airway. *Rev. Colomb. Anestesiol.* 2014;42(4):295-301.

[16] Lyaker MR, Davila VR, and Papadimos TJ. Excessive Dynamic Airway Collapse: An Unexpected Contributor to Respiratory Failure in a Surgical Patient *Case Reports in Anesthesiology* Volume 2015, Article ID 596857, 5 pages http://dx.doi.org/10.1155/2015/596857.

[17] Devaraj U, Rajagopala S, Kumar A et al. Undiagnosed Obstructive Sleep Apnea and Postoperative Outcomes: A Prospective Observational Study. *Respiration* 2017;94:18-25.

[18] Shu C, Lee P, Lin JW5, The Use of Sub-Mental Ultrasonography for Identifying Patients with Severe Obstructive Sleep Apnea. *PLoS ONE* 8(5): e62848. doi:10.1371/journal.pone.0062848.

[19] Liao P, Luo Q, Elsaid H, et al. Perioperative auto-titrated continuous positive airway pressure treatment in surgical patients with obstructive sleep apnea: a randomized controlled trial. *Anesthesiology*. 2013;119:837-47.

[20] Marik PE, and Desai H. Characteristics of Patients With the "Malignant Obesity Hypoventilation Syndrome" Admitted to an ICU. *Journal of Intensive Care Medicine* 2012: 28(2); 124-130.

[21] Ehilawa PI, Chisanga B, Smith P, Domiciliary Noninvasive Ventilation Reduces Re-Admissions in Persistent Hypercapnic Respiratory Failure due to COPD, But Are We Missing a Trick? *Thorax* 2019;74(Suppl 2):A195.

[22] El Solh AA, Aquilina A, Pineda L, et al. Noninvasive ventilation for prevention of post-extubation respiratory failure in obese Patients. *Eur. Respir. J.* 2006; 28: 588-595.

[23] Ferrer M, Sellarés J, Valencia M, et al. Non-invasive ventilation after extubation in hypercapnic patients with chronic respiratory disorders: randomised controlled trial. *Lancet*. 2009 Sep 26;374(9695):1082-8. doi: 10.1016/S0140-6736(09)61038-2. Epub 2009 Aug 12.

[24] Riad W, Vaez M, Raveendran R, et al. Neck circumference as a predictor of difficult intubation and difficult mask ventilation in morbidly obese patients A prospective observational study. *Eur. J. Anaesthesiol.* 2016; 33:244-249.

In: Sleep Medicine in Critical Care
Editors: Antonio M. Esquinas et al.
ISBN: 978-1-53617-768-8

Chapter 21

Difficult Weaning and Ventilator Dependent Patients: Key Practical Recommendations

Neeraj M. Shah*, MD and Patrick B. Murphy, MD
Lane Fox Respiratory Service,
Guy's and St Thomas' NHS Foundation Trust, London, UK
Centre for Human and Applied Physiological Sciences,
King's College London, London, UK
NIHR Biomedical Research Centre at Guy's
and St Thomas' NHS Foundation Trust
and King's College London, London, UK

Abstract

Weaning from mechanical ventilation is a key task for any intensivist. While the majority of patients will be liberated from invasive ventilation quickly, 20-30% will experience difficulty in weaning. These patients require a comprehensive physiological assessment to determine the cause of the weaning difficulty followed by a multidisciplinary approach to management. Complex weaning patients are likely to need optimisation of nutrition, physical rehabilitation and psychological health, as well as prevention of ventilator-associated pneumonias. This group of patients require a large amount of resources and are likely to require long-term care, which is best coordinated through specialist regional centres.

* Corresponding Author's E-mail: Neeraj.Shah@gstt.nhs.uk.

INTRODUCTION

Endotracheal intubation and invasive mechanical ventilation are associated with considerable morbidity, with increasing risk from increasing length of ventilation [1, 2]. Weaning from mechanical ventilation is therefore a crucial task for any critical care practitioner. Patients who are unable to wean rapidly have increased morbidity, mortality, long-term healthcare needs and require increased socioeconomic resources if they survive to discharge from critical care. The management of these patients requires a comprehensive, multidisciplinary strategy, which needs to be delivered over the prolonged period that these patients remain within a health care setting. This is a complex area of medicine requiring a strong understanding of the pathophysiology of respiratory failure and the barriers to weaning success as well as the social and logistical challenges faced when caring for patients requiring prolonged mechanical ventilation (PMV).

WEANING CLASSIFICATION

A barrier to both the collection and interpretation of data in patients who undergo weaning from invasive mechanical ventilation (IMV) has been the difficulty in classification of weaning. The initial classification system proposed by the international consensus conference (ICC) defined weaning by the time from 1st spontaneous breathing trial (SBT), which is not universally used in critical care units and failed to include those patients who were unable to be weaned from IMV [3-5]. There have been recent attempts to improve the classification by the weaning according to a new definition (WIND). The WIND classification categorises patients undergoing weaning from invasive ventilation into four groups; no weaning and 3 groups dependent on the time taken from initial liberation attempt [3]. Group 1 (simple weaning ~60%) consists of patients who are extubated after the first weaning attempt. Group 2 (difficult weaning ~20-30%) consists of patients who require up to three weaning attempts or as long as seven days to reach successful extubation. Group 3 (complex weaning ~10-15%) consists of patients who require more than three attempts or longer than seven days to reach extubation. The WIND classification further divides Group 3 into 3a (successful extubation after seven days of ventilation) and 3b (unsuccessful weaning) [4, 5].

Weaning failure is the requirement for reintubation following successful extubation, or death, within 48 hours of extubation. The prevalence of weaning failure has been reported as 30-40% [3, 6, 7].

THE WEANING PROCESS

There is considerable worldwide variation in weaning practice [8], but the overarching process of weaning remains the same. Weaning can be separated into four stages:

1) Treat underlying cause of respiratory failure (pre-weaning) – any attempt to wean without treating the underlying cause of respiratory failure is unlikely to be successful.
2) Assess the readiness to wean – readiness testing helps to identify patients who are ready to be liberated from mechanical ventilation to prevent extubation delay and also those who are not ready, to reduce the risk of weaning failure due to premature extubation.
3) Evaluate the response to a reduction in ventilatory support – spontaneous awakening trials by reducing sedation are followed by spontaneous breathing trials. A successful spontaneous breathing trial is suggestive of weaning success without post-extubation respiratory failure.
4) Extubation or decannulation.

Non-invasive ventilation (NIV) is increasingly used to supplement extubation to reduce the risk of post-extubation respiratory failure. The use of NIV appears to decrease hospital mortality, ICU length of stay and incidence of ventilator associated pneumonia [9, 10]. The evidence for NIV use is strongest in COPD patients, particularly those who are requiring difficult or complex weaning [11-13]. Its role in unselected patients with respiratory failure is less clear. Two large multicentre randomised trials have failed to demonstrate any additional benefit from the use of NIV to prevent post-extubation failure [14, 15]. High flow oxygen therapy with nasal cannula (HFNC) is a relatively recent intervention in the prevention of post-extubation failure. There appears to be added value from HFNC when compared with conventional oxygen therapy [16], and non-inferiority when compared with NIV [17]. The addition of HFNC to NIV has also been reported to lower the risk of reintubation, when compared with HFNC alone [18]. When interpreting these data it is important to be cognisant of the difference in delivery of HFNC and NIV. The former is technically simple with a low skill level required and has been successfully implemented in non-critical care environments and is usually well tolerated by patients. The latter requires a higher level of skill and may require the use of judicious sedation to optimise patient comfort with NIV delivered for <50% of the intervention period in some of the trials. Therefore, the skill mix of the unit delivering the weaning needs to be considered in addition to patient factors when devising local weaning strategies.

COMPLEX WEANING

Patients requiring complex weaning (Group 3) tend to suffer from poor outcomes [19]. Approximately half of patients requiring prolonged weaning remained dependant on invasive ventilation at one year [20, 21]. Their one-year mortality is as high as 40-75% [20-24]. Significantly, 42% of patients who were successfully extubated after prolonged weaning required reinstitution of mechanical ventilation [25]. These patients require a comprehensive management strategy involving the multidisciplinary team that encompasses all of the physiological, clinical and psychological factors that have an impact on the ability to wean successfully. The most common causes of prolonged weaning include persistence of the index condition causing respiratory failure, heart failure, chronic respiratory insufficiency, respiratory muscle weakness, psychological disturbance, poor sleep and recurring sepsis. The most common contributing factor to PMV is persistence of the process which led to initial admission to critical care and IMV. Without adequate correction of the cause of this initial insult, all other attempts at weaning are unlikely to be fruitful.

Patients struggling to wean should be considered for tracheostomy. Tracheostomy results in improved physiology, due to increase tidal volume and decreased airway resistance, compared with endotracheal intubation [26]. The optimal timing for conversion to tracheostomy remains unclear. Despite the known complications of prolonged endotracheal intubation, insertion of the tracheostomy itself involves risk. In addition, whilst early work appeared to suggest improved outcomes following early tracheostomy [27-30], a Cochrane review was unable to provide conclusive evidence to support early tracheostomy [31]. The majority of weaning failure units in the UK and Europe tend to convert to tracheostomy in patients who have not weaned from endotracheal intubation within two weeks [32, 33].

A structured approach is required to address the potential causes of weaning difficulty and ensure the patient's clinical condition is optimised for weaning success and ongoing rehabilitation.

Physiological

Physiological dependence on mechanical ventilation can be explained by persistent imbalance in the load-capacity-drive relationship of the respiratory system. Evaluation of the factors impacting on this relationship will aid identifying reversible causes of prolonged weaning.

Respiratory Muscle Load

Respiratory muscle load is the combination of elastic load (inversely proportional to compliance), resistive load (airway resistance to airflow) and threshold load (intrinsic positive end-expiratory pressure [PEEP]) [34]. Conditions that result in airflow limitation due to secretions and bronchospasm, such as COPD and asthma, lead to increased airways resistance and dynamic hyperinflation. This results in increased work of breathing that limits the ability to wean. To counter this, adequate bronchodilation therapy should be delivered to these patients. Obesity and chest wall deformity result in reduced chest wall compliance and therefore increased elastic load, which also increases the work of breathing, adding to the respiratory muscle load. Severe airflow resistance will lead to gas-trapping, which generates intrinsic PEEP, and an increased threshold load [35].

Respiratory Capacity

Capacity is a marker of inspiratory muscle strength and endurance [34]. Any condition causing respiratory muscle weakness will lead to reduced respiratory capacity. In critically unwell patients, this is most commonly seen in those suffering from critical care myopathy and electrolyte disturbances such as hypokalaemia [36]. In addition, pre-existing conditions such as the muscular dystrophies, motor neurone disease or spinal cord injury all result in pre-morbid respiratory muscle weakness and an increased risk of respiratory failure requiring invasive mechanical ventilation. All of these conditions increase the risk of the need for prolonged ventilation and extubation failure [37]. The key management strategy for respiratory muscle fatigue is rest [38]. To emphasise this, inspiratory muscle training during critical illness has not been demonstrated to improve weaning outcomes [39, 40]. Of interest, diaphragm fatigue does not appear to be a contributing factor to weaning failure [41-43].

Respiratory Drive

The respiratory centre within the medulla responds to changes in arterial pCO2, driving changes in pH, by altering the intensity of signals to the respiratory muscles; this is termed respiratory drive. It can be further influenced by higher cortical inputs and correlates strongly with perception of dyspnoea [44]. Acute conditions leading to respiratory failure such as Guillain-Barre Syndrome, spinal cord injury (above C3) and transverse myelitis, and chronic conditions such as motor neurone disease and myasthenia gravis cause reduced neural respiratory drive. In addition, the use of sedation, opiates, antiepileptics, neuromuscular blocking agents or aminoglycosides [45, 46] will also depress the respiratory centre and cause reduced drive. This reduced drive is associated with a need for prolonged weaning [47]. Caution is needed when ventilating patients with chronic respiratory failure when excessive ventilation to achieve normocapnia may lead to a reduction in respiratory drive frustrating weaning attempts.

Such patients should therefore be ventilated to their 'usual' CO_2 threshold, to maximise the drive to breathe when weaning.

Cardiac

Underlying cardiac disease has a significant influence on the risk of weaning failure [48, 49]. Positive end-expiratory pressure during invasive ventilation provides cardiac support, and its withdrawal during weaning can cause cardiac ischaemia or failure. Those who suffer from cardiac ischaemia or dysfunction following a spontaneous breathing trial are more likely to have an unsuccessful weaning attempt [50]. In patients who may be at risk for cardiac dysfunction, changes in $ScvO_2$ can be dynamically assessed; a fall in $ScvO_2$ can be due to an inadequate increase in cardiac output in response to added load occurring during weaning, which is associated with weaning failure [51]. B-type natriuretic peptide levels can be measured prior to a weaning attempt, to identify fluid overload, which would increase the risk of weaning failure. This can be managed using conventional diuretic therapy, particularly in those with left ventricular dysfunction [52, 53]. Cardiac function can be optimised with medical management of coronary procedures, to minimise the risk of weaning failure. The inotrope levosimendan may assist in the management of difficult to wean patients. There are small case series indicating potential benefit of levosimendan to assist weaning in those patients with identified left ventricular dysfunction [54]. Levosimendan may also have a direct effect on the respiratory musculature, with data demonstrating that it may have an enhancing effect on diaphragm contractility [55]. Subsequent clinical trial data has indicated that the delivery of levosimendan has a positive effect on respiratory parameters in patients undergoing IMV with increased tidal volume and minute ventilation during weaning trials [56].

Clinical

Ventilation Associated Pneumonia (VAP)

Prolonged weaning is associated with recurrent episodes of VAP which are associated with much of the morbidity of PMV. Attempts to reduce VAP are therefore vital in providing clinical stability during periods of weaning. Strategies to prevent VAP include minimising sedation, conversion to tracheostomy and cuff-down trials to promote bulbar function [57]. Optimal oral hygiene, using antiseptic mouthwash reduces the risk of VAP but has no impact on mortality [58]. Subglottic suction to remove supra-cuff secretions has been demonstrated to reduce the incidence of VAP, although, again, has no impact on mortality [59].

Physical Rehabilitation

ICU-acquired skeletal muscle weakness, due to catabolic activity during critical illness [60], is a risk factor for prolonged weaning [61] and is highly prevalent in the prolonged weaning population [62]. As skeletal muscle encompasses the respiratory musculature, physical reconditioning is an essential element of the management of weaning patients [63, 64]. A study investigating the combination of physical rehabilitation, sedation holds and occupational therapy reported improved outcomes with the intervention; however, the specific influence of physical rehabilitation was not separately analysed [65]. Although there is no strong evidence for the inclusion of physical rehabilitation, there is intuitive and conceptual perceived value and should be a part of the management strategy of any patient receiving prolonged invasive ventilation [66]. The widespread inclusion of early mobilisation to critically ill patients is not yet prevalent, despite its perceived importance [67, 68].

Nutrition

The value of good nutrition in critical care patients is clear, but the optimal nutrition strategy for prolonged weaning patients remains elusive. In fact, the optimal strategy for all critical care patients is unclear, with equivocal outcome data from trophic or full feeding [69, 70] and no consensus about the optimal calorie intake required [71, 72]. It appears that early feeding is particularly important in patients who go on to require prolonged ventilation [73]. Replacing trace elements such as magnesium enhance respiratory muscle function [74] but the impact of this on outcomes in prolonged weaning patients remains unclear [75].

Psychological

Critical illness survivors have a high prevalence of psychological morbidity [76]. This can influence on their ability to engage with the weaning process and can contribute to prolonged weaning. The use of biofeedback techniques may have value in managing prolonged weaning patients [77, 78] but a more recent study using cognitive behavioural therapy failed to demonstrate any benefit [79]. Despite the lack of evidence, it is intuitive that psychological wellbeing will impact on the patient's ability to engage in other approaches used to support weaning. Poor sleep quality is associated with poorer outcomes in critical care patients [80-82]. Although not studied in prolonged weaning patients specifically, non-pharmacological methods to improve sleep quality are likely to support the weaning process.

Logistical Factors in the Management of Prolonged Weaning

The management of prolonged weaning patients is complex, resource-heavy and expensive. Despite efforts to optimise the management of these patients by evidence-based protocols the outcomes in specialist prolonged mechanical ventilation centres remain superior [83]. These specialist centres have been demonstrated to be successful at liberating patients from invasive ventilation and are cost-effective [84-86]. Despite this, the long-term outcomes for these patients remains poor. In addition, some patients are unable to be liberated from mechanical ventilation regardless of receiving optimal care [86]. These patients may receive 24-hour tracheostomy ventilation, night-time ventilation via tracheostomy or are transitioned to non-invasive ventilation. Patients who require tracheostomy ventilation tend to reside in long-term care institutions, either specialised weaning centres or long-term care facilities in the community [87]. The quality of life for these patients is limited, with impact on care-givers, and comes at high cost. There is therefore an important need for comprehensive discussions with patients (if possible), care-givers and family members before deciding to commit to long-term invasive ventilation.

References

[1] Esteban A, Anzueto A, Frutos F, Alia I, Brochard L, Stewart TE, et al. Characteristics and outcomes in adult patients receiving mechanical ventilation: a 28-day international study. *JAMA*. 2002;287(3):345-55.

[2] Epstein SK, Ciubotaru RL, Wong JB. Effect of failed extubation on the outcome of mechanical ventilation. *Chest*. 1997;112(1):186-92.

[3] Boles JM, Bion J, Connors A, Herridge M, Marsh B, Melot C, et al. Weaning from mechanical ventilation. *Eur Respir J*. 2007;29(5): 1033-56.

[4] Beduneau G, Pham T, Schortgen F, Piquilloud L, Zogheib E, Jonas M, et al. Epidemiology of Weaning Outcome according to a New Definition. The WIND Study. *Am J Respir Crit Care Med*. 2017; 195(6):772-83.

[5] Jeong BH, Lee KY, Nam J, Ko MG, Na SJ, Suh GY, et al. Validation of a new WIND classification compared to ICC classification for weaning outcome. *Ann Intensive Care*. 2018;8(1):115.

[6] Mifsud Bonnici D, Sanctuary T, Warren A, Murphy PB, Steier J, Marino P, et al. Prospective observational cohort study of patients with weaning failure admitted to a specialist weaning, rehabilitation and home mechanical ventilation centre. *BMJ Open*. 2016;6(3): e010025.

[7] Davies MG, Quinnell TG, Oscroft NS, Clutterbuck SP, Shneerson JM, Smith IE. Hospital outcomes and long-term survival after referral to a specialized weaning unit. *Br J Anaesth*. 2017;118(4): 563-9.

[8] Burns KEA, Raptis S, Nisenbaum R, Rizvi L, Jones A, Bakshi J, et al. International Practice Variation in Weaning Critically Ill Adults from Invasive Mechanical Ventilation. *Ann Am Thorac Soc*. 2018;15 (4):494-502.

[9] Yeung J, Couper K, Ryan EG, Gates S, Hart N, Perkins GD. Non-invasive ventilation as a strategy for weaning from invasive mechanical ventilation: a systematic review and Bayesian meta-analysis. *Intensive Care Med*. 2018;44(12):2192-204.

[10] Burns KE, Adhikari NK, Keenan SP, Meade M. Use of non-invasive ventilation to wean critically ill adults off invasive ventilation: meta-analysis and systematic review. *BMJ*. 2009;338:b1574.

[11] Nava S, Ambrosino N, Clini E, Prato M, Orlando G, Vitacca M, et al. Noninvasive mechanical ventilation in the weaning of patients with respiratory failure due to chronic obstructive pulmonary disease. A randomized, controlled trial. *Ann Intern Med*. 1998;128(9):721-8.

[12] Girault C, Daudenthun I, Chevron V, Tamion F, Leroy J, Bonmarchand G. Noninvasive ventilation as a systematic extubation and weaning technique in acute-on-chronic respiratory failure: a prospective, randomized controlled study. *Am J Respir Crit Care Med*. 1999;160(1):86-92.

[13] Ferrer M, Esquinas A, Arancibia F, Bauer TT, Gonzalez G, Carrillo A, et al. Noninvasive ventilation during persistent weaning failure: a randomized controlled trial. *Am J Respir Crit Care Med*. 2003; 168(1):70-6.

[14] Esteban A, Frutos-Vivar F, Ferguson ND, Arabi Y, Apezteguia C, Gonzalez M, et al. Noninvasive positive-pressure ventilation for respiratory failure after extubation. *N Engl J Med*. 2004;350(24): 2452-60.

[15] Perkins GD, Mistry D, Gates S, Gao F, Snelson C, Hart N, et al. Effect of Protocolized Weaning With Early Extubation to Noninvasive Ventilation vs Invasive Weaning on Time to Liberation From Mechanical Ventilation Among Patients With Respiratory Failure: The Breathe Randomized Clinical Trial. *JAMA*. 2018;320(18):1881-8.

[16] Hernandez G, Vaquero C, Gonzalez P, Subira C, Frutos-Vivar F, Rialp G, et al. Effect of Postextubation High-Flow Nasal Cannula vs Conventional Oxygen Therapy on Reintubation in Low-Risk Patients: A Randomized Clinical Trial. *JAMA*. 2016;315(13):1354-61.

[17] Hernandez G, Vaquero C, Colinas L, Cuena R, Gonzalez P, Canabal A, et al. Effect of Postextubation High-Flow Nasal Cannula vs Noninvasive Ventilation on Reintubation and Postextubation Respiratory Failure in High-Risk Patients: A Randomized Clinical Trial. *JAMA*. 2016;316(15):1565-74.

[18] Thille AW, Muller G, Gacouin A, Coudroy R, Decavele M, Sonneville R, et al. Effect of Postextubation High-Flow Nasal Oxygen With Noninvasive Ventilation vs High-Flow Nasal Oxygen Alone on Reintubation Among Patients at High Risk of Extubation Failure: A Randomized Clinical Trial. *JAMA*. 2019.

[19] Hill AD, Fowler RA, Burns KE, Rose L, Pinto RL, Scales DC. Long-Term Outcomes and Health Care Utilization after Prolonged Mechanical Ventilation. *Ann Am Thorac Soc*. 2017;14(3):355-62.

[20] Keng LT, Chung KP, Lin SY, Liang SK, Cheng JC, Chen IC, et al. Significant Clinical Factors Associated with Long-term Mortality in Critical Cancer Patients Requiring Prolonged Mechanical Ventilation. *Sci Rep*. 2017;7(1):2148.

[21] Jubran A, Grant BJB, Duffner LA, Collins EG, Lanuza DM, Hoffman LA, et al. Long-Term Outcome after Prolonged Mechanical Ventilation. A Long-Term Acute-Care Hospital Study. *Am J Respir Crit Care Med*. 2019;199(12):1508-16.

[22] Saiphoklang N, Auttajaroon J. Incidence and outcome of weaning from mechanical ventilation in medical wards at Thammasat University Hospital. *PLoS One*. 2018;13(10):e0205106.

[23] Leroy G, Devos P, Lambiotte F, Thevenin D, Leroy O. One-year mortality in patients requiring prolonged mechanical ventilation: multicenter evaluation of the ProVent score. *Crit Care*. 2014;18(4): R155.

[24] Herer B. Outcomes of Tracheostomized Subjects Undergoing Prolonged Mechanical Ventilation in an Intermediate-Care Facility. *Respir Care*. 2018;63(3):282-8.

[25] Sansone GR, Frengley JD, Horland A, Vecchione JJ, Kaner RJ. Effects of Reinstitution of Prolonged Mechanical Ventilation on the Outcomes of 370 Patients in a Long-Term Acute Care Hospital. *J Intensive Care Med*. 2018;33(9):527-35.

[26] Lim CK, Ruan SY, Lin FC, Wu CL, Chang HT, Jerng JS, et al. Effect of Tracheostomy on Weaning Parameters in Difficult-to-Wean Mechanically Ventilated Patients: A Prospective Observational Study. *PLoS One*. 2015;10(9):e0138294.

[27] Boynton JH, Hawkins K, Eastridge BJ, O'Keefe GE. Tracheostomy timing and the duration of weaning in patients with acute respiratory failure. *Crit Care*. 2004;8(4):R261-7.

[28] Hsu CL, Chen KY, Chang CH, Jerng JS, Yu CJ, Yang PC. Timing of tracheostomy as a determinant of weaning success in critically ill patients: a retrospective study. *Crit Care*. 2005;9(1):R46-52.

[29] Alhajhusain A, Ali AW, Najmuddin A, Hussain K, Aqeel M, El-Solh AA. Timing of tracheotomy in mechanically ventilated critically ill morbidly obese patients. *Crit Care Res Pract*. 2014;2014:840638.

[30] Chen HC, Song L, Chang HC, Hsu MT. Factors related to tracheostomy timing and ventilator weaning: findings from a population in Northern Taiwan. *Clin Respir J.* 2018;12(1):97-104.

[31] Andriolo BN, Andriolo RB, Saconato H, Atallah AN, Valente O. Early versus late tracheostomy for critically ill patients. *Cochrane Database Syst Rev.* 2015;1:CD007271.

[32] Krishnan K, Elliot SC, Mallick A. The current practice of tracheostomy in the United Kingdom: a postal survey. *Anaesthesia.* 2005;60(4):360-4.

[33] Kluge S, Baumann HJ, Maier C, Klose H, Meyer A, Nierhaus A, et al. Tracheostomy in the intensive care unit: a nationwide survey. *Anesth Analg.* 2008;107(5):1639-43.

[34] Shah NMM, P. B. Hypercapnic Failure in Non-COPD. In: Heunks LMAD, A.; Windisch, W., editor. *Pulmonary Emergencies.* ERS Monograph. 74: ERS; 2016. p. 86-100.

[35] Ranieri VM, Dambrosio M, Brienza N. Intrinsic PEEP and cardiopulmonary interaction in patients with COPD and acute ventilatory failure. *Eur Respir J.* 1996;9(6):1283-92.

[36] Lee JW. *Fluid and electrolyte disturbances in critically ill patients.* Electrolyte Blood Press. 2010;8(2):72-81.

[37] Tsara V, Moisiadis N, Antoniadou M, Serasli E. Characteristics and outcome of patients with difficult weaning from mechanical ventilation: an 18 years' experience of a respiratory intermediate unit attached to a pulmonary department. *Hippokratia.* 2015;19(1):37-40.

[38] Moxham J. Respiratory muscle fatigue: mechanisms, evaluation and therapy. *Br J Anaesth.* 1990;65(1):43-53.

[39] Caruso P, Denari SD, Ruiz SA, Bernal KG, Manfrin GM, Friedrich C, et al. Inspiratory muscle training is ineffective in mechanically ventilated critically ill patients. *Clinics* (Sao Paulo). 2005;60(6):479-84.

[40] Martin AD, Smith BK, Davenport PD, Harman E, Gonzalez-Rothi RJ, Baz M, et al. Inspiratory muscle strength training improves weaning outcome in failure to wean patients: a randomized trial. *Crit Care.* 2011;15(2):R84.

[41] Yang L, Luo J, Bourdon J, Lin MC, Gottfried SB, Petrof BJ. Controlled mechanical ventilation leads to remodeling of the rat diaphragm. *Am J Respir Crit Care Med.* 2002;166(8):1135-40.

[42] Watson AC, Hughes PD, Louise Harris M, Hart N, Ware RJ, Wendon J, et al. Measurement of twitch transdiaphragmatic, esophageal, and endotracheal tube pressure with bilateral anterolateral magnetic phrenic nerve stimulation in patients in the intensive care unit. *Crit Care Med.* 2001;29(7):1325-31.

[43] Laghi F, Cattapan SE, Jubran A, Parthasarathy S, Warshawsky P, Choi YS, et al. Is weaning failure caused by low-frequency fatigue of the diaphragm? *Am J Respir Crit Care Med*. 2003;167(2):120-7.

[44] Jolley CJ, Luo YM, Steier J, Rafferty GF, Polkey MI, Moxham J. Neural respiratory drive and breathlessness in COPD. *Eur Respir J*. 2015;45(2):355-64.

[45] Paradelis AG, Triantaphyllidis C, Giala MM. Neuromuscular blocking activity of aminoglycoside antibiotics. *Methods Find Exp Clin Pharmacol*. 1980;2(1):45-51.

[46] Liu M, Kato M, Hashimoto Y. Neuromuscular blocking effects of the aminoglycoside antibiotics arbekacin, astromicin, isepamicin and netilmicin on the diaphragm and limb muscles in the rabbit. *Pharmacology*. 2001;63(3):142-6.

[47] Rialp G, Raurich JM, Llompart-Pou JA, Ayestaran I, Ibanez J. Central respiratory drive in patients with neuromuscular diseases. *Respir Care*. 2013;58(3):450-7.

[48] Lemaire F, Teboul JL, Cinotti L, Giotto G, Abrouk F, Steg G, et al. Acute left ventricular dysfunction during unsuccessful weaning from mechanical ventilation. *Anesthesiology*. 1988;69(2):171-9.

[49] Routsi C, Stanopoulos I, Kokkoris S, Sideris A, Zakynthinos S. Weaning failure of cardiovascular origin: how to suspect, detect and treat-a review of the literature. *Ann Intensive Care*. 2019;9(1):6.

[50] Vignon P. Cardiovascular failure and weaning. *Ann Transl Med*. 2018;6(18):354.

[51] Jubran A, Mathru M, Dries D, Tobin MJ. Continuous recordings of mixed venous oxygen saturation during weaning from mechanical ventilation and the ramifications thereof. *Am J Respir Crit Care Med*. 1998;158(6):1763-9.

[52] Mekontso Dessap A, Roche-Campo F, Kouatchet A, Tomicic V, Beduneau G, Sonneville R, et al. Natriuretic peptide-driven fluid management during ventilator weaning: a randomized controlled trial. *Am J Respir Crit Care Med*. 2012;186(12):1256-63.

[53] Mekontso-Dessap A, de Prost N, Girou E, Braconnier F, Lemaire F, Brun-Buisson C, et al. B-type natriuretic peptide and weaning from mechanical ventilation. *Intensive Care Med*. 2006;32(10):1529-36.

[54] Kaltsi I, Angelopoulos E, Tzanis G, Sideris A, Tyrovolas K, Kokkoris S, et al. Contribution of Levosimendan in Weaning from Mechanical Ventilation in Patients with Left Ventricular Dysfunction: A Pilot Study. *Crit Care Res Pract*. 2019;2019: 7169492.

[55] Doorduin J, Sinderby CA, Beck J, Stegeman DF, van Hees HW, van der Hoeven JG, et al. The calcium sensitizer levosimendan improves human diaphragm function. *Am J Respir Crit Care Med*. 2012;185 (1):90-5.

[56] Roesthuis L, van der Hoeven H, Sinderby C, Frenzel T, Ottenheijm C, Brochard L, et al. Effects of levosimendan on respiratory muscle function in patients weaning from mechanical ventilation. *Intensive Care Med*. 2019;45(10):1372-81.

[57] Lorente L, Blot S, Rello J. Evidence on measures for the prevention of ventilator-associated pneumonia. *Eur Respir J*. 2007;30(6):1193-207.

[58] Hua F, Xie H, Worthington HV, Furness S, Zhang Q, Li C. Oral hygiene care for critically ill patients to prevent ventilator-associated pneumonia. *Cochrane Database Syst Rev*. 2016;10:CD008367.

[59] Mao Z, Gao L, Wang G, Liu C, Zhao Y, Gu W, et al. Subglottic secretion suction for preventing ventilator-associated pneumonia: an updated meta-analysis and trial sequential analysis. *Crit Care*. 2016;20(1):353.

[60] Puthucheary ZA, Rawal J, McPhail M, Connolly B, Ratnayake G, Chan P, et al. Acute skeletal muscle wasting in critical illness. *JAMA*. 2013;310(15):1591-600.

[61] De Jonghe B, Bastuji-Garin S, Sharshar T, Outin H, Brochard L. Does ICU-acquired paresis lengthen weaning from mechanical ventilation? *Intensive Care Med*. 2004;30(6):1117-21.

[62] De Jonghe B, Sharshar T, Lefaucheur JP, Authier FJ, Durand-Zaleski I, Boussarsar M, et al. Paresis acquired in the intensive care unit: a prospective multicenter study. *JAMA*. 2002;288(22):2859-67.

[63] De Jonghe B, Bastuji-Garin S, Durand MC, Malissin I, Rodrigues P, Cerf C, et al. Respiratory weakness is associated with limb weakness and delayed weaning in critical illness. *Crit Care Med*. 2007;35(9): 2007-15.

[64] Chiang LL, Wang LY, Wu CP, Wu HD, Wu YT. Effects of physical training on functional status in patients with prolonged mechanical ventilation. *Phys Ther*. 2006;86(9):1271-81.

[65] Schweickert WD, Pohlman MC, Pohlman AS, Nigos C, Pawlik AJ, Esbrook CL, et al. Early physical and occupational therapy in mechanically ventilated, critically ill patients: a randomised controlled trial. *Lancet*. 2009;373(9678):1874-82.

[66] Taito S, Yamauchi K, Tsujimoto Y, Banno M, Tsujimoto H, Kataoka Y. Does enhanced physical rehabilitation following intensive care unit discharge improve outcomes in patients who received mechanical ventilation? A systematic review and meta-analysis. *BMJ Open*. 2019;9(6):e026075.

[67] Nydahl P, Ruhl AP, Bartoszek G, Dubb R, Filipovic S, Flohr HJ, et al. Early mobilization of mechanically ventilated patients: a 1-day point-prevalence study in Germany. *Crit Care Med*. 2014;42(5): 1178-86.

[68] Berney SC, Harrold M, Webb SA, Seppelt I, Patman S, Thomas PJ, et al. Intensive care unit mobility practices in Australia and New Zealand: a point prevalence study. *Crit Care Resusc*. 2013;15(4):260-5.

[69] Arabi YM, Tamim HM, Dhar GS, Al-Dawood A, Al-Sultan M, Sakkijha MH, et al. Permissive underfeeding and intensive insulin therapy in critically ill patients: a randomized controlled trial. *Am J Clin Nutr*. 2011;93(3):569-77.

[70] Needham DM, Dinglas VD, Bienvenu OJ, Colantuoni E, Wozniak AW, Rice TW, et al. One year outcomes in patients with acute lung injury randomised to initial

trophic or full enteral feeding: prospective follow-up of EDEN randomised trial. *BMJ*. 2013;346:f1532.

[71] Krishnan JA, Parce PB, Martinez A, Diette GB, Brower RG. Caloric intake in medical ICU patients: consistency of care with guidelines and relationship to clinical outcomes. *Chest*. 2003;124(1):297-305.

[72] Faisy C, Lerolle N, Dachraoui F, Savard JF, Abboud I, Tadie JM, et al. Impact of energy deficit calculated by a predictive method on outcome in medical patients requiring prolonged acute mechanical ventilation. *Br J Nutr*. 2009;101(7):1079-87.

[73] Wei X, Day AG, Ouellette-Kuntz H, Heyland DK. The Association Between Nutritional Adequacy and Long-Term Outcomes in Critically Ill Patients Requiring Prolonged Mechanical Ventilation: A Multicenter Cohort Study. *Crit Care Med*. 2015;43(8):1569-79.

[74] Dhingra S, Solven F, Wilson A, McCarthy DS. Hypomagnesemia and respiratory muscle power. *Am Rev Respir Dis*. 1984;129(3):497-8.

[75] Johnson D, Gallagher C, Cavanaugh M, Yip R, Mayers I. The lack of effect of routine magnesium administration on respiratory function in mechanically ventilated patients. *Chest*. 1993;104(2):536-41.

[76] Clancy O, Edginton T, Casarin A, Vizcaychipi MP. The psychological and neurocognitive consequences of critical illness. A pragmatic review of current evidence. *J Intensive Care Soc*. 2015;16(3):226-33.

[77] Corson JA, Grant JL, Moulton DP, Green RL, Dunkel PT. Use of biofeedback in weaning paralyzed patients from respirators. *Chest*. 1979;76(5):543-5.

[78] Holliday JE, Hyers TM. The reduction of weaning time from mechanical ventilation using tidal volume and relaxation biofeedback. *Am Rev Respir Dis*. 1990;141(5 Pt 1):1214-20.

[79] Wade DM, Mouncey PR, Richards-Belle A, Wulff J, Harrison DA, Sadique MZ, et al. Effect of a Nurse-Led Preventive Psychological Intervention on Symptoms of Posttraumatic Stress Disorder Among Critically Ill Patients: A Randomized Clinical Trial. *JAMA*. 2019;321(7):665-75.

[80] Little A, Ethier C, Ayas N, Thanachayanont T, Jiang D, Mehta S. A patient survey of sleep quality in the Intensive Care Unit. *Minerva Anestesiol*. 2012;78(4):406-14.

[81] Pisani MA, Friese RS, Gehlbach BK, Schwab RJ, Weinhouse GL, Jones SF. Sleep in the intensive care unit. *Am J Respir Crit Care Med*. 2015;191(7):731-8.

[82] Delaney LJ, Van Haren F, Lopez V. Sleeping on a problem: the impact of sleep disturbance on intensive care patients - a clinical review. *Ann Intensive Care*. 2015;5:3.

[83] Blackwood B, Alderdice F, Burns K, Cardwell C, Lavery G, O'Halloran P. Use of weaning protocols for reducing duration of mechanical ventilation in critically ill adult patients: Cochrane systematic review and meta-analysis. *BMJ*. 2011;342:c7237.

[84] Schonhofer B, Euteneuer S, Nava S, Suchi S, Kohler D. Survival of mechanically ventilated patients admitted to a specialised weaning centre. *Intensive Care Med.* 2002;28(7):908-16.

[85] Pilcher DV, Bailey MJ, Treacher DF, Hamid S, Williams AJ, Davidson AC. Outcomes, cost and long term survival of patients referred to a regional weaning centre. *Thorax*. 2005;60(3):187-92.

[86] Scheinhorn DJ, Hassenpflug MS, Votto JJ, Chao DC, Epstein SK, Doig GS, et al. Post-ICU mechanical ventilation at 23 long-term care hospitals: a multicenter outcomes study. *Chest*. 2007;131(1):85-93.

[87] Wise MP, Hart N, Davidson C, Fox R, Allen M, Elliott M, et al. Home mechanical ventilation. *BMJ*. 2011;342:d1687.

In: Sleep Medicine in Critical Care
Editors: Antonio M. Esquinas et al.
ISBN: 978-1-53617-768-8

Chapter 22

PROLONGED MECHANICAL VENTILATION: HOW TO DIAGNOSE AND TREAT SLEEP-RELATED BREATHING DISORDERS

Montserrat Diaz-Abad*, MD and Jennifer Y. So, MD
Department of Medicine, University of Maryland School of Medicine,
Baltimore, Maryland, US

ABSTRACT

There is an increasing number of patients with prolonged mechanical ventilation (PMV) with associated increased health care burdens and poor long-term outcomes. Sleep-disordered breathing (SDB) is very frequent in the general population but has been studied rarely in the PMV population. Based on a limited number of studies, the prevalence of SDB, mostly OSA and sleep-related hypoxemia in patients with PMV has been as high 95%. PSG with or without a capped tracheostomy is the most comprehensive testing modality, but other methods, such as polygraphy and nocturnal oximetry, can be considered to facilitate ventilator weaning and decannulation. Patients with SDB can be successfully decannulated and transitioned to positive airway pressure (PAP) therapy. Further study is needed to determine the impact of diagnosis and treatment of SDB in the short and long-term outcomes of this population. This chapter reviews the diagnosis and treatment of SDB in patients with PMV.

Keywords: prolonged mechanical ventilation, sleep-disordered breathing tracheostomy, decannulation, weaning

* Corresponding Author's E-mail: mdiaz@som.umaryland.edu.

INTRODUCTION

There is an is an increasing number of patients surviving prolonged intensive care unit (ICU) admissions who require long-term care due to prolonged mechanical ventilation (PMV) and tracheostomy. This is associated with increasing healthcare burden, cost to society, and health care organizational challenges related to the patients' debilitated state and poor long-term outcomes.

Sleep-related breathing disorders, also known as sleep-disordered breathing (SDB), encompass multiple disorders including obstructive sleep apnea (OSA), central sleep apnea and sleep-related hypoventilation/hypoxemia. OSA affects a large proportion of the population, and untreated OSA is associated with many comorbidities, including cardiovascular disease, leading to increase in healthcare utilization. While polysomnography (PSG) is the gold standard for diagnosing OSA, home sleep apnea test (HSAT) is an alternative for diagnosis in some populations, although this technique has its limitations.

While the prevalence of SDB has been studied in patients hospitalized in the acute care settings, both ICU and elsewhere, its prevalence in PMV population is not well studied. This chapter reviews the diagnosis and treatment of SDB in patients with PMV and tracheostomy.

PROLONGED MECHANICAL VENTILATION

With increasing life expectancy and technological advances, there is an increasing number of patients surviving critical illness and ICU care, often with significant disability and chronic severe illness. Many of these patients require PMV with tracheostomy due to inability to wean from ventilatory support. They often experience significant healthcare burden and cost, and face organizational and dispositional challenges related to their debilitated status and poor long-term outcomes, with high mortality and frequent residence in long-term care facilities [1].

There are several definitions for PMV, including the requirement of > 21 days of mechanical ventilation (MV) for > 6 hours/day, or the need for > 7 days of ventilation after 1 or 3 failed spontaneous weaning trials (SBTs) attempts. Prolonged hospitalization with deconditioning and muscle wasting or weakness and critical illness-associated diaphragmatic weakness are frequent complications in this patient population. Coordinated and multidisciplinary efforts are required to improve the medical care of these patients and to rehabilitate and achieve ventilator weaning success [1].

These patients often have increased ICU utilization and prolonged length of stay requiring transfer to various other health care settings. Patients may be transferred to intermediate care units or specialized respiratory units within acute care hospitals, and to long-term acute care hospitals (LTAC) located also within acute care hospitals or separately in rehabilitation hospitals. These programs provide multidisciplinary care directed at rehabilitation, care of resolving acute and chronic conditions and ventilator weaning [1]. Sheinhorn et al. studied a large series of 1,491 patients with PMV discharged to long-term acute care hospitals (LTACs) with average age 72 years and median length of stay 40 days (range 1-365 days). At LTAC discharge, 54% of patients were weaned from ventilators, 21% remained ventilator dependent and 25% had died. Disposition included 29% to home, 49% to rehabilitation and long-term care facilities and 20% to acute care hospitals. Less than one-third of patients were alive 1 year after LTAC admission [2].

Common ventilatory weaning modalities include progressive lengthening of SBTs, progressive decrease in pressure support levels and the use on noninvasive ventilation (NIV), which can be as effective as mechanical ventilation (MV) in reducing the work of breathing. The long-term outcomes are poor, but vary significantly based on patient population, settings of care, and resources available. After weaning from the ventilator, defined as at least 7 continuous days without ventilatory support, decannulation is the next step if a tracheostomy is present. Varied decannulation protocols exist, but there is no consensus to guide this process; thus, many patients who have successfully weaned maintain their tracheostomy in place [1].

SLEEP-DISORDERED BREATHING

The term SDB encompasses multiple disorders, most commonly OSA, as well as central sleep apnea and sleep-related hypoventilation/hypoxemia. OSA is a disorder characterized by repetitive partial or complete narrowing of the upper airway during sleep, which impairs ventilation and oxygenation and frequently leads to arousals, intrathoracic pressure swings and sympathetic activation. It is estimated to affect 14% of men and 5% of women, although prevalence varies across studies, due to varied definition and methodology used and the population studied. Obesity is the strongest risk factor for OSA - it can be present in 70-80% of patients evaluated for bariatric surgery. Untreated OSA may be associated with many comorbidities, including cardiovascular disease (treatment-resistant hypertension, congestive heart failure, coronary artery disease, atrial fibrillation, stroke), as well as insulin resistance, diabetes mellitus and neurologic conditions, which lead to increased healthcare utilization (Kapur 2017).

The diagnosis of OSA requires an obstructive respiratory disturbance index (RDI) (apneas + hypopneas + respiratory-effort related arousals) ≥5 events/hour associated with typical symptoms, or an obstructive RDI ≥ 15 events/hour even without symptoms on in-laboratory PSG as the gold standard diagnostic test. Diagnostic testing is performed along with a comprehensive sleep evaluation. Due to the limited access and cost associated with PSG, home HSAT can be utilized as an alternative for diagnosis in certain populations. These devices use different technologies and sensors to record different parameters. The most common HSATs are type III cardiopulmonary studies (e.g., polygraphy) which measure two respiratory variables such as airflow and respiratory effort, oxygen saturation, and one cardiac variable such as electrocardiogram or heart rate. The simplest HSAT is a type IV study that measures 1-2 parameters, typically a pulse oximetry. In addition to the risk of technical failure, and the limited variables being measured, most devices do not measure sleep, leading to use of total recording time instead of total sleep time as the denominator for the respiratory events leading to potential underestimation of SDB. In addition PSG, rather than HSAT should be used in patients with significant cardiopulmonary disease, respiratory muscle weakness, awake hypoventilation, among other conditions [3].

Diagnosis of Sleep-Disordered Breathing in Prolonged Mechanical Ventilation

Few studies have evaluated the prevalence of SDB in the PMV population. One study performed polygraphy in 15 patients average age 63 years discharged from the ICU after PMV and compared them to 10 healthy controls. Of note, the median duration of MV was 8 days (range 2-24) and only 1 patient had a tracheostomy in situ, therefore this may not represent the typical PMV population, especially those residing in LTACs. Admitting diagnosis included sepsis, abdominal perforation and major surgery, and patients were excluded if they had a past history or current suspicion of chronic respiratory failure or SDB. Of 10 patients that underwent spirometry, 1 had a normal study, while the rest had a restrictive ventilatory pattern with a median forced vital capacity of 41% (25-81). Only 1 patient was obese -body mass index (BMI) ≥ 30 kg/m^2. The polygraphy results were within normal limits in the control group. Eleven patients (73%) had an abnormal apnea-hypopnea index (AHI) ≥ 5 events/hour (5-34). Despite all patients receiving oxygen therapy as part of their clinical care, 13 (87%) patients experienced episodes of nocturnal oxygen desaturation, with 9 (60%) spending >2 hours with $SpO_2 < 90\%$, (range 5-34). The time spent in any type of SDB varied between 6% and 41% of the study night [4].

Another study performed PSG and subjective sleep quality assessments with questionnaires to evaluate sleep quality in 19 patients with PMV and tracheostomy in a specialized weaning unit. It demonstrated reduced sleep quality, and decreased total sleep time, sleep efficacy and rapid eye movement sleep with preserved slow wave sleep, but was unable to evaluate reliably for SDB due to continuous invasive MV with an open tracheostomy during the PSG [5].

Our group conducted a study of 19 patients average age 53 years with PMV > 21 days and tracheostomy with median duration MV 69 days (29-476) in an LTAC. Patients underwent an in-laboratory PSG to assess for the presence of SDB and also as part of the decannulation process. Mean BMI was 44.0 kg/m^2 and 17 (89%) patients were obese. Five patients (36%) had been admitted to the acute-care hospital with hypercapnic respiratory failure, but the majority had non-pulmonary related causes for the PMV. The study included clinically stable patients who had successfully weaned off MV for 7 days and were considered adequate candidates for decannulation after undergoing direct laryngoscopy, tracheostomy downsizing and 24-hour continuous tracheostomy capping. Patients were excluded if they had a prior history of SDB, prior home NIV or MV use, or if they would not be good candidates to use NIV. Patients underwent diagnostic PSG with the tracheostomy capped, except for 3 patients who had been decannulated a few days prior to the PSG. Five patients used supplemental oxygen 2-4 L/min via nasal cannula during the baseline sleep study. Eighteen patients (95%) demonstrated OSA, with median RDI 24.2 events/hour (5.9-82.0). Median time with SpO2 < 90% was 14 minutes (0-172). The five patients with end-tidal CO2 monitoring during the PSG did not show evidence of hypoventilation [6].

While there is limited information on the use of PSG to diagnose SDB and aid in PMV weaning and decannulation in adults, the use of sleep studies is more widespread in the pediatric population. A review of 148 children and 153 decannulation attempts over a 10-year period with 190 PSGs performed found PSG to a valuable tool to evaluate children with tracheostomy with and without home MV. Children had to tolerate 12 hours off MV during the day before undergoing an off-MV PSG. Normal gas exchange and absence of central apneas were important PSG predictors for successful MV discontinuation. Hypoxemia without hypoventilation that corrected with supplemental oxygen did not preclude ventilator weaning and/or decannulation. Most children had a favorable PSG and underwent decannulation. Not downsizing the tracheostomy tube was associated with an increased chance of an unfavorable capped PSG. The authors recommend a decannulation algorithm that includes endoscopic airway evaluation to rule out anatomical abnormalities such as granulomas and stenosis, downsizing the tracheostomy to the smallest and safest size, and daytime capping followed by an overnight capped PSG as a final confirmation prior to decannulation [7].

Other Diagnostic Options

While the above studies utilized PSG and polygraphy, a more accessible and low-cost alternative, such as an overnight pulse oximetry study could potentially be used in PMV patients to screen for OSA and sleep related hypoxemia when more advanced methods are not available or feasible. Although not specifically used in the PMV population, overnight pulse oximetry has been used in hospitalized patients with successful outcomes and accuracy comparable to PSG. One study evaluated the usefulness of screening for OSA in 754 obese patients (BMI > 30 kg/m^2) admitted to the medical services of a tertiary care hospital. Patients underwent screening for OSA with the STOP questionnaire followed by a pulmonary consultation, and underwent an overnight pulse oximetry study to detect the oxygen desaturation index (ODI - 4%) if there were no contraindications. Of the 149 patients who screened positive for OSA and completed the evaluation with an outpatient PSG after discharge, 129 (87%) were confirmed to have OSA; 84 patients (65%) had moderate to severe OSA, with AHI $\geq$ 15events/hour. An optimal cutoff point was determined to be ODI 4% $\geq$ 10 events/hour when AHI $\geq$ 10 events/hour. Furthermore, an ODI < 15 events/hour resulted in few false-positive diagnoses, whereas an ODI < 5 events/hour limited false negative diagnoses [8].

POTENTIAL FACTORS ASSOCIATED WITH THE PRESENCE OF SLEEP-DISORDERED BREATHING IN PROLONGED MECHANICAL VENTILATION

It is unclear why there is such a high prevalence of SDB in the PMV population in the few studies done so far. Obesity, which is the strongest risk factor for OSA, was predominant in only one study. Neuromuscular weakness may also contribute to the finding of SDB. Several neuromuscular problems have been described in the critically ill, and can contribute to respiratory muscle weakness, including critical care polyneuropathy and myopathy. Patients with reduced lung function and respiratory reserve from neuromuscular weakness, lung parenchymal diseases, cardiac disease and who are already hypoxemic can have severe oxygen desaturations with apneas and hypopneas [4].

An additional factor that has received little attention is the potential role of prolonged endotracheal intubation and/or tracheostomy in causing SDB. While tracheostomy is the definitive treatment for OSA as it bypasses the areas of upper airway obstruction, it can cause tracheal stenosis and tracheomalacia long-term, and can be a rare cause of OSA due to narrowing of the tracheal lumen. There is a report of 2 cases of severe OSA associated with collapse of the cervical trachea due to tracheomalacia at the site of a prior tracheostomy at tracheal rings 2-3 level. While some abnormal findings were noted on wake endoscopic exam, drug-induced sleep endoscopy with propofol was critical in demonstrating the real severity and location of the obstruction, raising the possibility that in some patients tracheal lumen narrowin may be missed if only an awake endoscopic airway exam is performed. One patient was treated surgically with tracheal reconstruction and the other with continuous positive airway pressure (CPAP) [9].

TREATMENT OF SLEEP-DISORDERED BREATHING IN PROLONGED MECHANICAL VENTILATION

SDB can be treated in PMV patients with successful outcomes leading to decannulation. In the above reference study of 19 patients, the 18 patients (95%) with diagnosed OSA had median RDI 24.2 events/hour (5.9-82.0) and 14 patients (78%) underwent successful PAP titration (12 patients with CPAP and 2 with bilevel PAP spontaneous mode) with a capped tracheostomy, except for the 3 recently decannulated patients. The other 4 patients were discharged prior to the titration study. Ten patients had a successful initial PAP titration, 2 required a second titration study and 2 were treated with autotitrating CPAP after the initial failed attempt. PAP titration significantly improved the median RDI to 0.9 events/hour (0.0-9.1), $p < 0.001$. All 14 patients who underwent a PAP titration study were started on PAP therapy during their LTAC stay and tolerated it well, except for 1 patient (RDI 5.9 events/hour) who was not decannulated due to unrelated medical conditions. The one patient who did not have SDB in this series (RDI 4.2 events/hour) was also not decannulated due to other medical conditions. All patients on PAP therapy were discharged on PAP, except for 1 patient transferred to an acute care facility. In total, 17 patients (89%) in this series were decannulated or remained decannulated. Regarding disposition, 10 patients were discharged home, 4 patients were transferred to an acute hospital, 3 patients went to another rehabilitation facility and 2 patients were discharged back to their previous nursing home [6].

While not directly treating diagnosed SDB, several groups have shown the feasibility and usefulness of using NIV with a capped tracheostomy in place to transition from MV to NIV and facilitate tracheostomy decannulation in patients with PMV. In a multicenter prospective study conducted in respiratory care units which included 231 chronically ill patients with PMV, weaning was performed with progressively longer SBTs. NIV was added when the duration of SBT could not be increased > 18 hours and use of this technique lead to successful PMV weaning in 40 patients. The transition to NIV occurred using a nasal or oronasal mask, and either with a tracheal button or a capped tracheostomy with a deflated cuff and a fenestrated inner cannula. When NIV was tolerated with effective ventilation the tracheostomy tube was removed. Of note, in the patients who required NIV to successfully wean, the proportion with a prior history of OSA and prior home CPAP/NIV use was higher compared to those who did not require NIV to wean [10].

CONCLUSION

There is an increasing number of patients with chronic critical illness and PMV with associated increased health care burdens and poor long-term outcomes. SDB is very frequent in the general population but it has been studied rarely in the PMV population. Based on a limited number of available studies, it has been demonstrated that there is a high prevalence of undiagnosed SDB, mostly OSA and sleep-related hypoxemia in patients with PMV. There is almost no data on measurements of nocturnal hypoventilation in these patients (e.g., transcutaneous or end-tidal CO_2) which would provide additional useful diagnostic information. PSG is the most comprehensive testing modality for these patients, but simpler testing such as polygraphy and nocturnal oximetry may also provide useful information. While used more broadly in the pediatric PMV population, sleep studies as part of weaning and a standardized decannulation protocol may be significantly underutilized in adults. The usefulness of incorporation evaluation for SDB in the PMV population requires more extensive study.

KEY POINTS

- There is an increasing number of patients with chronic critical illness and prolonged mechanical ventilation with associated increased health care burden and poor long-term outcomes
- The prevalence of sleep-disordered breathing is high in patients weaned from prolonged mechanical ventilation
- Sleep studies, including polysomnography, polygraphy and overnight oximetry may be useful tools to diagnose sleep-disordered breathing in this population and to facilitate ventilator weaning and tracheostomy decannulation
- Further study is needed to determine the impact of the diagnosis and treatment of sleep-disordered breathing in the short and long-term outcomes of the prolonged mechanical ventilation population

REFERENCES

[1] Ambrosino N., Vitacca M. "The patient needing prolonged mechanical ventilation: a narrative review." *Multidiscip Respir Med* 13, no.6 (2009) Published online 2018 Feb 26. doi: 10.1186/s40248-018-0118-7.

[2] Scheinhorn D. J., Hassenpflug M. S., Votto J. J., Chao D. C., Epstein S. K., Doig G. S., Knight E. B., Petrak R. "Ventilation Outcomes Study Group. Post-ICU

mechanical ventilation at 23 long-term care hospitals: a multicenter outcomes study." *Chest* 131, no.1 (2007):85-93. doi: 10.1378/chest.06-1081.

[3] Kapur V. K., Auckley D. H., Chowdhuri S., Kuhlmann D. C., Mehra R., Ramar K., Harrod C. G. "Clinical practice guideline for diagnostic testing for adult obstructive sleep apnea: an American Academy of Sleep Medicine clinical practice guideline." *J Clin Sleep Med* 13, no.3 (2017):479-504. Published online 2017 Mar 15. doi: 10.5664/jcsm.6506.

[4] Chishti A., Batchelor A. M., Bullock R. E., Fulton B., Gascoigne A. D., Baudouin S. V. "Sleep-related breathing disorders following discharge from intensive care." *Intensive Care Med* 26, no.4 (2000):426-33.

[5] Huttmann S. E., Wilms K., Hamm C., Magnet F. S., Windisch W., Storre J. H. "Assessment of Sleep in Patients Receiving Invasive Mechanical Ventilation in a Specialized Weaning Unit." *Lung* 195, no.3 (2017):361-369. doi: 10.1007/s00408-017-9988-2. Epub 2017 Mar 3.

[6] Diaz-Abad M., Verceles A. C., Brown J. E., Scharf S. M. "Sleep-disordered breathing may be under-recognized in patients who wean from prolonged mechanical ventilation." *Respir Care* 57, no.2 (2012):229-237. doi: 10.4187/respcare.01260. Epub 2011 Jul 12.

[7] Bashir A., Henningfeld J. K., Thompson N. E., D'Andrea L. A. "Polysomnography Provides Useful Clinical Information in the Liberation from Respiratory Technology: A Retrospective Review." *Pediatr Pulmonol* 53, no.11 (2018):1549-1558. doi: 10.1002/ppul.24164. Epub 2018 Sep 24.

[8] Sharma S., Mather P. J., Efird J. T., Kahn D., Shiue K. Y., Cheema M., Malloy R., Quan S. F. "Obstructive sleep apnea in obese hospitalized patients: a single center experience." *J Clin Sleep Med* 11, no.7 (2015):717-723. doi: 10.5664/jcsm.4842.

[9] Đanić D., Mrzljak Vučinić N., Đanić Hadžibegović A. "Obstructive sleep apnoea as a late complication after tracheostomy." *J Laryngol Otol* 133, no.7 (2019):632-635. doi: 10.1017/S0022215119001166. Epub 2019 Jun 14.

[10] Sancho J., Servera E., Jara-Palomares L., Barrot E., Sanchez-Oro-Gómez R., Gómez de Terreros F. J., Martín-Vicente M. J., Utrabo I., Núñez M. B., Binimelis A., Sala E., Zamora E., Segrelles G., Ortega-Gonzalez A., Masa F. "Noninvasive ventilation during the weaning process in chronically critically ill patients." *ERJ Open Res*. 28, no. 2(4) (2016). doi: 10.1183/23120541.00061-2016.

In: Sleep Medicine in Critical Care
Editors: Antonio M. Esquinas et al.
ISBN: 978-1-53617-768-8

Chapter 23

THE ROLE OF TRACHEOSTOMY IN SHORT- AND LONG-TERM MECHANICAL VENTILATION: IMPLICATIONS AND EFFECTS

Michalis Agrafiotis**[*]**, ***Anastassia Athanassiadou and Marianna Moysseos***
Department of Pulmonary Medicine, "Georgios Papanikolaou"
General Hospital of Thessaloniki, Exohi, Greece

ABSTRACT

Invasive mechanical ventilation via a tracheostomy tube (tracheostomy ventilation, TV) should be considered for critically ill patients with prolonged weaning course and for those with advanced chronic respiratory failure (e.g., patients with neuromuscular diseases, NMDs). Tracheostomy can be performed either with a surgical procedure or with various percutaneous dilatory procedures, the last being increasingly used in intensive care units (ICUs). In ICU patients early tracheostomy may expedite weaning and reduce sedation duration as well as the incidence of ventilator-associated pneumonia, although it is doubtful if it can also decrease mortality. Implementation of TV in patients with advanced chronic respiratory failure (commonly patients with NMDs) may lead to increased survival in some patients (e.g., younger patients with amyotrophic lateral sclerosis) although its effects on their health-related quality of life is unclear. TV in patients with chronic respiratory failure is associated with increased nursing requirements and caregiver burden.

Keywords: tracheostomy, weaning, amyotrophic lateral sclerosis, Duchenne muscular dystrophy, sedation

[*] Corresponding Author's E-mail: m.agrafiotis@gmail.com.

INTRODUCTION

Tracheostomy is a commonly performed procedure aiming at bypassing the vocal cords and the upper airway by establishing an artificial airway through a surgically created stoma (opening) in the cervical trachea. The stoma is maintained by insertion of an artificial tube through it. The main indications for a tracheostomy are: 1) upper airway obstruction (e.g., tumor, foreign body, trauma/surgery, infection) 2) provision of long-term mechanical ventilation (MV) post-critical illness or in cases of advanced chronic respiratory failure (commonly patients with neuromuscular diseases, NMDs) and 3) secretion clearance [1–3].

Advances in the management of critical illness and chronic respiratory failure (especially in patients with neuromuscular diseases, NMDs) have led to an increasing number of patients considered nowadays "ventilator-dependent". Tracheostomy ventilation (TV) should be considered in critically ill patients with prolonged weaning from MV and for those with reversible NMDs (e.g., Guillain Barre syndrome) [4]. Patients with chronic respiratory failure, particularly those with NMDs, are also candidates for TV, especially at advanced disease stages [4, 5]. In both cases, however, apart from providing an airway for the delivery of the required ventilatory dose, tracheostomy also facilitates secretion clearance.

There are several techniques for performing a tracheostomy although these can be generally categorized into two groups: the "open" or "surgical" technique (ST) and the various "percutaneous" or "percutaneous dilatory" techniques (PDT) which have become lately very popular in intensive care units (ICUs). These approaches differ in several aspects and have been compared in various clinical trials and systematic reviews. A recent systematic review of randomized controlled trials (RCTs) comparing ST against PDT in critically ill patients identified 24 papers for a total of 1795 procedures (ST 869; PDT 926). Overall no significant risk difference (RD) was observed in the rate of life-threatening complications and in mortality; however, PDT was associated with a significantly higher risk for technical difficulties (RD 0.04) and a lower risk for stoma infection (RD -0.05) [6]. Likewise, in a synthesis of data from comparative randomized and non-randomized studies (29 studies, 5473 subjects), no difference was observed between ST and PDT in the risk for tracheal stenosis and major bleeding; however, the risk for wound infection was higher for ST as compared to the Ciaglia PDT [7]. Last, by synthesizing data from randomized and quasi-randomized controlled trials (20 papers, 1652 subjects) Brass et al. observed no difference in the procedure-related mortality rates and in the risk for intraoperative and postoperative life-threatening adverse events; PDT lowered the risk for wound infection by 76% and the risk for unfavorable scaring by 75% but no significant difference was observed in the rates of major bleeding, tube occlusion, accidental decannulation and difficulty in tube exchange; however, the overall quality of evidence was poor [8].

TRACHEOSTOMY IN CRITICALLY ILL PATIENTS

Acute respiratory failure necessitating invasive MV is very common and among ICU patients who require invasive MV for >48 hours, 34% will need tracheostomy to accommodate prolonged ventilation needs [9]. Several advantages of tracheostomy in critically ill patients have been proposed, including improved patient comfort and safety, lower work of breathing, less need for sedation, improved oral care and hygiene, facilitation of oral intake and improved long term laryngeal function. Importantly, some experts have speculated that earlier tracheostomy might lead to faster weaning from MV, lower mortality and morbidity, lower rates of pneumonia and shorter ICU and hospital stay; however, controversy exists regarding the definition of "early" tracheostomy timing and the patient groups who might benefit from it [2, 4, 10, 11]. On the other hand, tracheostomy procedures are not without complications such as bleeding, pneumothorax, airway injuries, stomal infection, scarring and swallowing disorders [12].

A randomized controlled trial (RCT) recruited adult critically ill patients from 12 Italian medical and surgical ICUs to compare the effects of early vs. late tracheostomy on clinical outcomes. Forty-eight hours after enrollment, patients with worsening respiratory failure, but no pneumonia (Clinical Pulmonary Infection Score, CPIS < 6) were randomized to early tracheostomy (6-8 days after intubation; n = 209) vs. late tracheostomy (13-15 days after intubation; n = 210); all procedures were percutaneous, and the rate of ventilator-associated pneumonia (VAP) at 28 days was the primary outcome [13]. No significant difference in VAP incidence was observed between the early and the late tracheostomy group (14 vs. 21%, respectively). The number of ventilator-free were significantly higher in the early tracheostomy group (11 vs. 6) and significantly more patients were successfully weaned in the early tracheostomy as opposed to the late tracheostomy group (77 vs. 68%, respectively); however survival at 28 days was not different between the two groups (74 vs. 68%, respectively). Based on data from 292 patients who were discharged from hospital alive (144 from the early and 148 from the late group) no significant difference was noted at the 1-year survival rate (50% vs. 43%, respectively). In addition, no difference was noted in the rates of perioperative and postoperative events between the two groups; stomal inflammation was the most common adverse event and occurred equally between the two groups (15%). The authors concluded that early tracheostomy is not associated with a lower incidence of VAP although it may improve the number of ventilator-free and ICU-free days and weaning outcomes; however the study was criticized for using CPIS for the diagnosis of VAP [10, 13].

Trouillet et al. conducted a single-center prospective RCT to investigate whether early tracheostomy is associated with improved outcomes in cardiac surgical patients requiring prolonged respiratory support [14]. Patients remaining on MV 4 days after surgery were randomized to early tracheostomy (before day 5; n = 107) or prolonged intubation (n = 109); all tracheostomies were performed with the Ciaglia PDT and eventually 27% of the patients in the prolonged intubation group also underwent tracheostomies because of requirements for prolonged respiratory support. No difference was observed between the early tracheostomy and the prolonged intubation group in the average number of the ventilator-free days at 60 days which was the primary study outcome (30.4 vs. 28.3 days, respectively). In addition, no difference was noted between the two groups in the number of ventilator-free days at 28 and 90 days, the mortality rates, the durations of ICU and hospital stay, the rates of VAP, stomal, sternal and bloodstream infections and the percentages of patients receiving catecholamines or antibiotics. Patients in the early tracheostomy group had significantly lower rates of unscheduled extubation/decannulation (3 vs. 16%, respectively), reintubation/ recannulation (16 vs. 33%, respectively) and use of noninvasive ventilation (10 vs. 25%, respectively). Importantly, patients in the early tracheostomy group had a significantly lower number of days in intravenous sedation (6.4 vs. 9.6 days) and more sedation-free days within the first 4 weeks (19 vs. 15.5 days, respectively). No differences were observed in health-related quality of life (HRQL) and in long-term survival for a median follow-up of 2 years [14].

Zheng et al. conducted a prospective single-center RCT to investigate the effects of early tracheostomy on the outcomes of surgical patients [15]. Patients were randomized to early tracheostomy (at day 3; n = 58) or late tracheostomy (day 15, if still required; n = 61). All procedures were percutaneous, and the number of ventilator-free days at 28 days was the primary outcome variable. This study observed a significantly higher number of ventilator-free days for the early as opposed to the late group (9.57 vs. 7.38, respectively). In addition, sedation-free and ICU-free days were also significantly increased in the early as opposed to the late group (20.8 vs. 17.1 days and 8 vs. 3 days, respectively). Patients in the early group had significantly higher rates of successful weaning and ICU discharge when compared to the late tracheostomy group (74.1 vs. 55.7% and 67.2 vs. 47.5%, respectively) and lower rates of VAP (29.3% vs. 49.2%, respectively). However, no difference was noted between the two groups in the cumulative mortality rates at 60 days [15].

Bosel et al. randomized patients with ischemic or hemorrhagic stroke and an expected ventilation of at least 2 weeks to early tracheostomy (<3 days; n = 60) or late tracheostomy (between day 7 and 14, if not extubated earlier; n = 60) [16]. The length of ICU stay was the primary study endpoint, and all patients underwent percutaneous procedures. This study observed no difference in the median number of days of ICU stay between the early and late group (17 vs. 18 days, respectively). On the other hand, patients in the early group had significant lower ICU and 6-month mortality as compared to the late group (3 vs. 14% and 26 vs. 60%, respectively) and reduced use of sedatives (62 vs. 42% of ICU stay, respectively) [16].

The TracMan trial was a multicenter RCT that recruited 909 mechanically ventilated adult patients from 70 general and 2 cardiothoracic ICUs in the United Kingdom. Patients were recruited within the first 4 days of MV, if the treating physician considered them likely to require at least 7 additional days of MV and were subsequently randomized to early (<4 days; n = 455) or late tracheostomy (>10 days if tracheostomy was still indicated; n = 454) [17]. Finally, 91.9% of patients from the early tracheostomy group, but only 45.5% of patients from the late tracheostomy group underwent the procedure; all-cause mortality at 30 days post-randomization was the primary study outcome and 90% of the procedures were percutaneous. The 30-day all-cause mortality did not differ between the early and the late tracheostomy group (30.8 vs. 31.5%, respectively); no differences were also noted in the total duration of respiratory support (13.6 vs. 15.2 days, respectively), the median duration of ICU stay (13 vs. 13.1 days, respectively) and the 2-year survival rates (51 vs. 53.7%, respectively); however, the median number of days on which sedatives were given was significantly smaller for the early group (5 vs. 8 days, respectively). The incidence of procedural complications did not differ between the early and the late group (5.5 vs. 7.8%, respectively), with bleeding being the most common (3.1 vs. 3.9%, respectively). This study did not investigate the role of tracheostomy timing on VAP incidence although the percentages of antibiotic use did not differ between the two groups. The main finding of this study was that early tracheostomy does not improve clinically relevant outcomes [17].

Siempos et al. performed a systematic review and meta-analysis of randomized and quasi-randomized controlled trials comparing early vs. late or no tracheostomy (prolonged intubation) in critically ill patients [18]. A tracheostomy procedure was considered "late" if it was performed at least 1 week after MV initiation. All-cause ICU mortality and VAP incidence were the two primary outcomes assessed by the authors. This review identified 15 relevant articles, of which 13 provided mortality data for a total of 2434 participants; data for VAP incidence were also available from 13 trials (1599 participants); both surgical and percutaneous techniques were used. Overall, this review demonstrated that all-cause ICU mortality did not differ between the early and the late or no tracheostomy group (25 vs. 28%, respectively). On the other hand, VAP incidence was significantly lower in the early tracheostomy group as opposed to the late or no tracheostomy group (38.7% vs. 47.5%, respectively). These results persisted when sensitivity analyses were carried out using only trials with a low risk of bias. The rates of periprocedural complications did not differ between the two groups. Post-hoc data analyses also indicated that early tracheostomy is associated with a shorter length of ICU stay (mean difference 9.1 days) and a shorter MV duration (mean difference 3.6 days) but did not improve the length of hospital stay, the duration of sedation, long-term disability and 1-year mortality [18]. On the other hand, a more recent systematic review and meta-analysis, which defined early tracheostomy as a procedure performed ≤10 days after translaryngeal intubation, synthesized data from 9 RCTs for a total of 2040 subjects. This review demonstrated no difference between the early and the late group in mortality rates, duration of MV and length of ICU stay; nevertheless, early tracheostomy was associated with a significantly shorter duration of sedative use (weighted mean difference 6 days) [19].

Two other meta-analyses have focused on brain-injured and trauma patients. McCredie et al. synthesized data from 10 randomized and quasi-randomized trials for a total of 503 brain-injured patients [20]. Early tracheostomy (<10 days) was associated with a significantly lower duration of MV (average difference 2.7 days) and length of ICU stay (average difference 2.6 days), but did not improve short-term mortality; long-term mortality was significantly improved (risk ratio, RR 0.57), but this result did not persist in sensitivity analysis [20]. Cai et al. also synthesized data from 6 RCTs and 14 non-RCTs involving 7751 trauma patients [21]. Early tracheostomy (<7 days) was associated with a lower risk for pneumonia (RR 0.83), although mortality rates were not influenced by tracheostomy timing (11.5 vs. 11.6%, respectively); however, early tracheostomy was associated with significantly lower length of hospital and ICU stay (mean difference 1.2 days and 3.1 days, respectively) and a shorter duration of MV (mean difference 2.9 days) [21].

The accumulated data indicate that early tracheostomy may expedite weaning, reduce sedation requirement and probably decrease the incidence of VAP although it may not be associated with a lower mortality. Further large-scale studies and trials targeting specific populations, e.g., trauma or neurosurgical patients, are warranted to clarify the effects of the early tracheostomy strategy on various outcomes.

Tracheostomy in Patients with Chronic Respiratory Failure

Several NMDs (e.g., Duchenne muscular dystrophy, DMD; amyotrophic lateral sclerosis, ALS) are characterized by a progressive decline in respiratory muscle strength necessitating initiation of noninvasive positive pressure ventilation (NIV) during sleep hours. However, as the disease progresses, the ventilator-free breathing time is significantly reduced and ventilatory needs extend into the daytime. In a addition, progressive respiratory muscle weakness is associated with impaired cough and failure to clear secretions from the airways. Thus, at advanced disease stages, when ventilator use is extended beyond 16-20 hours per day and/or when peak cough flow (PCF) is <160 L/min several practitioners and patients/caregivers would consider TV as a therapeutic option [5]. According to the Eurovent study, which surveyed home mechanical ventilation practices in 16 European countries for >20000 users between 2001 and 2002, patients with NMDs were more likely to require prolonged ventilatory support (≥6 years) and to sustain tracheostomy procedures [22]. Importantly, the transition to invasive ventilation via tracheostomy might also be an option for unweanable ICU patients with chronic respiratory failure (e.g., chronic obstructive pulmonary disease, COPD) [4]. However, the use of invasive tracheostomy tubes has been associated with several shortcomings such as voice loss, disturbed self-image, airway injuries and increased requirements for chronic care [5]. In addition, the decision for transition to invasive ventilation via tracheostomy can be influenced by various factors including practitioner's and caregiver's attitudes, patient sex, country, model of care funding and presence of spouse or marital status [23].

Toussaint et al. also reported data from 42 end-stage DMD patients with chronic respiratory failure treated with mouthpiece ventilation (MPV) for a follow-up period of 7 years; their survival rates at 1, 3, 5 and 7 years were 88, 57, 58 and 51%, respectively, which were higher compared to historical controls treated with TV [24]. By comparing TV (n = 16) to MPV (n = 26) in DMD over a 5 year follow-up period, Soudon et al. observed a 50% mortality for tracheostomized patients vs. 38.5% for patients treated noninvasively. Causes of death did not roughly differ between the two groups, however 63% of patients managed with TV sustained severe complications including tracheal injury, mucus hypersecretion and chest infections; on the other hand, weight loss and requirement for enteral feeding were more common in MPV users [25]. In addition, according to data from a prospective cohort of 150 DMD patients treated with MV, swallowing disorders and cardiac disease, but not TV were associated with a higher risk of death [26].

By prospectively analyzing a database of 1260 ALS patients, of whom 134 (10.6%) underwent tracheostomy, Chio et al. observed a <1 year (253 days) median survival, with only 42.6% of the patients being alive at the first year [27]. Sancho et al. also followed 116 ALS patients over a 9-year period; during this period, 76 patients had an indication of tracheostomy and 38 (50%) agreed to the procedure. The 1-year survival rate of patients with an indication of tracheostomy was 78.9% for a total mean survival of 10.4 months; patients who refused tracheostomy had a significantly worse survival (0.83 months) [28]. In a retrospective review of 60 tracheostomized ALS patients, median post-tracheostomy survival was 21 months, with 65% of the patients being alive at the 1st year [29]. In a retrospective study of 431 Dutch ALS patients from a single-center, patients who were initially treated with NIV before transitioning to TV had significantly better survival (1734 days) as compared to those treated exclusively by TV (1031 days), those who received NIV only (788 days) and those who received no treatment (699 days). The 1-year survival rate was 83%, for patients on NIV/TV, 80% for TV, 73% for NIV and 68% for no treatment [30]. Similarly, based on a retrospective study of 160 Japanese ALS patients, of whom 52 (32.5%) underwent tracheostomy, median survival was higher for patients on TV (74 months), as opposed to patients on NIV (48 months) and non-ventilated patients (32 months); however, the survival benefit from TV was more clear in younger patients (<65 years old) [31]. Likewise, according to data from a prospective Italian study of 279 ALS patients, of whom 87 (31%) underwent tracheostomy, median survival was significantly better in tracheostomized patients (47 months) as opposed to non-tracheostomized patients (31 months), but this advantage was lost in patients >60 years old [32]. Similarly, in the study by Vianello et al. median survival after tracheostomy was significantly shorter in patients >60 years old (hazard ratio, HR 16.5) as opposed to younger patients (HR 32.5) [29].

How TV may affect patient and caregiver quality of life has also been extensively investigated. According to an earlier survey which interrogated 168 ventilatory-dependent patients with at least 1-month experience in both NIV and tracheostomy ventilation (TV), noninvasive management was considered more convenient and more preferable in terms of speech, appearance and comfort [33]. By studying a mixed population of patients treated with TV (n = 77), Marchese et al. reported that survival in patients with NMDs was significantly higher as compared to patients with pulmonary and thoracic wall diseases. In addition, the majority of patients (83%) were satisfied with TV and would choose it again (90%) as a life-sustaining option. On the other hand, only 55% of the caregivers (including all caregivers who were parents of the patient) were satisfied with the patient's choice and would encourage them to choose TV again, while 38% reported that having to care for a patient on TV was stressful and affected significantly their lifestyle [34]. In another study investigating HRQL in patients who had sustained tracheostomy following unsuccessful weaning (32 with lung disease; 14 with NMDs) HRQL, as assessed by the Severe Respiratory Insufficiency Questionnaire (SRI) varied greatly across different individuals; however, patients with NMDs had higher nursing requirements and significantly better SRI scores compared to patients with lung diseases (58 vs. 48); the site of care (home vs. chronic care facility) did not influence HRQL [35]. Based on data from 25 unweanable patients on TV (11 with NMDs; 14 with COPD), the same group reported that 42.9% of COPD patients and 18.2% of NMD patients would not choose tracheostomy again "in hindsight" even if the alternative was death. In addition, 85.7% of COPD patients and 45.5% of NMD patients were unsatisfied by their mobility, and the majority of the patients (84%) required technical aids for communication [36]. In a retrospective study by Vianello et al., Beck Depression Inventory (BDI) scores were obtained from 13 tracheostomized ALS patients and a moderate-to-severe level of depression was observed for the entire group (mean BDI 19.2) [29]. When these patients were compared to 14 controls, no differences were observed in BDI and short-form Life Satisfaction Index-11 (LSI-11) scores; 11 out of the 13 patients were satisfied with their treatment and said they would choose it again [29]. By using the Profile of Mood States (POMS) and the Munich Quality of Life Dimensions List (MLDL) a German study investigated patient and primary caregiver quality-of-life (QOL) in a group of ALS patients under NIV (n = 32) and TV(n = 21) [37]. Overall, no difference in POMS and MLDL scores was observed between the NIV and TV groups for both patients and caregivers. Importantly, 94% of the NIV patients and 80% of the TV patients would choose ventilation again as a treatment and would advise other patients to do so; on the other hand, 97% of the NIV caregivers but only 75% of the TV caregivers would advise a patient to choose ventilation again. Similarly, 94% of the NIV caregivers but only 50% of the TV caregivers would opt for ventilation if they had to make the decision for themselves. Interestingly, when asked directly, 30% of TV caregivers considered their QOL worse than that of the patient they cared for [37]. On the other hand, by comparing TV (n = 16) against MPV (n = 16) in patients with ALS, Nicolini et al. demonstrated similar improvements in life expectancy for both groups; however, the TV group displayed great improvements in arterial blood gases while the MPV group greater improvements in HRQL scores [38].

To conclude tracheostomy in NMDs (and other patients with chronic respiratory failure) may improve survival in some cases (for instance, younger patients with ALS) but the evidence is controversial regarding its effects on HRQL. However, the caregiver burden and nursing requirements are increased.

Key Points

- The main indications for tracheostomy are upper airway obstruction, requirement for prolonged MV and secretion removal.
- Critically ill patients and patients with chronic respiratory failure (especially those with NMDs) are the most common candidates for TV.
- The surgical and the various percutaneous tracheostomy techniques do not differ in terms of mortality and percentages of life-threatening complications. However, the latter are preferred for critically ill patients.
- Early tracheostomy in critically ill patients may improve weaning outcomes, decrease sedation use and possibly reduce the incidence of VAP although it is unclear if it can reduce mortality.
- In patients with progressive NMDs (and other causes of chronic respiratory failure) tracheostomy may improve survival, but its effects on HRQL are unclear. However, caregivers of tracheostomy patients commonly complain of burden overload and reduced QOL.

References

[1] Durbin, CG. Indications for and timing of tracheostomy. *Respir Care*, 2005, 50(4), 483–7.

[2] Durbin, CG. Tracheostomy: why, when, and how. *Respir Care*, 2010, 55(8), 1056–68.

[3] Mitchell, RB; Hussey, HM; Setzen, G; et al., Clinical consensus statement: tracheostomy care. *Otolaryngol Head Neck Surg*, 2013, 148(1), 6–20.

[4] Trouillet, JL; Collange, O; Belafia, F; et al., Tracheotomy in the intensive care unit: guidelines from a French expert panel: the French Intensive Care Society and the French Society of Anaesthesia and Intensive Care Medicine. *Anaesthesia Critical Care & Pain Medicine*, 2018, 37(3), 281–94.

[5] Agrafiotis, M; Nikolaou, K; Siopi, D; et al. (November 5th 2018). Open-circuit mouthpiece ventilation: indications, evidence and practicalities. In: *Noninvasive ventilation in medicine - recent updates* (Mayank Vats eds). IntechOpen, DOI: 10.5772/intechopen.73243. Available from: https: //www.intechopen.com/books/ noninvasive-ventilation-in-medicine-recent-updates/open-circuit-mouthpiece-ventilation-indications-evidence-and-practicalities.

[6] Klotz, R; Probst, P; Deininger, M; et al., Percutaneous versus surgical strategy for tracheostomy: a systematic review and meta-analysis of perioperative and postoperative complications. *Langenbecks Arch Surg*, 2018, 403(2), 137–49.

[7] Dempsey, GA; Morton, B; Hammell, C; et al., Long-Term Outcome Following Tracheostomy in Critical Care: A Systematic Review. *Crit Care Med*, 2016, 44(3), 617–28.

[8] Brass, P; Hellmich, M; Ladra, A; et al., Percutaneous techniques versus surgical techniques for tracheostomy. *Cochrane Database Syst Rev*, 2016, 7, CD008045.

[9] Quality, OLAMVITESI, 2-month mortality and functional status of critically ill adult patients receiving prolonged mechanical ventilation. *Chest*, 2002, 121(2), 549–58.

[10] Cheung, NH; Napolitano, LM. Tracheostomy: epidemiology, indications, timing, technique, and outcomes. *Respir Care*, 2014, 59(6), 895–915, discussion 916.

[11] Groves, DS; Durbin, CG. Tracheostomy in the critically ill: indications, timing and techniques. *Curr Opin Crit Care*, 2007, 13(1), 90–7.

[12] François, B; Clavel, M; Desachy, A; et al., Complications of tracheostomy performed in the ICU: subthyroid tracheostomy vs surgical cricothyroidotomy. *Chest*, 2003, 123(1), 151–8.

[13] Terragni, PP; Antonelli, M; Fumagalli, R; et al., Early vs late tracheotomy for prevention of pneumonia in mechanically ventilated adult ICU patients: a randomized controlled trial. *JAMA*, 2010, 303(15), 1483–9.

[14] Trouillet, JL; Luyt, CE; Guiguet, M; et al., Early percutaneous tracheotomy versus prolonged intubation of mechanically ventilated patients after cardiac surgery: a randomized trial. *Ann Intern Med*, 2011, 154(6), 373–83.

[15] Zheng, Y; Sui, F; Chen, XK; et al., Early versus late percutaneous dilational tracheostomy in critically ill patients anticipated requiring prolonged mechanical ventilation. *Chin Med J (Engl)*, 2012, 125(11), 1925–30.

[16] Bösel, J; Schiller, P; Hook, Y; et al., Stroke-related Early Tracheostomy versus Prolonged Orotracheal Intubation in Neurocritical Care Trial (SETPOINT): a randomized pilot trial. *Stroke*, 2013, 44(1), 21–8.

[17] Young, D; Harrison, DA; Cuthbertson, BH; et al., Effect of early vs late tracheostomy placement on survival in patients receiving mechanical ventilation: the TracMan randomized trial. *JAMA*, 2013, 309(20), 2121–9.

[18] Siempos, II; Ntaidou, TK; Filippidis, FT; et al., Effect of early versus late or no tracheostomy on mortality and pneumonia of critically ill patients receiving mechanical ventilation: a systematic review and meta-analysis. *Lancet Respir Med*, 2015, 3(2), 150–8.

[19] Meng, L; Wang, C; Li, J; et al., Early vs late tracheostomy in critically ill patients: a systematic review and meta-analysis. *Clin Respir J*, 2016, 10(6), 684–92.

[20] McCredie, VA; Alali, AS; Scales, DC; et al., Effect of Early Versus Late Tracheostomy or Prolonged Intubation in Critically Ill Patients with Acute Brain Injury: A Systematic Review and Meta-Analysis. *Neurocrit Care*, 2017, 26(1), 14–25.

[21] Cai, SQ; Hu, JW; Liu, D; et al., The influence of tracheostomy timing on outcomes in trauma patients: A meta-analysis. *Injury*, 2017, 48(4), 866–73.

[22] Lloyd-Owen, SJ; Donaldson, GC; Ambrosino, N; et al., Patterns of home mechanical ventilation use in Europe: results from the Eurovent survey. *Eur Respir J*, 2005, 25(6), 1025–31.

[23] Turner, MR; Faull, C; McDermott, CJ; et al., Tracheostomy in motor neurone disease. *Pract Neurol*, 2019, 19(6), 467–75.

[24] Toussaint, M; Steens, M; Wasteels, G; et al., Diurnal ventilation via mouthpiece: survival in end-stage Duchenne patients. *Eur Respir J*, 2006, 28(3), 549–55.

[25] Soudon, P; Steens, M; Toussaint, M. A comparison of invasive versus noninvasive full-time mechanical ventilation in Duchenne muscular dystrophy. *Chron Respir Dis*, 2008, 5(2), 87–93.

[26] Boussaïd, G; Lofaso, F; Santos, DB; et al., Impact of invasive ventilation on survival when non-invasive ventilation is ineffective in patients with Duchenne muscular dystrophy: A prospective cohort. *Respir Med*, 2016, 115, 26–32.

[27] Chiò, A; Calvo, A; Ghiglione, P; et al., Tracheostomy in amyotrophic lateral sclerosis: a 10-year population-based study in Italy. *J Neurol Neurosurg Psychiatry*, 2010, 81(10), 1141–3.

[28] Sancho, J; Servera, E; Díaz, JL; et al., Home tracheotomy mechanical ventilation in patients with amyotrophic lateral sclerosis: causes, complications and 1-year survival. *Thorax*, 2011, 66(11), 948–52.

[29] Vianello, A; Arcaro, G; Palmieri, A; et al., Survival and quality of life after tracheostomy for acute respiratory failure in patients with amyotrophic lateral sclerosis. *J Crit Care*, 2011, 26(3), 329.e7–14.

[30] Dreyer, P; Lorenzen, CK; Schou, L; et al., Survival in ALS with home mechanical ventilation non-invasively and invasively: a 15-year cohort study in west Denmark. *Amyotroph Lateral Scler Frontotemporal Degener*, 2014, 15(1-2), 62–7.

[31] Tagami, M; Kimura, F; Nakajima, H; et al., Tracheostomy and invasive ventilation in Japanese ALS patients: decision-making and survival analysis: 1990-2010. *J Neurol Sci*, 2014, 344(1-2), 158–64.

[32] Spataro, R; Bono, V; Marchese; S et al., Tracheostomy mechanical ventilation in patients with amyotrophic lateral sclerosis: clinical features and survival analysis. *J Neurol Sci*, 2012, 323(1-2), 66–70.

[33] Bach, JR. A comparison of long-term ventilatory support alternatives from the perspective of the patient and care giver. *Chest*, 1993, 104(6), 1702–6.

[34] Marchese, S; Lo Coco, D; Lo Coco, A. Outcome and attitudes toward home tracheostomy ventilation of consecutive patients: a 10-year experience. *Respir Med*, 2008, 102(3), 430–6.

[35] Huttmann, SE; Windisch, W; Storre, JH. Invasive home mechanical ventilation: living conditions and health-related quality of life. *Respiration*, 2015, 89(4), 312–21.

[36] Huttmann, SE; Magnet, FS; Karagiannidis, C; et al., Quality of life and life satisfaction are severely impaired in patients with long-term invasive ventilation following ICU treatment and unsuccessful weaning. *Ann Intensive Care*, 2018, 8(1), 38.

[37] Kaub-Wittemer, D; Steinbüchel, N; Wasner, M; et al., Quality of life and psychosocial issues in ventilated patients with amyotrophic lateral sclerosis and their caregivers. *J Pain Symptom Manage*, 2003, 26(4), 890–6.

[38] Nicolini, A; Parrinello, L; Grecchi, B; et al., Diurnal mouthpiece ventilation and nocturnal non-invasive ventilation versus tracheostomy invasive ventilation in patients with amyotrophic lateral sclerosis. *Panminerva Med*, 2019, May 30. doi: 10.23736/S0031-0808.19.03644-9.

In: Sleep Medicine in Critical Care
Editors: Antonio M. Esquinas et al.
ISBN: 978-1-53617-768-8

Chapter 24

SLEEP DISORDERED BREATHING DISORDERS: IMPLICATIONS FOR PATIENT, FAMILY, PHYSICIANS AND OTHER CAREGIVERS

Rexford Muza*[*], *MD
Sleep Disorders Centre, Guy's Hospital, Great Maze Pond, London, UK

ABSTRACT

Sleep disordered breathing disorders and in particular obstructive sleep apnoea, are very common. In fact obstructive sleep apnoea is now one of the commoner chronic respiratory condition. This condition has significant and serious implications on the health outcomes of affected individuals. It also has negative social consequences. As most adults with obstructive sleep apnoea share a bed with their partners or spouses, it will directly affect them during the night and it will also have a bearing on their overall wellbeing. The effects of sleep disordered breathing disordered will further cascade down to the family and society. The burden of sleep disordered breathing disorders is huge and going forwards specialist clinics are unlikely to be able to cope with health demands of the affected individuals. A joint collaborative approach with primary care might be needed.

INTRODUCTION

Sleep disordered breathing disorders are quite prevalent in our modern societies. Physicians and patients alike are now increasingly aware of them. The number of patients

[*] Corresponding Author: Sleep and Respiratory Physician, MbChB, MMED MED, MRCP, FRCP, ESRS certified somnonologist. E-mail: Rexford.Muza@gstt.nhs.uk.

presenting to sleep clinics with symptoms related to sleep disordered breathing is increasing in parallel with the obesity epidemic. The categories of sleep disordered breathing include obstructive sleep apnoea, central sleep apnoea, sleep related hypoventilation syndromes and sleep related hypoxaemia disorders (Table 1). Of these disorders, the commonest one is obstructive sleep apnoea (OSA). Obstructive sleep apnoea is characterized by intermittent episodes of pharyngeal collapse and airflow interruption leading to intermittent episodes of oxygen desaturation and increased respiratory effort. This leads to repeated arousals and sleep fragmentation. Over the past few decades our understanding of sleep disordered breathing disorders and their associated co-morbidities has expanded hugely. Obstructive sleep apnoea is now one of the commoner chronic respiratory conditions which has important social consequences as well as very significant adverse health outcomes in the affected individuals. Sleep disordered breathing disorders negatively impact on the patient's health and wellbeing. As a good number of adults have bed partners, symptoms relating to their condition such as noisy breathing and fidgetiness can be quite disruptive to their partners. Treatments which may involve a positive airway pressure device, albeit helpful, might be a further intrusion into the partners' life. This chapter will mostly address obstructive sleep apnoea with occasional mentioning of other sleep disordered breathing disorders.

Table 1. Sleep-related hypoventilation disorders

Obstructive sleep apnoea (OSA)
Central sleep apnoea (CSA) syndromes
Sleep-related hypoventilation disorders
Sleep-related hypoxaemia disorder

IMPLICATION OF SLEEP DISORDERED BREATHING DISORDERS ON THE PATIENT

Health Implications of Obstructive Sleep Apnoea for the Patient

Sleep disordered breathing disorders are associated with quite significant symptomatology. Symptoms of obstructive sleep apnoea can be quite debilitating for the patient (Table 2). Central sleep apnoea can also be quite symptomatic. Symptoms of central will depend on the type (Table 3).

Sleep disordered breathing disorders, and in particular obstructive sleep apnoea, are associated with quite a number of clinically very significant long term health consequences including cardiovascular conditions such as hypertension, atrial fibrillation, coronary heart disease, heart failure as well as stroke (Shahar, et al., 2001). The patient is therefore not only saddled with the OSA and its symptoms but will also have to deal with the symptoms and consequences of its comorbid conditions (Figure1). Clinical outcomes in patients with the obesity hypoventilation syndrome are also very poor.

Table 2. Common symptoms of Obstructive Sleep Apnoea

Snoring
Spousal/partner observed apnoeas
Gasping or choking during sleep
Excessive daytime sleepiness
Daytime fatigue
Insomnia/fragmented sleep
Restlessness in sleep
Non-restorative sleep
Morning headaches
Poor concentration levels/mental fog
Memory impairment
Irritability/mood changes
Nocturia

Table 3. Central Sleep Apnoea Syndromes

Eucapnic/Hypocapnic	**Hypercapnic**
• Primary CSA • Cheyne Stokes Respiration • CSA due to Medical disorder (no CSR) • CSA due to High Altitude Periodic Breathing • Treatment Emergent CSA (Complex Sleep Apnoea) • CAs dues to medication or substance use/abuse	• Central Drive Abnormalities • Neuromuscular Disorders • Chest Wall Disorders

Night sleep can be disrupted by the choking episodes leading to sleep maintenance insomnia. The sleep disordered breathing can also act as a driver of other parasomnias. Physical effects include restlessness, excessive sweating at night, dryness of the mouth on waking and morning headaches. Daytime functionality is compromised by the excessive sleepiness, fatigue and poor concentration levels/ brain fog.

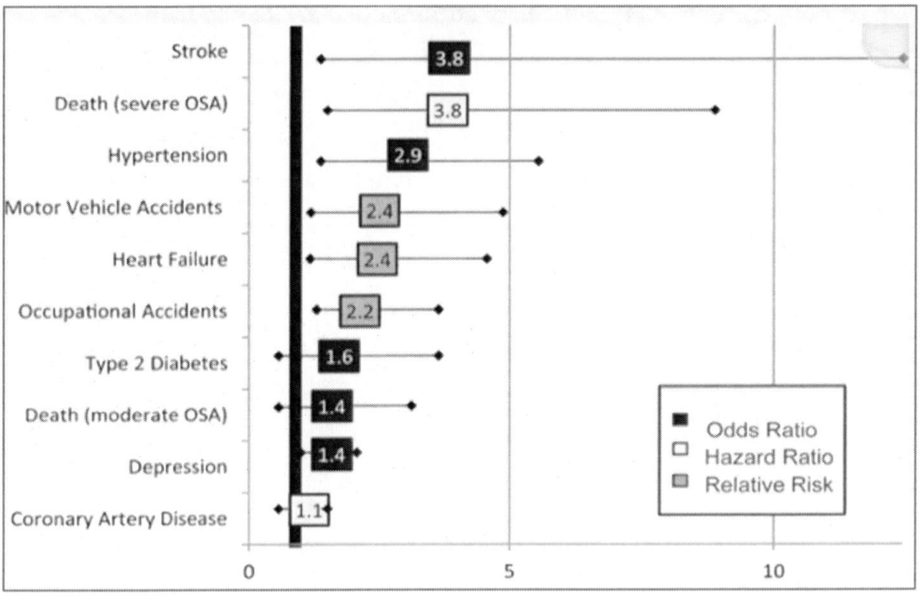

Figure 1. Adverse outcomes associated with obstructive sleep apnoea – From Knauert et al. (Knauert M, 2015).

Obstructive Sleep Apnoea and Hypertension

In healthy individuals blood pressure normally decreases during sleep. Absence of this phenomenon (non-dipping) is known to be associated with significant cardiovascular risk (Boggia, 2007; Eguchi, 2009; Ohkubo, 2002). This non dipping phenomena is found in patients with obstructive sleep apnoea. Numerous studies have now demonstrated that obstructive sleep apnoea is an independent risk factor for hypertension (Young, et al., 2008; Peppard, et al., 2000; Nieto, et al., 2000; Lavie & Hoffstein, 2000; Davis, et al., 2000). In hypertension clinics and sleep clinics it is now well recognized that a significant number of patients with hypertension have obstructive sleep apnoea. The aetiology of systemic hypertension in obstructive sleep apnoea patients has been debated quite extensively. Sympathetic over activation has been suggested as a possible mechanistic factor. Way back in the mid-1980s, in the pre-CPAP (Continuous Positive Airway Pressure) era, Fletcher and co-workers measured urinary catecholamines in 8 subjects with severe symptomatic sleep apnoea as well as hypertension before and after tracheostomy (Fletcher, et al., 1987). Interestingly following tracheostomy, catecholamines in these 8 patients returned to control levels. Similar findings were also reported by other workers (Jennum, et al., 1989; Lapinski, et al., 1993; Marrone, et al., 1993; Dimsdale, et al., 1995). Subsequently similar findings were reported in the CPAP era (Ziegler, et al., 2001). Thirty eight patients with obstructive sleep apnoea were prospectively treated with either nasal CPAP or placebo CPAP. Both plasma and urinary catecholamine levels fell by nearly 50% in the CPAP group while remaining at baseline in the placebo group. Back in the late 1980s' Hedner and colleagues demonstrated that apnoea related hypoxia and hypercapnia was associated with increased muscle sympathetic nerve activity (Hedner, et al., 1988). It was subsequently shown that the sympathetic traffic was elevated during daytime wakefulness in patients with obstructive sleep apnoea (Carlson, et al., 1993).

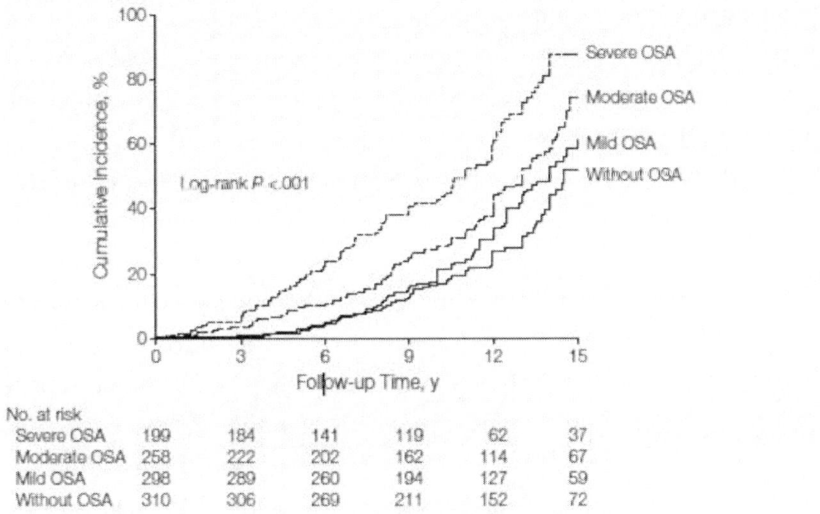

OSA indicates obstructive sleep apnea. Severity of OSA was defined by the apnea-hypopnea index (AHI) as mild OSA (AHI, 5.0-14.9), moderate OSA (AHI, 15.0-29.9), and severe OSA (AHI, ≥30.0). *P* value reflects an overall log-rank χ^2_3 test, providing an overall survival difference among the 4 study groups.

Figure 2. Cumulative Incidence of Hypertension In Participants Without OSA and Untreated Patients With OSA. (Figure from Marin et al.)

Narkiewicz and colleagues (Narkiewicz, et al., 1999) demonstrated that nocturnal CPAP decreased daytime sympathetic traffic in patients with obstructive sleep apnoea. In addition to the central nervous system facilitation leading to the sustained blood pressure there also seems to be other reasons for the increased vascular reactivity and hence the increased vascular tone (Carlson, et al., 1996; Duchna, et al., 2000). Carlson et al. demonstrated this increased vascular resistance in patients with obstructive sleep apnoea; a diminished responsiveness to the vasodilator effect of acetylcholine in individuals with obstructive sleep apnoea was demonstrated. Marin and colleagues elegantly demonstrated the cumulative incidence of hypertension in individuals with untreated OSA compared to individuals without OSA (Figure 2) (Marin, et al., 2012). In patients with treatment resistant hypertension it is important to exclude obstructive sleep apnoea as a contributory factor (Gonçalves, et al., 2007).

Obstructive Sleep Apnoea and Atrial Fibrillation

Obstructive sleep apnoea and atrial fibrillation (AF) are two fairly common conditions, particularly in the aging population. It has been reported that in patients with OSA, the prevalence of AF is up to 5%, (Mehra, et al., 2006). On the other hand the prevalence of OSA in patients diagnosed with AF has been put at 32% to 39%. (Albuquerque FN, 2012; Bitter T, 2009; Gami AS, 2004). The AF might possibly be induced by the repetitive sympathetic surges as well as the OSA associated hypertension and perhaps to some extent the structural remodeling of the atria. The structural remodeling of the cardiac chambers in patients with OSA might be due to the exaggerated intrathoracic pressure swings (Orban M, 2008; Camen G, 2013). Alterations in the sympathetic as well as the parasympathetic regulations has been described in OSA patients (Leung, 2009). Intermittent hypoxia results in sympathetic system surges, but this is unlikely to be the only contributory mechanism to the AF (May AM, 2017). Recognition of OSA can be quite important in the management of treatment refractory AF. The ORBIT–AF (Outcomes Registry for Better Informed Treatment of Atrial Fibrillation), looked at over a 10 000 patients with AF, and noted that those with co-morbid OSA had significantly more severe AF symptoms and were more likely to be on a rhythm control agent. Patients with AF and co-morbid OSA were at an increased risk of recurrent AF following an incident episode (Holmqvist F, 2015) and had worse outcomes following catheter ablation (Kanagala R, 2003; Naruse Y, 2013; Ng CY, 2011). OSA is associated with other arrhythmias such as pauses and bradycardia (Simantirakis EN, 2004), higher incidence of ventricular arrhythmias (Simantirakis EN, 2004) and also an increased risk of sudden death (Mehra, et al., 2006).

Obstructive Sleep Apnoea and Heart Failure

Sleep apnoea, and in particular central sleep apnoea, is quite common in patients with heart failure (Oldenburg, et al., 2007; Oldenburg & Teerlink, 2015; Lafranchi, et al., 2003). In patients with heart failure, the presence of sleep apnoea is associated with an increased risk of adverse outcomes, including an increased risk of mortality. The poorer outcomes could well be due to the recurrent activation of the sympathetic nervous system following apnoeas (Gami AS, 2004), as well as the intrathoracic pressure swings which may increase preload and afterload (Bradley, et al., 2001). Additionally sleep apnoea also worsens systemic hypertension (Logan, et al., 2003), increases the risk of arrhythmias including sudden death and also increases the risk of coronary events (Perker, et al., J). The CANPAP (Canadian Continuous Positive Airway Pressure for Patients with Central Sleep Apnoea and Heart Failure) which investigated the effect of CPAP treatment in patients with heart failure and central sleep apnoea showed no benefit from CPAP therapy although the post hoc analysis suggested a reduction in mortality in the "responders" in whom CPAP therapy resulted in a significant improvement of the apnoea hypopnea index (AHI) (Bradley, et al., 2005). The SERVE-HF (Treatment of Sleep-Disordered Breathing with Predominant Central Sleep Apnoea by Adaptive Servo Ventilation in Patients with Heart Failure) using adaptive servo ventilation (ASV) failed to demonstrate any survival benefit from this form of therapy, and in fact showed an increase in cardiovascular mortality (Cowie, et al., 2015)

Obstructive Sleep Apnoea and Ischaemic Heart Disease

Patients with obstructive sleep apnoea are at increased risk of ischaemic heart disease (Peppard, et al., 2000; Gottlieb, et al., 2010). The presumed mechanism behind this includes the increased sympathetic activity, oxidative stress as well as endothelial dysfunction (Patt, et al., 2010; Phillips, et al., 2004). The predilection for hypertension in patients with OSA patients is another contributory mechanism as is their pro-coagulant state (Phillips, et al., 2004) as well as the metabolic dysregulation (Ip, et al., 2002; Botros, et al., 2009). Table 4 summarizes the proposed mechanisms contributory to an increased incidence of ischaemic heart disease in patients with OSA.

Table 4. Mechanisms which promote Ischaemic Heart Disease in OSA

Increased sympathetic drive
Oxidative stress
Increased predilection for hypertension
Endothelial Dysfunction
Pro-coagulant state
Metabolic dysregulation

Obstructive Sleep Apnoea and Pulmonary Hypertension

Pulmonary hypertension is present in 10-20% of patients with obstructive sleep apnoea (MInai, et al., 2009). Hypoxia as well as hypercapnia can acutely cause pulmonary arteriolar vasoconstriction. Chronic hypoxia will lead to pulmonary vascular remodeling, subsequently leading to established irreversible pulmonary hypertension. The pulmonary hypertension secondary to OSA tends to be mild but the presence of the sleep apnoea in patients with severe pulmonary hypertension is associated with an increased mortality (Yamakawa, et al., 2002).

Obstructive Sleep Apnoea and Stroke

Unsurprisingly OSA is also associated with an increased incidence of cerebrovascular disease (Redline, et al., 2010). The same mechanisms which are behind increased coronary artery disease as described above do apply for cerebrovascular disease. Lipford and co-workers explored the relationship between OSA and stroke (Lipford, et al., 2015). They found out that those with OSA had a 4–6 fold higher odds of cardio-embolic stroke compared to those without OSA after taking into account relevant variables individually in statistical models. Specifically, after taking into account AF, there was a 4.5-fold higher odds of cardio-embolic stroke in OSA versus those with a lower apnoea hypopnea index (AHI). Although a greater degree of hypoxia was observed in those with cardio-embolic strokes compared to other stroke subtypes, the relationship was not statistically significant. They concluded that there is a strong magnitude of association of OSA and cardio-embolic stroke relative to other stroke subtypes and that this relationship may not be appreciably confounded by AF. A few other mechanisms are at play in the causation of stroke in patients with sleep apnoea .Several other studies have also confirmed the relationship between OSA and increased stroke risk. It is now appreciated that multiple factors work in concert to increase the risk of stroke in patients with sleep apnoea (Figure 3).

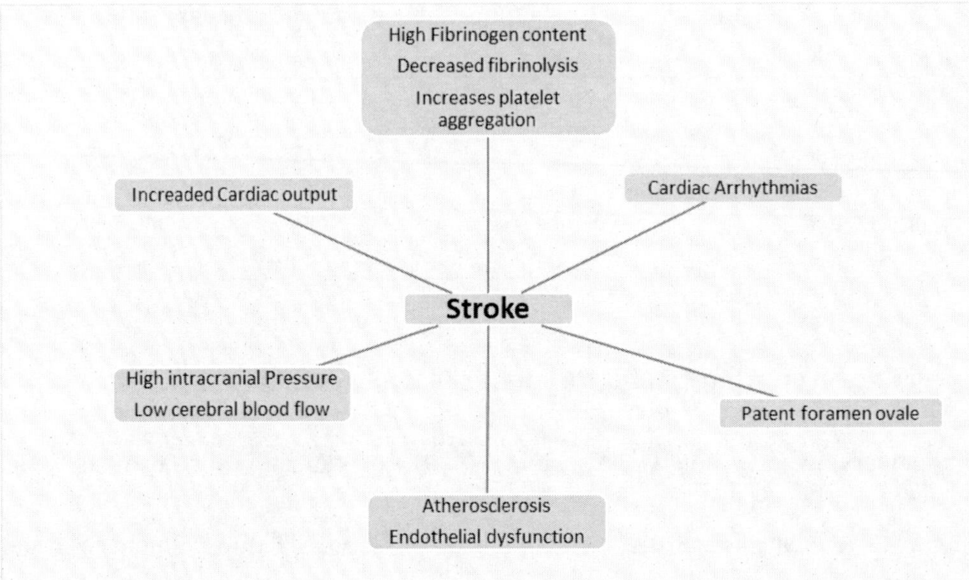

Figure 3. Factors leading to stroke in patients with sleep apnoea Adapted from Yaggi and Mohsenin Lancet Neurol 2004

Obstructive Sleep Apnoea and Diabetes

Patients with OSA are also at an increased risk of diabetes (Botros, et al., 2009). In fact the relationship between OSA and type 2 diabetes seems to be bidirectional (Framnes & Arble, 2018). Worldwide the incidence of both OSA and diabetes is increasing. A number of cross sectional studies have demonstrated an independent association between the severity of OSA and insulin resistance. Reutrakul and Mokhlesi (Reutrakul & Mokhlesi, 2017) proposed multiple mechanistic pathways which may be contributory to the development of diabetes in patients with OSA which include intermittent hypoxia, sleep fragmentation, sleep restriction, oxidative stress, systemic inflammation, activation of the HPA axis and alteration of circulating adipokines (Figure 2). This leads to β-cell activation and insulin resistance and ultimately type 2 diabetes. Untreated OSA has been shown to be associated with poorer glycaemic control in type 2 diabetes.

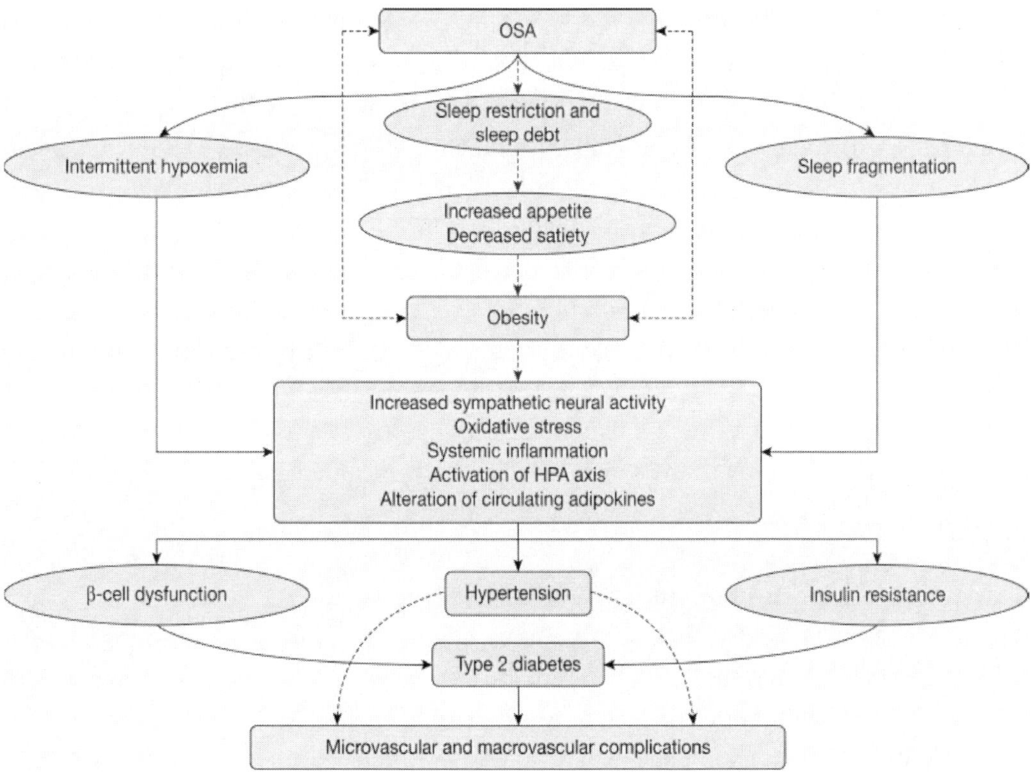

Figure 4. OSA and Diabetes. HPA = hypothalamic-pituitary –axis (Image from Reutrakul and Mokhlesi).

Obstructive Sleep Apnoea and the Liver

Non-alcoholic fatty liver disease (NAFLD) affects an estimated 25% of the global population, with prevalence increasing up to 75% in populations with obesity (Estes, et al., 2018). NAFLD can be defined as simple hepatic steatosis, or non-alcoholic steatohepatitis (NASH), which is a potentially progressive process that includes fibrosis. NASH is associated with the consequent risks of cirrhosis and hepatocellular carcinoma, and is the fastest growing indication for liver transplant, again likely associated with the increasing prevalence of obesity (Mishra & Younossi, 2012). In the past decade there has been a good number of publications that have associated the severity of OSA with the development of NAFLD. Prevalence estimates of NAFLD in OSA range from 60-99% (Kallwitz, et al., 2007; Qi, et al., 2016). NASH estimates are more conservative at 27-44%, (Jullian-Desayes, et al., 2016). In 2005 Tanne´ et al. studied 163 subjects with suspected OSA through liver function tests (LFTs) as well as liver biopsy (Tanne', et al., 2005). They concluded that severe OSA was independently associated with elevated LFTs, insulin resistance, liver necrosis, and fibrosis. In 2007 Joue and colleagues (Joue, et al., 2007) also concluded that OSA was an independent risk factor for elevated LFTs but not for NASH. In the same year Kallwitz and co-workers also showed a link between OSA and elevated LFTs (ALT). In a study involving 200 subjects undergoing bariatric surgery by Campos et al., previously diagnosed OSA was associated with a fourfold increased risk for the presence of NASH (Campos, et al., 2008). Further studies also confirmed the link between the severity of OSA hypoxic burden and the development of NASH(Mishra, et al., 2008; Polotsky, et al., 2009; Utitsky, et al., 2010; Aron-Wisnewsky, et al., 2012; Pulixi, et al., 2014; Agrawal, et al., 2015). The same mechanistic pathway of intermittent hypoxia, oxidative stress, mitochondrial dysfunction, inflammation and activation of the sympathetic nervous system is believed to be at play.

Obstructive Sleep Apnoea and the Metabolic Syndrome

The metabolic syndrome, which is comprised of visceral obesity, dyslipidaemia, hyperglycaemia, and hypertension is now one of the major public-health challenges worldwide. It is often found in patients with OSA (Aurora RN, 2013; Parish JM, 2007). It is now well accepted that OSA is an independent risk factor for the development of the metabolic disorders. Having OSA increases risk of having the metabolic syndrome and its various components; (Pamidi S, 2012) and with increasing OSA severity, the number of metabolic syndrome features increases independently of body mass index (Peled N, 2007).

Obstructive Sleep Apnoea and the Kidney

Table 5. Author / Subjects Diagnostic method/sleep apnoea threshold Main Findings

(Millman RP, 1985)	29 males on haemodialysis	Polysomnography	41% with sleep apnoea symptoms
(Kimmel PL, 1989)	26 patients with ESRD	Polysomnography Disordered breathing events > 30 per session	Sleep apnoea symptomatic group (22): sleep apnoea found in 7% Sleep apnoea asymptomatic group: None had sleep apnoea
(Nicholl DD, 2012)	254 patients (nephrology clinic)	Ambulatory sleep recorder Respiratory disturbance index >15	Sleep apnoea, predominantly OSA in (eGFR >60 mUmin) group (55): 27% Sleep apnoea in CKD (eGFR < 60 mUmin, not on dialysis) group(124): 41%) Sleep apnoea in ESRD on haemodialysis group (75): 57% (p = 0.002) Nocturnal hypoxia found in 50% of CKD and ESRD (P < 0.001)
(Markou N, 2006)	35 dialysis independent CKD patients	Polysomnography AHI > 5	Sleep apnoea, mainly obstructive found in 54.3% In non-diabetic subjects, AHI correlated with Urea (r = 0.608. p = 0.001) Creatinine (r = -0.50, p = 0'012)
(Sakaguchi Y, 2011)	100 dialysis independent CKD patients	Type 3 portable monitor AHI > 5	OSA found in 65% Multivariate variate logistic regression analysis: A decrease of 10mUmin/1.73m² in eGFR associated with 42% increase in odds of the likelihood of OSA (p = 0.02)

The relationship between obstructive sleep apnoea and the kidney is an interesting one and is likely to be bi-directional. There are studies which have shown the increased prevalence of sleep disordered breathing in patients with chronic kidney disease (Table 5) and on the other hand there have also been studies which have shown an increased prevalence of CKD in patients with sleep disordered breathing (Table 6). Factors which can contribute to the increased incidence of OSA in patients with end stage renal disease (ESRD) include altered chemo-reflex responsiveness secondary to metabolic acidosis which may lead to respiratory system / breathing instability, pharyngeal narrowing due to pharyngeal wall oedema from fluid overload and possible ureamic myopathy / neuropathy involving the upper airway dilator muscles. It appears like the kidney is not spared from the injurious effects of nocturnal hypoxia associated with sleep disordered breathing. Tubulointerstitial injury is the final common pathway in ESRD (Eckardt KU, 2005; M., 2006). Ahmed and colleagues (Ahmed SB, 2011) showed that compared to control subjects, patients with nocturnal hypoxia were at a significant risk for accelerated kidney function loss but in their study severe OSA was not associated with increased risk of accelerated loss of kidney function using a multivariate adjusted model of logistic regression. As with other organs the pathological mechanisms linked to kidney injury are believed to be related to the nocturnal hypoxia, oxidative stress (DJ., 2000; J., 2001), increased sympathetic tone (Ritz E, 1998; Neumann J, 2004) and a contribution from the OSA associated hypertension.

Table 6. Author/ Subjects Diagnostic method/ sleep apnoea threshold Main Findings

Author	Design	Diagnostic Method/Sleep Apnoea Threshold	Main Findings
(Iseki K, 2008)	Retrospec-tive	Polysomnography AHI ≥5	Prevalence of CKD in the sleep-related breathing disorder: 30.5% Prevalence of CKD in control:b9.1% ($p < 0.001$) Adjusted odds ratio:n4.542($p < 0.0001$) AHI is not a significant determinant for CKD in sleep-related breathing disorder patients
(Agrawal V, 2009)	Cross-sectional	Polysomnography AHI ≥5	Serum creatinine in control group: 0.8mg/dl Serum creatinine in OSA group: 0.9 mg/Dl ($p = 0.013$) No major difference in albuminuria between groups
(Kanbay A, 2012)	Cross-sectional Retrospec-tive	Polysomnography AHI ≥5	Mean eGFR in negative group: 50mL/min Mean eGFR in mild OSA (AHI+5-15):44.8Ml/min Mean eGFR in moderate OSA (AHI = 15-30): 40.8mL/min Mean eGFR in severe OSA (AHI > 30): 38.8mL/min $p < 0.001$ for trend

OSA AND MORTALITY

There has been a number of studies which have demonstrated an increased mortality risk in patients with OSA both generally and more specifically from cardiovascular causes (Young T, 2008). The increased OSA-associated mortality was more apparent in individuals under the age of 50 (Lavie P, 2005).

OBSTRUCTIVE SLEEP APNOEA AND SEXUAL FUNCTION

Reduced sexual drive and erectile dysfunction is common in patients with sleep apnoea. Way back in 1990, Hirshkowitz et al. (Hirshkowitz M, 1990) reported that 43.8%

of patients with erectile dysfunction had an apnoea index ≥5/hr. Since then a number of studies have shown an association between sleep apnoea and erectile dysfunction (Hoyos CM, 2015; Teloken PE, 2006; Margel D, 2004; Heruti R, 2005; Goncalves MA, 2005; Budweiser S, 2009; Zias N, 2009). In a long-term nationwide population-based cohort study in Taiwan (Chia-Min Chen, 2015) the incident rate of erectile dysfunction was significantly higher in probable sleep apnoea patients as compared with the corresponding control subjects. Patients with OSA also frequently complain of sexual dysfunction (Hirshkowitz M, 1990; Margel D, 2004). A prevalence study analyzing 1025 males with erectile dysfunction showed that 91% of these individuals had at least mild OSA (Hirshkowitz M, 1990). Sexual dysfunction may contribute to the emotional distress (Shiri R, 2007), problems in sexual relationship and impaired quality of life experienced by some patients with OSA (Martin-Morales A, 2007).

Obstructive Sleep Apnoea and Mood Disorder/ Neuropsychiatric Disorders

Depressive symptoms seem to be common in people with obstructive sleep apnoea (Kendzerska T, 2017). In an early study, Kales and colleagues reported on high levels of psychological distress in 50 patients with severe OSA (Kales A, 1985). Their view was that the depression was a consequence rather than a cause of the OSA. The patients' reported symptoms mostly focused on their physical vulnerability. Subsequent to that a few other studies demonstrated the higher incidence of depression in the OSA groups compared to controls even after controlling for obesity (Harris M, 2009; Basta M, 2008; Peppard PE, 2006; Chen YH, 2013; Chen YH, 2013). In some series the prevalence of depression in patients with OSA ranged from 20 to about 40%. In a study with a large sample size (>1000), and over a long follow up period (~10 years), Kendzerska and colleagues demonstrated that OSA and its measures, such as the apnoea hypopnea index, were not related to the risk of hospitalization for depression.

Worryingly, the features cognitive deficits and vigilance impairment in patients with OSA are similar to those of patients with central nervous system organic damage (Bawden FC, 2011; Stranks EK, 2016). These include verbal performance, attention, memory, learning, psychomotor coordination, and other executive functions

Obstructive Sleep Apnoea and Perioperative Risk

There has been a number of studies which have repeatedly shown that OSA is associated with poor peri-operative outcomes. Table 7 lists some of the commoner OSA associated postoperative complications. Patients with OSA are at an increased risk of emergent intubation; absolute increases of 3 - 5% were reported across a variety of surgery types (Memtsoudis S, 2011; Mokhlesi B, 2013).

Table 7. Obstructive Sleep Apnoea Associated Postoperative Complications

Respiratory Failure
Re-intubation
Intensive care unit transfer
Aspiration Pneumonia
Myocardial infarction
Cardiac death
Atrial Fibrillation
Poor wound healing
Prolonged length of hospital stay
Stroke

Furthermore, rates of aspiration pneumonia and atrial fibrillation were also increased in patients with OSA. In studies were polysomnography was used to confirm the diagnosis of OSA, the OSA was associated with more than a doubling of the risk of respiratory failure, re-intubation, intensive care unit transfer and a one day increase in length of hospital stay (Kaw R, 2012). OSA and obesity hypoventilation syndrome (OHS) related respiratory compromise is worsened by post-operative sedation, opiate analgesia as well as the supine position. In a report by Abdelsatter et al. (Abdelsattar ZM, 2015), the adjusted odds ratio for any cardiopulmonary complication in treated versus untreated OSA was 1.8 (95% CI 1.3-2.7, $p < 0.001$), with most of the difference accounted for by post-operative myocardial infarction and re-intubation (Abdelsattar ZM, 2015). Unfortunately the study had some methodological issues which limited its generalizability. In a more recent study by Matthew at al (Matthew, et al., 2019) they demonstrated that among the at-risk individuals undergoing major non-cardiac surgery, unrecognized severe OSA was significantly associated with increased risk of 30-day postoperative cardiovascular complications (Figure 5).

To minimize risk of perioperative complications it therefore good clinical practice to screen the at risk patients for OSA before anaesthesia. This undoubtedly has costs implications. Furthermore, individuals with OSA/OHS are likely to have delays/cancellation of their surgical procedures while awaiting commencement of appropriate OSA therapy.

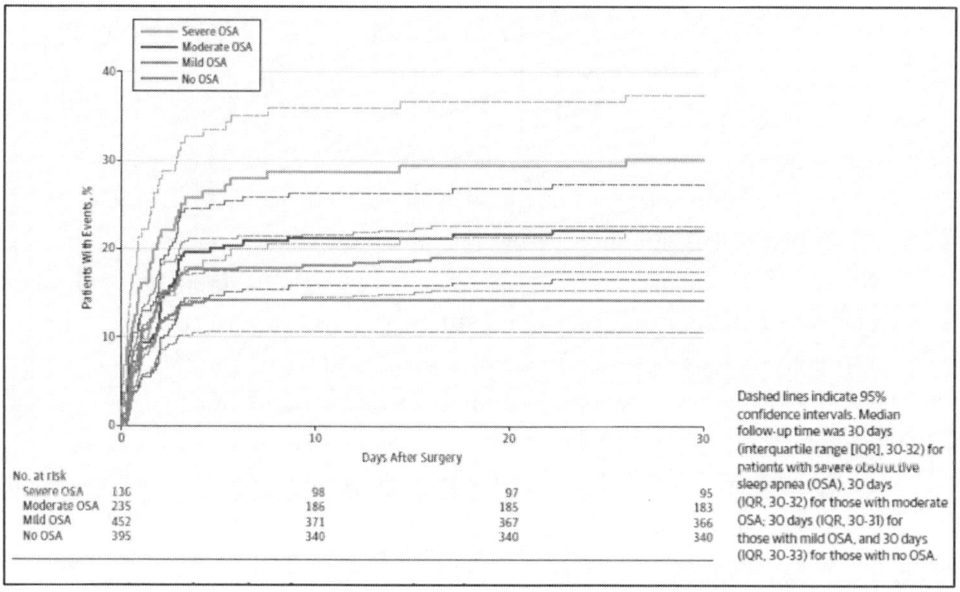

Figure 5. Kaplan-Meier Estimates of the Primary Composite Outcome (Death, Myocardial Injury, Congestive Heart Failure, Thromboembolism, New Atrial Fibrillation, and Stroke at 30 Days After Surgery). Adapted from Matthew et al.

Social Implications of Obstructive Sleep Apnoea on the Patient

Symptoms of OSA (Table 1) do not only affect the patient, but also affect their partners and family. In fact the patient might not be aware of some of the symptoms which are witnessed by their partners such as the loud snoring and the apnoes. Their day time symptoms (Table 8) will impact on their interaction with their families and their work colleagues as well as their social acquaintances.

Table 8. Wake symptoms of obstructive sleep apnoea

Dry mouth on waking
Morning headaches
Sleepiness
Fatigue/anergia
Non-refreshed on waking
Mental fog
Concentration difficulties/decreased attention and vigilance
Psychomotor and executive dysfunction
Poor co-ordination
Poor memory
Altered affect – depressed mood, irritability
Heartburn
Loss of sex drive

Sleep Disordered Breathing and the Work Place

Obstructive sleep apnoea is a common cause of excessive daytime sleepiness and impaired vigilance and concentration levels at the workplace. This may have safety implications at the workplace. Affected individuals are not as productive as their unaffected workmates. It is common to see patients presenting in the sleep clinics after receiving warnings from their supervisors because they would have been found asleep at work. It might be suspected that they are slothful or even on drugs. Sleep disordered breathing disorders such as obstructive sleep apnoea assume more importance in safety critical occupations where utmost levels of vigilance are required all the time such as in the aviation industry, public transportation etc. There has been quite a few major catastrophic events in the work place where sleepiness might have been contributory. Lindberg and colleagues noted that survey respondents reporting both snoring and excessive daytime sleepiness over a ten-year period were at a greater risk for workplace accidents; the odds ratio was 3.1 (1.5–6.4) (Lindberg E., 2001). A limitation of the Lindberg study was that they only categorized subjects based on snoring and daytime sleepiness; polysomnography was not performed to confirm the diagnosis of OSA. In addition, their study was a retrospective study that relied on patient self-reports of errors made. However, it seems reasonable to assume that many of those reporting snoring and excessive daytime sleepiness were reporting symptoms that resulted from OSA. Omachi and colleagues (Omachi T.A., 2009) found that individuals suffering from OSA symptoms and reporting excessive daytime sleepiness, experience a significantly greater risk of workplace disability than those with no OSA and no daytime sleepiness. Another group evaluated the relationship between severity of OSA by polysomnographic measures and sleepiness as well as job satisfaction, in individuals with and without OSA (Guglielmi O., 2014). They found that subjective sleepiness in OSA patients did influence job satisfaction and burnout regardless of OSA severity by polysomnographic parameters. The same group reported in another paper also that absenteeism and productivity were worse among OSA patients (Jurado-Gamez B., 2015). From all the studies published this far, it is clear that OSA is associated with impaired productivity at work and an increased risk of accidents.

OSA and Driving

It is well recognized that obstructive sleep apnoea is related to an increased risk of road traffic accidents (S Tregear, 2009; George, 2007; Karimi, et al., 2013). It has been estimated that individuals with OSA have a tenfold increased risk of road traffic accidents compared to individuals without OSA. The excessive daytime sleepiness and

OSA associated cognitive deficits are contributory to the increased incidence of road traffic accidents (Philip, 2005; Barbe, 1998). In the United Kingdom it is a legal requirement that patients with obstructive sleep apnoea should inform the Driver and Vehicle Licencing Agency (DVLA) of the diagnosis of OSA if they hold a driving licence of any type. The affected individuals will be able to resume driving when they are on appropriate therapy and are no longer sleepy during the day.

OSA AND TRAVELLING

Some planning is needed before travelling. Affected individuals will need to check on availability of power supply to run their positive airway pressure (PAP) machine. Practical considerations such as extra equipment or spares (extension leads, masks and plug adapters) should be taken into account. A covering letter from the sleep clinic explaining the PAP machine is useful for customs and security clearance. If flying, it might also be useful to check with the airline if they are able to provide power for the machine during long haul flights.

IMPLICATIONS OF SLEEP DISORDERED BREATHING DISORDERS ON PARTNERS AND FAMILY

Effect of Untreated OSA on partners

Symptoms of obstructive such as snoring, chocking and gasping are heard/witnessed by their bed partners. It has been reported that partners of patients who snore are three times more likely to experience sleep initiation and sleep maintenance insomnia as well as non-refreshing sleep as compared to the general population (Ulfberg J, 2000). They are also twice as likely to report fatigue and daytime sleepiness compared to the general population. Patients with OSA very frequently come to the sleep clinic at the behest of their partners troubled by their \snoring. In a study involving 37 patients with OSA, Virkkula and colleagues observed that 55% of the partners reported that snoring disturbed their sleep every night or almost every night (Virkkula P, 2005). Disruption of partner's sleep can be from the snoring, the apnoeas, and the restless sleep (McArdle N, 2001). Partners can become quite anxious and alarmed by the patient's apnoeas (Henry D, 2013; Luyster FS, 2016). The frightening apnoeas can be the main reason some partners insist that the patient seeks medical attention. The sleep disruptive effect of OSA symptoms on partners has been well demonstrated polysomnographically (Beninati W, 1999; Sharief I, 2008; Smith AKA, 2009). Partner's sleep statics including sleep latency, sleep stage distribution, sleep efficiency, arousal index, the amount of wake after sleep onset (WASO) and total sleep time (TST) are all affected when sleeping next to an individual with OSA. In one study in which 10 wives of patients with suspected OSA had polysomnography at the same time as their husbands, a reduced sleep efficiency (median sleep efficiency of 74%) and an increased arousal index (arousal index of 21) was demonstrated. Interestingly the altered sleep architecture and sleep statistics can remain even on the night they are not sleeping with the patient. In a study by Smith et al. (Smith AKA, 2009) involving 17 wives who normally shared a bed with husbands with untreated OSA, they recorded an increased amount of wake after sleep onset, a higher percentage of the least restorative stage N1 sleep and increased alpha intrusion into slow wave sleep during an in-laboratory polysomnography without their husbands compared to the wives of individuals without OSA.

Partners of individuals who snore regularly give them the elbow treatment or try and roll them to the side to stop them from snoring. Some resort to earplugs and some use sleeping pills or change their sleep schedule (Luyster FS, 2016). They may also sleep in separate rooms (Henry D, 2013; Luyster FS, 2016; Cartwright RD, 1987). One study showed that spouses of husbands with untreated OSA were 2.9 times more likely to sleep apart from them as compared to wives of men who do not regularly snore (Billmann SJ, 2002). Intrusive snoring can lead to relationship problems and as such should not be dismissed lightly.

Obstructive sleep apnoea affects the affected individual's quality of life as well as the quality of lives of their partners. MacAdle and colleagues (McArdle N, 2001) showed that the general health related quality of life was significantly worse among partners of patients with untreated OSA compared to the general population. Doherty at al (Doherty LS, 2003) also reported similar findings. When they compared the quality of life of 55 partners of patients with OSA prior to CPAP therapy, a significant number of partners reported anxiety symptoms (50%) and depressive symptoms (18%) before CPAP therapy initiation.

Living with a partner who has obstructive sleep apnoea can be quite challenging. In an article aptly titled "Listening for his breath:" Henry and colleagues gave an account of the responses obtained from interviewing spouses living with patients with untreated OSA (Henry D, 2013). Patients with sleep apnoea are often fatigued and not able to contribute as much as they should to the domestic chores. They are also less likely to engage in activities such as watching movies or going out to theatres due to their sleepiness. Affected individuals can easily fall asleep while on holidays and at times even at important functions such as weddings. This can be quite frustrating to partners and families. As obstructive sleep apnoea and other sleep related breathing disorders have significant symptoms as well as multi-morbidity, partners may end up being more like caregivers rather than wives / husbands. Akin to looking after an infant they might be subconsciously on the lookout for their partners while they are asleep especially when concerned about apnoeas. They might end up feeling like a parent rather than a spouse. They might have to take the extra responsibility of instituting and supervising dietary changes and other necessary life style changes. They may feel empathetic towards the patient but equally it is possible they may feel frustrated trapped in a relationship were their night sleep is very much disturbed and daytime functionality is also compromised. In consultations clinicians can sometimes pick up on this frustration by the less than endearing terms they might use to describe their partners' symptoms such " I can't sleep all night because he snores like a wild pig". Furthermore, the sexual relationship can be affected.

In a 2004 population based study, Strawbridge and colleagues looked at the impact of spouses' sleep on partners. Their study revealed poorer physical and mental health, poorer well-being and social involvement as well as poorer marital quality in spouses of OSA sufferers. There is no doubt that OSA has a significant impact on partners' and families' lives.

Effect of OSA Therapies on Partners' Sleep and Daytime Functioning

Generally the introduction of CPAP is well received by partners of patients with OSA. But there is also no doubt that the bedroom dynamics changes with the introduction of the PAP machine. Some partners report sleep disturbances relating to the PAP machine. The leaking and hissing from the machine can be quite disruptive. Sometimes the partners have to wake up and try to reposition the mask. The sleeping arrangement and sleeping position has to be changed to accommodate the CPAP machine. As previously mentioned travelling has to take the CPAP machine into consideration.

CPAP therapy usually has beneficial effects on the quality of sleep of partners of patients with OSA (Luyster FS, 2016; Beninati W, 1999). Siccoli and colleagues reported significant improvements in sleep quality, daytime alertness, mood, quality of life and personal relationships in patients on CPAP who had moderate to severe OSA compared to patients on sham CPAP (Siccoli MM, 2008). Doherty and colleagues assessed 45 partners of patients with OSA treated with CPAP for six weeks and noted less daytime sleepiness, anxiety symptoms and better quality of life in the 36-item short-form health survey (SF36) domains of role-physical, role-emotion, social functioning, mental health, and vitality compared to before CPAP treatment (Doherty LS, 2003). In another study assessing 54 partners of patients with OSA before and after CPAP therapy, it was noted that there was significant improvement in the quality of life as measured by the SF-36 and the sleep apnoea quality of life index (SAQLI) (Parish JM, 2003). There were significant improvements in daytime sleepiness as well as the SAQLI. The role-physical, vitality, social functioning and marital health domains of the SF36 were also improved. CPAP also had a positive effect on partner's depressive symptoms as well as their sexual functioning (Luyster FS, 2016). CPAP might also have a positive impact on marital health but did not seem to improve bed sharing (McFadyen T, 2001).

Oral appliance can usefully reduce snoring and are usually less cumbersome compared to CPAP. Izci and colleagues showed that partners of patients who continued to use their oral appliances had greater improvement in sleep quality as compared to partners of patients who discontinued use of the appliances (Izci B, 2005). Bed sharing was also improved with the use of an oral appliance. In another study involving 121 patients using oral appliances it was noted that 64% of their partners reported an improvement in their sleep after three months of treatment (Bates C, 2006). A positive impact on general well-being, mental energy, sleep quality as well as decreased daytime sleepiness and less disturbed sleep was reported after one year of treatment with an oral appliance (Tegelberg A, 2011).

There has not been many studies looking at the impact of OSA surgical procedures on partners of patients with OSA. In one study there was a significant reduction in anxiety and depressive symptoms among partners of OSA patients treated with radiofrequency tissue ablation.

Table 9. List of problems experienced by partners of patients with OSA

Sleep Initiation and sleep maintenance insomnia
Daytime sleepiness
Reduced bed sharing
Marital dissatisfaction
Reduced sexual functioning
Reduced vitality and day time fatigue
Reduced social involvement
Anxiety
Depressive symptoms
Frustration

Table 10. Partner Domains affected by a patient with SDB

Physical Health
Mental Health
General well being
Social involvement
Marital health

OSA is one of those conditions which is lived with and shared by the patients and their bed partners. The snoring more often than not bothers the bed partner, caregiver or family members more than the patient. Similarly the apnoeas are mostly witnessed by others. The partner's support or lack of it may play a significant role on how patients may accommodate to PAP therapies. Tarasuik and colleagues showed that living with a partner improved acceptance of CPAP therapy amongst OSA patients on average or high income but not amongst low income patients (Tarasiuk A, 2012). Patients with a new diagnosis of OSA who live alone struggle to accommodate to CPAP when compared to those living with a partner (Lewis KE, 2004). During the CPAP initiation process bed sharing with a partner can help improve CPAP uptake (Cartwright, 2008). Those who are married or live with a partner are also more likely to remain complaint with CPAP therapy (Gagnadoux F, 2011). Partner encouragement, positive and collaborative support, can greatly enhance PAP therapy uptake and adherence (Simon-Tuval T, 2009; Cartwright, 2008; Brin YS, 2005; Baron KG, 2011). On the other hand, a critical partner who displays negative emotions does not help PAP therapy uptake (Stålkrantz A, 2012). Positive partner support in the diagnostic process, CPAP education and initiation process greatly facilitates CPAP acceptance and compliance (Broström A, 2010).

Impact of OSA on family

Loud snoring can be domestically quite disruptive. The snoring can keep the whole house awake. In severe cases it can even disturb neighbours. They have even been accounts of snoring even scaring away the domestic pets such as cats. Patients may not participate in family activities as they are too tired or too sleepy. All the negative effects of OSA on the patient will cascade down to the partners and family,

OSA; Implication on Physicians and Care givers

Sleep apnoea is now one of the most prevalent chronic respiratory conditions. We also now have a better understanding of its implication on the patient in relation to adverse outcomes as well as its social implications. There has been a massive increase in reported cases of sleep apnoea in most health care settings but there are still a lot more who are undiagnosed and therefore not on treatment. At the same time, there has been a huge variety of positive airway pressure machines and other non-invasive ventilators which have hit the market. The physicians and the care givers will need to keep abreast of the diagnostic and treatment methods of sleep disordered breathing. The magnitude of the problem means that the specialist clinics are unlikely to be able to cope with the burden alone for much longer. It is therefore imperative that the primary care physicians should regularly undergo appropriate training to enable them to work more fluidly with the specialist units in the management of this public health problem. Caring for the patients with sleep disordered breathing can be challenging if the patient has learning difficulties. In patients with Down's syndrome for instance, sleep apnoea is quite common but patients might struggle to accommodate to it. In such cases care-giver input will be crucial. Similarly patients with some psychiatric conditions might need greater care-giver input.

Conclusion

Amongst other sleep disordered breathing conditions, obstructive sleep apnoea is a very common chronic medical problem which has serious health implications for the affected individual. It also has very important social consequences. Domestic life and interpersonal relationships can be affected by the condition. As such, it has a negative impact on the affected individual, their partners and families. Its management can be quite challenging and costly given its varied clinical associations. Going forward, there will need to be a better collaborative way of managing it amongst care givers.

References

Abdelsattar ZM, Hendren S, Wong SL, Campbell DA Jr, Ramachandran SK. The impact of untreated obstructive sleep apnea on cardiopulmonary complications in general and vascular surgery: a cohort study,. *Sleep,* Volume 38, pp. 1205-10.

Agrawal V, Vanhecke TE, Rai B, Franklin BA, Sangal RB, McCullough PA. Albuminuria and renal function in obese adults evaluated for obstructive sleep apnea. *Nephron Clin Pract.,* Volume 113, pp. c140-7.

Agrawal S1, Duseja A, Aggarwal A, Das A, Mehta M, Dhiman RK, Chawla Y. Obstructive sleep apnoea is an important predictor of hepatic fibrosis in patients with non alcoholic fatty liver disease in a tertiary care center. *Hepatol Int,* Volume 9, pp. 283-291.

Ahmed SB, Ronksley PE, Hemmelgarn BR, Tsai WH, Manns BJ, Tonelli M, Klarenbach SW, Chin R, Clement FM, Hanly JP. Nocturnal Hypoxia and Loss of Kidney Function. *PLoS ONE,* 6(4), p. e19029.

Alberti KG, Eckel RH, Grundy SM, Zimmet PZ, Cleeman JI, Donato KA, Fruchart JC, James WP, Loria CM, Smith SC. Harmonizing the metabolic syndrome: Jr International Diabetes Federation Task Force on Epidemiology and Prevention; Hational Heart, Lung, and Blood Institute; American Heart Association; World Heart Federation; International Atherosclerosis Society; International Association for the Study o. *Circulation,* 120(16), pp. 1640-1645.

Albuquerque FN, Calvin AD, Sert Kuniyoshi FM, Konecny T, Lopez-Jimenez, Pressman GS, Kara T, Friedman P, Ammash N, MD, Somers VK, MD, Caples SM. Sleep-

Disordered Breathing and Excessive Daytime Sleepiness in Patients With Atrial Fibrillation. *Chest,* . 141(4): 967–973

Aron-Wisnewsky J, Minville C, Tordjman J, Lévy P, Bouillot JL, Basdevant A, Bedossa P, Clément K, Pépin JL. Chronic intermittent hypoxia is a major trigger for non-alcoholic fatty liver disease in morbid obese. *J Hepatol,* Volume 56, pp. 225-233.

Aurora RN, Punjabi NM. Obstructive sleep apnoea and type 2 diabetes mellitus: a bidirectional association. *Lancet Respir Med,* Volume 1, pp. 329-338.

Barbé, Pericás J, Muñoz A, Findley L, Antó JM, Agustí AG. Automobile accidents in patients with sleep apnea syndrome. An epidemiological and mechanistic study. *Am. J. Respir. Crit. Care Med.,* 158(1), pp. 18-22.

Baron KG, Smith TW, Berg CA, Czajkowski LA, Gunn H, Jones CR. Spousal involvement in CPAP adherence among patients with obstructive sleep apnea. *Sleep Breath.,* 15(3), pp. 525-534.

Basta M, Lin H, Pejovic S, Sarrigiannidis A, Bixler E, Vgontzas AN. Lack of regular exercise, depression, and degree of apnea are predictors of excessive daytime sleepiness in patients with sleep apnea: sex differences. *J Clin Sleep Med,* Volume 4, pp. 19-25.

Bates CJ, McDonald JP. Patients' and sleeping partners' experience of treatment for sleep-related breathing disorders with a mandibular repositioning splint. *Br Dent J.,* 200(2), pp. 95-101.

Bawden FC, Oliveira CA, Caramelli P. Impact of obstructive sleep apnoea on cognitive performance. *Arq Neuropsiquiatr.,* 69(4), pp. 585-9.

Beninati W, Harris CD, Herold DL, Shepard JW Jr. The effect of snoring and obstructive sleep apnea on the sleep quality of bed partners. *Mayo Clin Proc.,* 74(10), pp. 955-958.

Betteridge DJ. What is oxidative stress?. *Metabolism.,* Volume 49, pp. 3-8.

Billmann SJ, Ware JS. Marital satisfaction of wives of untreated sleep apneic men. *Sleep Med,* 3(1), pp. 55-59.

Bitter T, Langer C, Vogt J, Lange M, Horstkotte D, Oldenburg O. Sleep-disordered breathing in patients with atrial fibrillation and normal systolic left ventricular function. *Dtsch Arztebl Int.,* Volume 106, pp. 164-170.

Boggia J, Li Y, Thijs L, Hansen TW, Kikuya M, Björklund-Bodegård K, Richart T, Ohkubo T, Kuznetsova T, Torp-Pedersen C, Lind L, Ibsen H, Imai Y, Wang J, Sandoya E, O'Brien E, Staessen JA. Prognostic accuracy of day versus night ambulatory blood pressure: a cohort study. *Lancet,* 370(9594), pp. 1219-1229.

Botros N, Concato J, Mohsenin V, Selim B, Doctor K, Yaggi HK. Obstructive sleep apnea as a risk factor for type 2 diabetes. *Am J Med,* Volume 122, pp. 1122-1127.

Bradley TD, Hall MJ, Ando S, Floras JS. 2001. Hemodynamic effects of simulated obstructive heart failure. *Chest,* Volume 119, pp. 1827-1835.

Bradley TD, Logan AG, Kimoff RJ, Sériès F, Morrison D, Ferguson K, Belenkie I, Pfeifer M, Fleetham J, Hanly P, Smilovitch M, Tomlinson, CANPAP Investigators. Continous positive airway pressure for central sleep apnea and heart failure. *N Engl J Med,* Volume 353, pp. 2025-2033.

Brin YS, Reuveni H, Greenberg S, Tal A, Tarasiuk A. Determinants affecting initiation of continuous positive airway pressure treatment. *Isr Med Assoc J.,* 7(1), pp. 13-18.

Broström A, Nilsen P, Johansson P, Ulander M, Strömberg A, Svanborg E, Fridlund B. Putative facilitators and barriers for adherence to CPAP treatment in patients with obstructive sleep apnea syndrome: a qualitative content analysis. *Sleep Med.,* 11(2), pp. 126-130.

Budweiser S, Enderlein S, Jörres RA, Hitzl AP, Wieland WF, Pfeifer M, Arzt M. Sleep apnea is an independent correlate of erectile and sexual dysfunction. *J Sex Med,* 6(11), pp. 3147-57.

Camen G, Clarenbach CF, Sto¨whas A, Rossi VA, Sievi NA, Stradling JR, Kohler M. The effects of simulated obstructive apnea and hypopnea on arrhythmic potential in healthy subjects. *Eur J Appl Physiol.,* Volume 113, pp. 489-496.

Campos GM, Bambha K, Vittinghoff E, Rabl C, Posselt AM, Ciovica R, Tiwari U, Ferrel L, Pabst M, Bass NM, Merriman RB. A clinical scoring system for predicting nonalcoholic steatohepatitis in morbidly abese patients. *Hepatology,* Volume 47, pp. 1916-1923.

Carlson JT, Hedner J, Elam M, Ejnell H, Sellgren J, Wallin BG. Augmented resting sympathetic activity in awake patients with obstructive sleep apnea. *Chest,* Volume 103, pp. 1763-68.

Carlson JT, Rangemark C, Hedner JA. Attenuated endothelium-dependent vascular relaxation in patients with sleep apnoea. *J Hypertension,* Volume 14, pp. 577-584.

Cartwright RD, Knight S. Silent partners: the wives of sleep apneic patients. *Sleep,* 10(3), pp. 244-248.

Cartwright, R. Sleeping together: a pilot study of the effects of shared sleeping on adherence to CPAP treatment in obstructive sleep apnea. *J Clin Sleep Med.,* 4(2), pp. 123-127.

Chan MTV, Wang CY, Seet E, Tam S, Lai HY, Chew EFF, Wu WKK, Cheng BCP, Lam CKM, Short TG, Hui DSC, Chung F. Association of Unrecognised Obstructive Sleep Apnoea With Postoperative Cardivascular Events in PatientsUndergoing MajorNoncardiac Surgery. *JAMA,* 321(18), pp. 1788-1798.

Chen YH, Keller JK, Kang JH, Hsieh HJ, Lin HC. Obstructive sleep apnea and the subsequent risk of depressive disorder: a population-based follow-up study. *J Clin Sleep Med,* Volume 9, pp. 417-423.

Chen CM, Tsai MJ, Wei PJ, Su YC, Yang CJ, Wu MN, Hsu CY, Hwang SJ, Chong IW, Huang MS. Erectile Dysfunctionin Patients with SleepApnea - A Nationwide Population-Based Study. *PLoS One.,* 10(7), p. e0132510.

Cowie MR, Woehrle H, Wegscheider K, Angermann C, d'Ortho M, Erdmann E, Levy P, Simonds AK, Somers VK, Zannad F, Teschler H. Adaptive servo-ventilation for central sleep apnea in sysltolic heart failure. *N Engl J Med,* Volume 373, pp. 1095-1105.

Davies CW, Crosby JH, Mullins RL, Barbour C, Davies RJ, Stradling JR. Case control study of 24-hour ambulatory blood pressure in patients with obstructive sleep apnoea and normal matched control subjects. *Thorax,* 55(9), pp. 736-40.

Dimsdale JE, Coy J, Ziegler MG, Ancoli-Israel S, Clausen J. The effects of sleep apnea on plasma and urinary catecholamines. *Sleep,* Volume 18, pp. 377-381.

Doherty LS, Kiely JL, Lawless G, McNicholas WT. Impact of nasal continuous positive airway pressure therapy on the quality of life of bed partners of patients with obstructive sleep apnea syndrome. *Chest,* 124(6), pp. 2209-2214.

Duchna HW, Guilleminault C, Stoohs RA, Faul JL, Moreno H, Hoffman BB, Blaschke TF. Vascular reactivity in OSA syndrome 2000; 161:187-91. *Am J Respir Crit Care Med,* Volume 161, pp. 187-91.

Eckardt KU, Bernhardt WM, Weidemann A, Warnecke C, Rosenberger C, Wiesener MS, Willam C. Role of hypoxia in the pathogenesis of renal disease. 2005;99:S46–51. *Kidney Int Suppl.,* Volume 99, pp. S46-51.

Eguchi K, Ishikawa J, Hoshide S, Pickering TG, Schwartz JE, Shimada K, Kario K. Night time blood pressure variability is a strong predictor for cardiovascular events in patients with type 2 diabetes. *Am J Hypertens,* Volume 1, pp. 46-51.

Estes C, Razavi H, Loomba R, Younossi Z, Sanyal AJ. Modelling the epidemic of nonalcoholic fatty liver disease demonstrates ann exponential increase in burden os disease. *Hepatology,* Volume 67, pp. 123-133.

Fletcher EC, Miller J, Schaaf JW, Fletcher JG. Urinary catecholamines before and after tracheostomy in patients with obstructive sleep apnea and hypertensive. *Sleep,* Volume 10, pp. 35-44.

Framnes SN, Arble DM. The Bidirectional Relationship Between Obstructive Sleep Apnea and Metabolic Disease. *Front Endocrinol,* 400(9).

Gagnadoux F, Le Vaillant M, Goupil F, Pigeanne T, Chollet S, Masson P, Humeau MP, Bizieux-Thaminy A, Meslier N. Influence of marital status and employment status on long-term adherence with continuous positive airway pressure in sleep apnea patients. *PLoS One,* 6(8), p. e22503.

Galle J. Oxidative stress in chronic renal failure. *Nephrol Dial Transplant,* Volume 16, pp. 2135-7.

Gami AS, Pressman G, Caples SM, Kanagala R, Gard JJ, Davison DE, Malouf JF, Ammash NM, Friedman PA, Somers VK. Association of atrial fibrillation and obstructive sleep apnea. *Circulation,* Volume 110, pp. 364-367.

Gami AS, Olson EJ, Shen WK, Wright RS, Ballman KV, Hodge DO, Herges RM, Howard DE, Somers VK. Obstructive sleep apnea and the risk of sudden cardiac death: a longitudinal study of 10701 adults. *J Am Coll Cardiol,* Volume 62, pp. 610-616.

George CF. Am J Respir Crit Care Med. *Sleep apnea, alertness, and motor vehicle crashes.,* Volume 176, pp. 954-6.

Gonçalves MA, Guilleminault C, Ramos E, Palha A, Paiva T. Erectile dysfunction, obstructive sleep apnea syndrome and nasal CPAP treatment. *Sleep Med.,* 6(4), pp. 333-9.

Gonçalves SC, Martinez D, Gus M, de Abreu-Silva EO, Bertoluci C, Dutra I, Branchi T, Moreira LB, Fuchs SC, de Oliveira AC, Fuchs FD. Obstructive sleep apnea and resistant hypertension: a case-control study. *Chest,* Volume 132, p. 1858–1862.

Gottlieb DJ, Yenokyan G, Newman AB, O'Connor GT, Punjabi NM, Quan SF, Redline S, Resnick HE, Tong EK, Diener-West M, Shahar E. Prospective study of obstuctive sleep apnea and incident coronary heart disease and heart failure : the sleep Heart Health Study. *Circulation,* Volume 122, pp. 352-360.

Guglielmi O, Jurado-Gámez B, Gude F, Buela-Casal G. Job stress, burnout, and job satisfaction in sleep apnea patients. *Sleep Med.,* Volume 15, p. 1025–1030.

Harris M1, Glozier N, Ratnavadivel R, Grunstein RR. Obstructive sleep apnea and depression. *Sleep Med Rev,* Volume 13, p. 437–444.

Hedner J, Ejnell H, Sellgren J, Hedner T, Wallin G. Is high and fluctuating muscle nerve sympathetic activity in the sleep apnea syndrome of pathogenetic importance for the development of hypertension?. *J. Hypertension,* Volume 6, pp. S529-531.

Henry D, Rosenthal L. "Listening for his breath:" The significance of gender and partner reporting on the diagnosis, management, and treatment of obstructive sleep apnea. *Soc Sci Med.,* Volume 79, pp. 48-56.

Heruti R, Shochat T, Tekes-Manova D, Ashkenazi I, Justo D. Association between erectile dysfunction and sleep disorders measured by self-assessment questionnaires in adult men. *J Sex Med,* 2(4), pp. 543-50.

Hirshkowitz M, Karacan I, Arcasoy MO, Acik G, Narter EM, Williams RL. Prevalence of sleep apnea in men with erectile dysfunction. 1990;36(3):232–4. *Urology.,* 36(3), pp. 232-4.

Holmqvist F, Guan N, Zhu Z, Kowey PR, Allen LA, Fonarow GC, Hylek EM, Mahaffey KW, Freeman JV, Chang P, Holmes DN, Peterson ED, Piccini JP, Gersh BJ. *ORBIT-AF Investigators . Impact of obstructive sleep apnea and continuous positive airway pressure therapyon outcomes in paients with atrial fibrillation - results from the Outcomes Registry for Better Informed Treatment of Atrial Fibrillation (ORBIT-AF),* Volume 169, pp. 647-654.

Hoyos CM, Melehan KL, Phillips CL, Grustein RR, Liu PY. To ED or not to ED—Is erectile dysfunction in obstructive sleep apnea related to endothelial dysfunction?. *Sleep Med Rev.,* Volume 20, pp. 5-14.

Ip MS, Lam B, Ng MM, Lam WK, Tsang KW, Lam KS. Obstructive sleep apnea is independently associated with insulin resistance. *Am J RespirCrit Care Med,* Volume 165, pp. 670-676.

Iseki K, Tohyama K, Matsumoto T, Nakamura H. High Prevalence of chronic kidney disease among patients with sleep related breathing disorder (SRBD). *Hypertens Res.,* Volume 31, pp. 249-55.

Izci B, McDonald JP, Coleman EL, Mackay TW, Douglas NJ, Engleman HM. Clinical audit of subjects with snoring & sleep apnoea/hypopnoea syndrome fitted with mandibular repositioning splint. *Respir Med.,* 99(3), pp. 337-246.

Jennum P, Wildschiodtz G, Christensen NJ, Schwartz T. Blood pressure, catecholamines and pancreatic polypeptide in OSA with and without nCPAP treatment. *Am J Hyperten,* Volume 2, pp. 847-852.

Jouët P, Sabaté JM, Maillard D, Msika S, Mechler C, Ledoux S, Harnois F, Coffin B. Relationship between obstructive sleep apnea and liver abnormalities in morbidity obese patients: a prospective study. *Obes Surg,* Volume 17, pp. 478-485.

Jullian-Desayes I, Tamisier R, Zarski JP, Aron-Wisnewsky J, Launois-Rollinat SH, Trocme C, Levy P, Joyeux-Faure M, Pepin JL. Impact of effective versus sham continuous positive airway pressure on liver injury in obstructive sleep apnoea: Data from randomised trials. *Respirology,* 21(2), pp. 378-385.

Jurado-Gamez B, Guglielmi O, Gude F, Buela-Casal G. Workplace accidents, absenteeism and productivity in patients with sleep apnea. *Arch Bronconeumol.,* Volume 51, pp. 213-218.

Kales A, Caldwell AB, Cadieux RJ, Vela-Bueno A, Ruch LG, Mayes SD. Severe obstructive sleep apnea--II: associated psychopathology and psychosocial consequences. *J Chronic Dis,* Volume 38, pp. 427-434.

Kallwitz ER, Herdegen J, Madura J, Jakate S, Cotler SJ. Liver enzymes and histology in obese patients with obstructive sleep apnea. *J Clin Gastroenterol,* 41(10), pp. 918-921.

Kallwitz ER, Herdegen J, Madura J, Jakate S, Cotler SJ. Liver enzymes and histology in obese patients with obstructive sleep apnea. *J Clin Gastroenterol,* Volume 41, pp. 1916-1923.

Kanagala R, Murali NS, Friedman PA, Ammash NM, Gersh BJ, Ballman KV, . Shamsuzzaman ASM, Somers VK. Obstructive sleep apnea and the recurrence of atrial fibrillation. *Circulation,* Volume 107, pp. 2589-2594.

Kanbay A, Buyukoglan H, Ozdogan N, Kaya E, Oymak F, Gulmez I, Demir R, Kokturk O, Covic A. Obstructive sleep apnea syndrome is related to the progression of chronic kidney disease. *Int Urol Nephrol.,* Volume 44, pp. 535-9.

Karimi M, Eder DN, Eskandari D, Zou D, Hedner JA, Grote L. *Impaired vigilance and increased accident rate in public transportation operators is associated with sleep disorders.* 2013:208–214. pp. 208-214.

Kaw R, Pasupuleti V, Walke E, Ramaswamy A, Foldvary-Schafer N. Postoperative complications in patients with obstructive sleep apnea. *Chest,* Volume 141, pp. 436-41.

Kendzerska T, Gershon AS, Hawker GA, Tomlinson GA, Leung RS. Obstructive sleep apnoea is not a risk factor for incident hospitalised depression: a historical cohort study. *Eur Respir J 2017,* Volume 49, p. 1601361.

Kimmel PL, Miller G, Mendelson WB. Sleep apnea syndrome in chronic renal disease. *Am J Med.,* Volume 86, pp. 308-14.

Knauert M, Naika S, Gillespie B, Kryger M. Clinical consequences and economic costs of untreated obstructive sleep apnea syndrome. *World J Oto* 1(1), pp. 17-27.

Lafranchi PA, Somers VK, Braghiroli A, Corra U, Eleuteri E, Giannuzzi P. Central sleep apnea in left ventricular dysfunction: prevalence and implications for arrhythmic risk. *Circulation,* Volume 107, pp. 727-732.

LaGrotte C, Fernandez-Mendoza J, Calhoun SL, Liao D, Bixler EO, Vgontzas AN. The relative association of obstructive sleep apnea, obesity and excessive daytime sleepiness with incident depression: a longitudinal, population-based study. *Int J Obes (Lond),* Volume 40, pp. 1397-1404.

Lapiński M, Przybylowski T, Lewandowski J, Januszewicz A, Wocial B, Kowalski J, Droszcz W, Januszewicz W. Diurnal blood pressure rhythm and urinary catecholamine excretion in obstructive sleep apnea and essential hypertension. *J Hypertension,* 11(S5), pp. S292-293.

Lavie P, Lavie L, Herer P. *All cause mortality in men with sleep apnoea syndrome: declining mortality rates with age.,* Volume 27, pp. 1-7.

Lavie P, Hoffstein V. Obstructive sleep apnea syndrome as a risk factor for hypertension: a population study. *BMJ,* Volume 320, pp. 479-482.

Leung RS. Sleep-disordered breathing: autonomic mechanisms and arrhythmias. *Prog Cardiovasc Dis.,* Volume 51, p. 324–338.

Lewis KE, Seale L, Bartle IE, Watkins AJ, Ebden P. Early predictors of CPAP use for the treatment of obstructive sleep apnea. *Sleep,* 27(1), pp. 134-138.

Lindberg E, Carter N, Gislason T, Janson C. Role of snoring and daytime sleepiness in occupational accidents. *Am J Respir Crit Care Med.,* Volume 164, pp. 2031-2035.

Lipford MC, Flemming KD, Calvin AD, Mandrekar J, Brown RD, Somers VK, Caples SM. Associations between cardioembolic stroke and obstructive sleep apnea. *Sleep,* Volume 38, pp. 1699-1705.

Logan AG, Tkacova R, Perlikowski SM, Leung RS, Tisler A, Floras JS, Bradley TD. Refractory hypertension and sleep apnoea: effect of CPAP on blood pressure and baroreflex. *Eur Respir J,* Volume 21, pp. 241-247.

Luyster FS, Dunbar-Jacob J, Aloia MS, Martire LM, Buysse DJ, Strollo PJ. Patient and partner experiences with obstructive sleep apnea and cpap treatment: a qualitative analysis. *Behav Sleep Med.,* 14(1), pp. 67-84.

Margel D, Cohen M, Livne PM, Pillar G. Severe, but not mild, obstructive sleep apnea syndrome is associated with erectile dysfunction. *Urology,* 63(3), pp. 545-549.

Marin JM, Agusti A, Villar I. Association Between Treated and Untreated Obstructive Sleep Apnea and Risk of Hypertension. *JAMA,* 2169-2176(307 (20)).

Markou N, Kanakaki M, Myrianthefs P, Hadjiyanakos D, Vlassopoulos D, Damianos A, Siamopoulos K, Vasiliou M, Konstantopoulos S. Sleep-disordered breathing in nondialyzed patients with chronic renal failure. *Lung,* Volume 184, pp. 43-9.

Marrone O, Riccobono L, Salvaggio A, Mirabella A, Bonanno A, Bonsignore MR. Catecholamines and blood pressure in obstructive sleep apnea syndrome. *Chest,* Volume 103, pp. 722-727.

Martin-Morales A, Meijide F, García N, Artes M, Muñoz A. Efficacy of vardenafil and influence on self-esteem and self confidence in patients with severe erectile dysfunction. *J. Sex. Med.,* 4(2), pp. 440-447.

May AM, Van Wagoner DR. Mehra R. OSA and cardiac arrhythmo-genesis: mechanistic insights. *Chest,* Volume 151, pp. 225-241.

McArdle N, Kingshott R, Engleman H, Mackay T, Douglas N. Partners of patients with sleep apnoea/hypopnoea syndrome: effect of CPAP treatment on sleep quality and quality of life. *Thorax,* 56(7), pp. 513-518.

McFadyen TA, Espie CA, McArdle N, Douglas NJ, Engleman HM. Controlled, prospective trial of psychosocial function before and after continuous positive airway pressure therapy. *Eur Respir J,* 18(6), pp. 996-1002.

Mehra R, Benjamin EJ, Shahar E, Gottlieb DJ, Nawabit R, Kirchner HL, Sahadevan J, Redline S. Association of nocturnal arrhythmias with sleep-disordered breathing: the Sleep Heart Health Study. *Am J Respir Crit Care Med.,* Volume 173, p. 910–916.

Memtsoudis S, Liu SS, Ma Y, Chiu YL, Walz JM, Gaber-Baylis LK, Mazumdar M. Perioperative pulmonary outcomes in patients with sleep apnea after noncardiac surgery,. *Anesth Analg,* Volume 112, pp. 112-21.

Millman RP, Kimmel PL, Shore ET, Wasserstein AG. Sleep apnea in hemodialysis patients: the lack of testosterone effect on its pathogenesis. *Nephron,* Volume 40, pp. 407-10.

Minai OA, Ricaurte B, Kaw R, Hammel J, Mansour M, McCarthy K, Golish JA, Stoller JK. Frequency and impact of pulmonary hypertension in patients with obstructive sleep apnea syndrome. *Am J Cardiol,* Volume 104, pp. 1300-1306.

Mishra A, Younossi ZM. Epidemiology and natural History of Non-alcoholic Fatty Liver disease. *J Clin Exp Hepatol,* 2(2), pp. 135-144.

Mishra P, Nugent C, Afendy A, Bai C, Bhatia P, Afendy M, Fang Y, Elariny H, Goodman Z, Younossi ZM. Apnoeic-hypopnoeic episodes during obstructive sleep apnoea are associated with histological nonalcoholic steatohepatitis. *Liver Int,* Volume 28, pp. 1080-1086.

Mokhlesi B, Hovda MD, Vekhter B, Arora VM, Chung F, Meltzer DO. Sleep-disordered breathing and postoperative outcomes after elective surgery: analysis of the nationwide inpatient sample. *Chest,* Volume 144, pp. 903-14.

Naguka M. Chronic hypoxia and tubulointerstitial injury: a final common pathway to end-stage renal failure. *J Am Soc Nephrol.,* Volume 17, pp. 17-25.

Narkiewicz K, Kato M, Phillips BG, Pesek CA, Davison DE, Somers VK. Nocturnal CPAP decreases daytime sympathetic traffic in OSA. *Circulation,* 2335(100), p. 2332.

Naruse Y, Tada H, Satoh M, Yanagihara M, Tsuneoka H, HirataY, Ito Y, Kuroki K, Machino T, Yamasaki H, Igarashi M, Sekiguchi Y, Sato A, Aonuma K. Concomitant obstructive sleep apnea increases the recurrence of atrial fibrillation following radiofrequency catheter ablation of atrial fibrillation: clinical impact of continuous positive airway pressure therapy,. *Heart Rhythm,* Volume 10, pp. 331-337.

Neumann J, Ligtenberg G, Klein II, Koomans HA, Blankestijn PJ. Sympathetic hyperactivity in chronic kidney disease: pathogenesis, clinical relevance, and treatment. 2004;65:1568–76. *Kidney Int.,* Volume 65, pp. 1568-76.

Ng CY, Liu T, Shehata M, Stevens S, Chugh SS, Wang X. Meta-analysis of obstructive sleep apnea as predictor of atrial fibrillation recurrence after catheter ablation. *Am J Cardiol.,* Volume 108, pp. 47-51.

Nicholl DDM, Ahmed SB, Loewen AHS, Hemmelgarn BR, Sola DY, Beecroft JM, Turin TC, Hanly PJ. Declining kidney function increases the prevalence of sleep apnea and nocturnal hypoxia. *Chest,* Volume 141, pp. 1422-30.

Nieto FJ, YoungTB, Lind BK. Association of sleep-disordered breathing, sleep apnea, and hypertension in a large community based study. *JAMA,* Volume 283, pp. 1829-1836.

Ohayon MM. The effects of breathing-related sleep disorders on mood disturbances in the general population. *J Clin Psychiatry,* Volume 64, pp. 1195-1200.

Ohkubo T, Atsushi H, Junko Y, Masahiro K, Kaori O, Mari M, Mitsunobu M, Junichiro H, Haruhisa H, Tsutomu A, Ichiro T, Hirosi S, Shigeru H, Yutaka I. Prognostic significance of the nocturnal decline in blood pressure in individuals with and without high 24-h blood pressure: the Ohasama study. *J Hypertens,* 20(11), pp. 2183-2189.

Oldenburg O, Lamp B, Faber L, Teschler H, Horstkotte D, Töpfer V. Sleep Disordered breathingin patients with symptomatic heart failure: a contemporary study of prevalence in and characteristics of 700 patients. *Eur J Heart Fail,* Volume 9, pp. 251-257.

Oldenburg O, Teerlink JR. Screening for sleep-disordered breathing in patients hospitalised for jheart failure. *JACC Heart Fail,* Volume 3, pp. 732-733.

Omachi TA, Claman DM, Blanc PD, Eisner MD. Obstructive sleep apnea: a risk factor for work disability. *Sleep,* Volume 32, pp. 791-798.

Orban M, Bruce CJ, Pressman GS, Leinveber P, Romero-Corral A, Korinek J, KonecnyT, Villarraga HR, Kara T, Caples SM, Somers VK. Dynamic changes of left ventricular performance and left atrial volume induced by the mueller maneuver in healthy young adults and implications for obstructive sleep apnoea, atrial fibrillation, and heart failure. *Am J Cardiol.,* Volume 102, pp. 1557-1561.

Pamidi S, Wroblewski K, Broussard J, Day A, Hanlon EC, Abraham V, Tasali E. Obstructive sleep apnea in young lean men: impact on insulin sensitivity and secretion. *Diabetes Care,* 35(11), pp. 2384-23-89.

Parish JM, Adam T, Facchiano F. Relationship of metabolic syndrome and obstructive sleep apnea. *J Clin Sleep Med.,* Volume 3, pp. 467-472.

Parish JM, Lyng PJ. Quality of life in bed partners of patients with obstructive sleep apnea or hypopnea after treatment with continuous positive airway pressure. *Chest,* 124(3), pp. 942-947.

Patel N, Donahue C, Shenoy A, Patel A, El-Sherif N. Obstuctive Sleep apnea and arrhymia. *Int J CArdiol,* Volume 228, pp. 967-970.

Patt BT, Jarjoura D, Haddad DN, Sen CK, Roy S, Flavahan NA, Khayat RN. Endothelial dysfunction in the microcirculation of patients with obstructive sleep apnea. *Am J Respir Crit Care Med,* Volume 182, pp. 1540-1545.

Peled N, Kassirer M, Shitrit D, Kogan Y, Shlomi D, Berliner AS, Kramer MR. The association of OSA with insulin resistance, inflammation and metabolic syndrome. *Respir Med,* 101(8), pp. 1696-1701.

Peppard PE, Szklo-Coxe M, Hla KM, Young T. Longitudinal association of sleep-related breathing disorder and depression. *Arch Intern Med,* Volume 166, pp. 1709-1715.

Peppard PE, Young T, Palta M, Skatrud J. Prospective study of the association between sleep-disordered breathing and hypertension. *New Engl J Med,* 342(19), pp. 1378-84.

Perker Y, Carlson J, Hedner J. Increased incidence of coronary artery disease in sleep apnoea: a long term follow up. *Eur Respir,* 2006(28), pp. 596-602.

Philip P. Sleepiness of occupational drivers. *Ind. Health,* 43(1), pp. 30-33.

Phillips CL, McEwen BJ, Morel-Kopp MC, Yee BJ, Sullivan DR, Ward CM, Tofler GH, Grunstein RR. Effects of continous positive airway pressure on coagulability in obstructive sleep apnea: a randomised, placebo-controlled crossover study. *Thorax,* Volume 67, pp. 639-644.

Phillips SA, Olson EB, Morgan BJ, Lombard JH. Chronic intermittent hypoxia impairs endothelium-dependent dilation in rat cerebral and skeletal muscle resistance arteries. *AM J Physiol Heart Circ Physiol,* Volume 286, pp. H388-H393.

Polotsky VY, Patil SP, Savransky V, Laffan A, Fonti S, Frame LA, Steele KE, Schweizter MA, Clark JM, Torbenson MS, Schwartz AR. Obstructive sleep apnea, insulin resistance, and steatohepatitis in severe obesity. *Am J Respir Crit Care Med,* Volume 179, pp. 228-234.

Pulixi EA, Tobaldini E, Battezzati PM, D'Ingianna P, Borroni V, Fracanzani AL, Maggioni M, Pelusi S, Bulgheroni M, Zuin M, Fargion S, Montano N, Valenti L. Risk of obstructive sleep apnea with daytime sleepness is associated with liver damage in non-mobidily obese patients with non-alcoholic fatty liver disease. *Plos One,* Volume 9, p. e96349.

Qi JC, Huang JC, Lin QC, Zhao JM, Lin X, Chen LD, Huang JF, Chen X. Relationship between obstructive sleep apnea and nonalcoholic fatty liver disease in nonobese adults. *Sleep Breath,* 20(2), pp. 529-535.

Redline S, Yenokyan G, Gottlieb DJ, Shahar E, O'Connor GT, Resnick HE, Diener-West M, Sanders MH, Wolf PA, Geraghty EM, Ali T, Lebowitz M, Punjabi NM. Obstructive sleep apnea-hypopnea and incident stroke: the Sleep Health Study. *Am J Respir Crit Care Med,* Volume 182, pp. 269-277.

Reutrakul S, Mokhlesi B. Obstructive Sleep apnea and diabetes: A state of the art Review. *Chest,* Volume 152, pp. 1070-1086.

Ritz E, Amann K, Fliser D. The sympathetic nervous system and the kidney: its importance in renal diseases. *Blood Press Suppl,* Volume 3, pp. 14-9.

Sakaguchi Y, Shoji T, Kawabata H, Niihata K, Suzuki A, Kaneko T, Okada N, Isaka Y, Rakugi H, Tsubakihara Y. High prevalence of obstructive sleep apnea and its association with renal function among nondialysis chronic kidney disease patients in Japan: a cross-sectional study. *Clin J Am Soc Nephrol,* Volume 6, pp. 995-1000.

Shahar E, Whitney CW, Redline S, Lee ET, Newman AB, Nieto FJ, O'Connor GT, Boland LL, Schwartz JE, Samet JM. Sleep-Disordered breathind and cardiovascular disease: cross-sectional results of the Sleep Heart Health Study. *AM J Respir Crit Care Med,* Volume 163, pp. 19-25.

Sharief I, Silva GE, Goodwin JL, Quan SF. Effect of sleep disordered breathing on the sleep of bed partners in the sleep heart health study. *Sleep,* 31(10), pp. 1449-1456.

Shiri R, Koskimäki J, Tammela T, Häkkinen J, Auvinen A, Hakama M. Bidirectional relationship between depression and erectile dysfunction. *J. Urol.,* 177(2), pp. 669-673.

Siccoli MM, Pepperell JCT, Kohler M, Craig SE, Davies RJO, StradlingJR. Effects of continuous positive airway pressure on quality of life in patients with moderate to severe obstructive sleep apnea: data from a randomized controlled trial. *Sleep,* 31(11), pp. 1551-1558.

Simantirakis EN, Schiza SI, Marketou ME, Chrysostomakis SI, Chlouverakis GI, Klapsinos NC, Siafakas NS, Vardas PESevere bradyarrhythmias in patients with sleep apnoea: the effect of continuous positive airway pressure treatment: a long-term evaluation using an insertable loop recorder. *Eur Heart J.,* Volume 25, pp. 1070-1076.

Simon-Tuval T, Reuveni H, Greenberg-Dotan S, Oksenberg A, Tal A, Tarasiuk A. Low socioeconomic status is a risk factor for CPAP acceptance among adult OSAS patients requiring treatment. *Sleep,* 32(4), pp. 545-552.

Smith AKA, Togeiro SMG, Tufik S, Roizenblatt S. Disturbed sleep and musculoskeletal pain in the bed partner of patients with obstructive sleep apnea. *Sleep Med.,* 10(8), pp. 904-912.

Stålkrantz A, Broström A, Wiberg J, Svanborg E, Malm D. Everyday life for the spouses of patients with untreated OSA syndrome. *Scand J Caring Sci.,* 26(2), p. 324–332.

Stranks EK, Crowe SF. The Cognitive Effects of Obstructive Sleep Apnea: An Updated Meta-analysis. *Arch Clin Neuropsychol.,* 31(2), pp. 186-93.

Tanné F, Gagnadoux F, Chazouillères O, Fleury B, Wendum D, Lasnier E, Lebeau B, Poupon R, Serfaty L. Chronic liver injury during obstructive sleep apnea. *Hepatology,* Volume 41, pp. 1290-1296.

Tarasiuk A, Reznor G, Greenberg-Dotan S, Reuveni H. Financial incentive increases CPAP acceptance in patients from low socioeconomic background. *PLoS One.,* 7(3), p. e33178.

Tegelberg A, Nohlert E, Bergman LE, Andrén A. Bed partners' and patients' experiences after treatment of obstructive sleep apnoea with an oral appliance. *Swed Dent J.,* 36(1), pp. 35-44.

Teloken PE, Smith EB, Lodowsky C, Freedom T, Mulhall JP. Defining association between sleep apnea syndrome and erectile dysfunction. *Urology,* 67(5), pp. 1033-7.

Tregear S, Reston J, Schoelles K, Phillips B. Obstructive sleep apnea and risk of motor vehicle crash: systematic review and meta-analysis. *J Clin Sleep Med,* 5(6), pp. 573-581.

Ulfberg J, Carter N, Talbäck M, Edling C. Adverse health effects among women living with heavy snorers. *Health Care Women Int.,* 21(2), pp. 81-90.

Utitsky A, Ananthakrishnan AN, Komorowski R, Wallace J, Surapaneni SN, Franco J, Saeian K, Gawrieh S. A noninvasive clinical scoring model predicts risk of nonalcoholic steatohepatitis in mobidly obese patients. *Obes Surg,* Volume 20, pp. 685-691.

Virkkula P, Bachour A, Hytönen M, Malmberg H, Salmi T, Maasilta. Patient-and bed partner-reported symptoms, smoking, and nasal resistance in sleep-disordered breathing. *Chest,* 128(4), pp. 2176-2182.

Yaggi H, Mohsenin V. Obstructive sleep apnoea and stroke. *Lancet Neurol.* 2004 Jun;3(6):333-42.

Yamakawa H, Shiomi T, Sasanabe R, Hasegawa R, Ootake K, Banno K, Wakayama H, Katada M, Kobayashi T. Pulmonary hypertension in patients with sleep apnea syndrome. *Psychiatry Clin Neurosci,* Volume 56, pp. 311-312.

Young T, Finn L, Peppard PE, Szklo-Coxe M, Austin D, Nieto FJ, Stubbs R, Hla KM. *Sleep-disordered-Breathing and mortality; Eighteen-year follow-up of Wisconsin Sleep Cohort.,* Volume 31, pp. 1071-1078.

Young T, Finn L, Peppard PE, Szklo-Coxe, Austin D, Nieto FJ, Stubbs R, Hla KM. Sleep disordered breathing and mortality: eighteen-year follow-up of the Wisconsin sleep cohort. *Sleep,* 31(8), pp. 1071-8.

Zias N, Bezwada V, Gilman S, Chroneou A. Obstructive sleep apnea and erectile dysfunction: still a neglected risk factor?. *Sleep Breath.,* 13(1), pp. 3-10.

Ziegler MG, Mills PJ, Loredo JS, Ancoli-Israel S, Dimsdale JE. Effect of continuous positive airway pressure and placebo treatment on sympathetic nervous activity in patients with obstructive sleep apena. *Chest,* Volume 120, pp. 887-893.

About the Editors

Antonio M. Esquinas is a 54 year old critical care MD in Intensive Unit at Hospital Morales Meseguer, Murcia (Spain). He holds a PhD in Medicine (University of Murcia) and BA in Pulmonary and Critical Care Medicine (University of Granada). He has taken part in many academic and research activities in the field of mechanical ventilation, with special focus on Noninvasive Mechanical Ventilation and weaning from mechanical ventilation, COPD exacerbation and acute hypoxemic respiratory failure.

Furthermore, Antonio M. Esquinas MD, PhD has contributed to research as author of 648 articles indexed, 550 chapters and as editor in chief of 55 books edited in the field of related mechanical ventilation, invasive (weaning mechanical ventilation) and noninvasive ventilation approach in acute hypoxemic and chronic respiratory failure (COPD, idiopathic pulmonary fibrosis, sleep breathing disorders) in pulmonary, critical care and sleep medicine.

He is recognized as International Fellow from the American College Chest Physicians (FCCP), International Fellow American Association Respiratory Care (AARC) and Fellow Noninvasive Ventilation by International Association of Noninvasive Ventilation. Besides, Antonio M. is an active member in many educational postgraduate programs in pulmonary and critical care as he is the Director of International School of Noninvasive Ventilation and of the program of Fellowship Noninvasive Ventilation, as well as President of the International Association of Noninvasive Ventilation.

Joerg Steier's training in medicine commenced at the University of Leipzig in Saxony. Following graduation, he worked on his MD thesis entitled "Transthoracic Echocardiography in Pulmonary Hypertension" and gathered work experience in Zurich, at the University of Alabama in Birmingham and in Bavaria. His respiratory training led him to the Western German Lung Centre at the University of Essen. His interest in respiratory physiology and sleep-disordered breathing brought him to London on a long-term research fellowship of the European Respiratory Society (ERS). His studies concluded in the PhD thesis on "Sleep-Disordered Breathing and the Respiratory Muscles" at King's College London. The projects with the London Respiratory Physiology group resulted in research publications with involvement in an impact case and the development of new intellectual property. His work in the field of respiratory and sleep physiology has evolved into collaborations across six continents. Professor Steier works as Consultant at Guy's & St Thomas' NHS Foundation Trust in the Lane Fox Unit, a tertiary service for weaning and non-invasive ventilation. He is also placed at the British Sleep Society (BSS) accredited Sleep Disorders Centre of King's Health Partners. He was awarded the chair for Respiratory and Sleep Medicine at King's College London. He is member of the executive committee of the British Sleep Society (BSS), task force member of the ERS, and currently serves as President of the BSS.

Behrouz Jafari is currently Director of VALBHCS Sleep Program and Associate Professor of Medicine at the Section of Pulmonary and Critical Care Medicine in University of California, Irvine.